MANUAL OF C
WITH ANNOTAT

MW01170737

NC

Amy P. McLellan

MANUAL OF CLINICAL PROBLEMS IN ONCOLOGY
WITH ANNOTATED KEY REFERENCES

CAROL S. PORTLOCK, M.D.
Associate Professor of Medicine, Division of Medical Oncology, Yale University School of Medicine, New Haven, Connecticut

DONALD R. GOFFINET, M.D.
Associate Professor of Radiology, Division of Radiation Therapy, Stanford University School of Medicine, Stanford, California

LITTLE, BROWN AND COMPANY   BOSTON

CONTENTS

Clinical oncology is a rapidly developing area of medicine with few rigid rules and much controversy. We have attempted here to set forth an objective examination of common problems encountered in the clinic. This manual is not meant to be a "cookbook of management," or a comprehensive treatise on medical, surgical, and radiation oncology. Instead, it is an up-to-date reference guide for clinicians, whether they are medical students, house officers, general practitioners, internists, surgeons, or oncology specialists.

Care has been taken to organize the manual in a clinically useful format. Specific problems of diagnosis, treatment, and general patient management are grouped separately. In addition, those chapters that discuss specific diseases are divided into two parts (Part III presenting each disease as a primary or regional malignancy, Part IV, as a relapsing or metastatic malignancy) in order to highlight the different clinical problems faced in the management of localized and disseminated malignancies. Pathophysiology, natural history, and "standard" management approaches are discussed with a view to the dynamism and rapid advances of clinical and laboratory research. References have been selected for their individual contribution to the field and their illustration of important topics. We have not avoided controversy and areas of uncertainty; rather, we have attempted to discuss the data objectively and to provide references for the reader's own scrutiny.

We would like to give special thanks to our secretaries, Ms. Jeanne Reardon and Ms. Mary Lou Rose for their expert assistance.

PART I. ONCOLOGIC EMERGENCIES

1. TRACHEAL OBSTRUCTION

Tracheal obstruction may result from postintubation or posttracheotomy cicatricial stenosis. Stenosis may also occur after laryngeal trauma, may be caused by tracheomalacia (loss of wall rigidity) or, infrequently, may arise from such infectious diseases as tuberculosis. The trachea may also be involved by papillomatosis, in which multiple benign papillomas involve the mucosal surface and produce tracheal obstruction. Primary malignant neoplasms of the trachea are usually either squamous carcinomas, arising in the lower third of the trachea, or adenoid cystic carcinomas originating in mucous glands in the upper third. The trachea may also be directly invaded by such neoplasms as squamous carcinomas of the esophagus and lung and anaplastic thyroid carcinomas.

Common symptoms or signs of tracheal neoplasms include hemoptysis, wheezing, and chronic cough, associated with progressive and insidious dyspnea. If a tracheoesophageal fistula has developed, aspiration, pneumonia, and rapidly increasing dyspnea also occur.

A chest radiograph should be obtained to rule out tracheal invasion by a primary pulmonary or mediastinal neoplasm. Over-penetrated radiographs of the trachea and surrounding soft tissues, plus oblique cervical radiographs, may aid in localizing the mass. Tracheal tomograms are useful in delineating the extent of involvement. Computerized axial tomography may aid in estimating both the extent of the lesion and the degree of tracheal obstruction.

The tracheal lesion may be visualized and biopsied bronchoscopically, but when the airway is markedly narrowed, this procedure should be deferred until the time of resection, in order to avoid postendoscopic edema and possible complete obstruction. Localized stenotic areas in the trachea may be dilated endoscopically, or if they severely limit the airway, may be managed by resection and end-to-end anastomosis. However, tracheal obstruction by a malignant tumor presents a formidable treatment problem. Since the obstructive lesion often arises in the mid- or upper trachea, a standard tracheostomy through the second or third tracheal ring may not be possible. Even gentle manipulation of an occluding tumor may produce hemorrhage or increased edema, with occlusion of the airway and death.

Obstructing tracheal lesions are most often treated surgically, either by primary resection or by endoscopic resection or cryosurgery. The technique most commonly used for tracheal tumors is primary resection and, ideally, end-to-end tracheal reconstruction. Maximum lengths of 3.5 to 6.0 cm and 2 to 4 cm may be resected from the superior and inferior trachea, respectively, and will still allow an end-to-end anastomosis to be performed. Transbronchoscopic cryosurgery has had limited clinical use, although two patients with severe airway obstruction ($>90\%$) were successfully palliated by this technique. In a few instances, obstructing tracheal lesions have been treated under direct visualization with a laser beam, but there has been only limited clinical experience with this technique.

With inoperable or incompletely resected tracheal lesions or for external tracheal compression from contiguous masses, radiation therapy is indicated. If there is high-grade tracheal obstruction, corticosteroids (Decadron, 16 mg/day in divided doses) are begun prior to the initiation of radiation therapy. Total radiation doses (at standard fractionations of 180–200 rads daily, 900–1000 rads a week) range from 4000–5000 rads in 5 weeks for lymphomas to 6000–7000 rads in 6 to 7 weeks for solid tumors. The spinal cord must be protected, so that it receives no more than 4000–4500 rads during the course of treatment to the trachea.

The results of treating primary tracheal carcinomas are poor. Fewer than one-third of these neoplasms may be primarily resected and reconstructed, and only a few patients survive free of disease, even in the more favorable (operable) group. Radiotherapy may delay growth and provide palliation but has produced few long-term survivors.

D.G.

Gorenstein A, Neel H, Sanderson D: Transbronchoscopic cryosurgery of respi-
    ratory structures: Experimental and clinical studies. Ann Otol 85:670–678,
    1976.
    *Animal experiments are described. In the humans discussed, 5 of 6 with
    endobronchial tumors achieved palliation.*
Grillo H: Circumferential resection and reconstruction of the mediastinal and
    cervical trachea. Ann Surg 162:374–388, 1966.
    Techniques and limits of procedures are described.
Grillo H: Surgery of the Trachea. Curr Probl Surg. Chicago, Year Book, July
    1970.
    This publication is a definitive monograph on surgical approaches.
Laforet E, Berger R, Vaughan C: Carcinoma obstructing the trachea: Treat-
    ment by laser resection. N Engl J Med 1579–1584, 1976.
    This article consists of case reports.
Sise JG, Crichlow RW: Obstruction due to malignant tumors. Semin Oncol
    5:213–224, 1978.
    Tracheal obstruction is discussed here.

2. SUPERIOR VENA CAVA SYNDROME

The superior vena cava syndrome (SVC) is caused by a mediastinal mass (either primary or metastatic) or by a contiguous pulmonary mass invading the mediastinum, which impairs the venous drainage of the head and neck and the upper thoracic area. The thin-walled superior vena cava, enclosed by the rigid thorax and situated near the trachea and lymph nodes, is especially vulnerable to neoplastic compression. The SVC syndrome is due to a malignant tumor in at least 80% of cases and occurs in 3% to 8% of patients with lung cancers and/or lymphomas. At least 75% of malignant SVC obstructions are caused by lung cancer. Another 15% to 20% are due to lymphomas, usually a diffuse histiocytic lymphoma. SVC obstruction is rarely seen in either Hodgkin's disease or the nodular subtypes of non-Hodgkin's lymphomas. Finally, mediastinal metastases from a variety of primary sites less frequently cause malignant caval obstruction. Benign causes of SVC compression, such as goiter, aortic aneurysms, granulomatous infections, and fibrosing mediastinitis, are rare.

This potentially life-threatening emergency may have an insidious onset but when fully developed results in cervicofacial edema; plethora; dilated veins over the thorax, face, and neck; and occasionally stridor, if laryngeal edema is present. Since obstruction of the great vessels in the mediastinum diminishes cardiac venous return, dyspnea and easy fatigability may also be noted. These signs may be accompanied by headache, altered consciousness, and decreased visual acuity or visual blurring. Upper extremity edema, Horner's syndrome, and vocal cord paralysis are uncommon signs of the SVC syndrome (9.5%, 3.5%, and 2.3% of patients, respectively).

A chest radiograph will usually reveal a mediastinal mass, which may be further delineated by mediastinal tomograms. If necessary, the level of SVC obstruction may be demonstrated by contrast venacavography. However, Tc99m scintillation scans may also adequately demonstrate the area of obstruction and provide follow-up information without the necessity of injecting contrast media.

The full clinical picture of dilated neck veins, facial edema, and dyspnea is usually striking. Lesser degrees of venous obstruction may be more difficult to detect, however, without careful examination of the cervical veins, especially to note whether they remain abnormally engorged with the patient upright. Funduscopic examination may also reveal dilated retinal veins and conjunctival edema.

Since the fully established SVC syndrome is potentially life-threatening, treatment should begin as soon as possible. Cytologic examination of sputum (63% accuracy), bronchoscopy, biopsy (62% accuracy), and cervical or supraclavicular lymph node biopsies (84% accuracy when nodes are palpable) are the least invasive ways to make a definitive diagnosis; however, if these give negative results, the initiation of treatment should not be delayed. Mediastinoscopy may be necessary but may be hazardous due to the presence of dilated and engorged cervical veins. Mediastinoscopy is reported to provide the diagnosis in 81% of patients.

If all these studies have been performed and a tissue diagnosis still has not been made, needle biopsy of an accessible mass may be considered. Occasionally, when all other diagnostic procedures are unrewarding, thoracotomy is indicated to obtain suitable tissue after the SVC syndrome has subsided; in the series of Perez et al. the diagnosis of a malignancy was confirmed in 100% of patients subjected to a thoracotomy.

Radiation therapy is the treatment of choice for SVC obstruction and should begin as soon as the syndrome is detected. A mid-plane radiation dose of 400 rads on each of the first 3 days, followed by reduction of the daily dose rate to 180–200 rads per day, for a total dose of 5000–6000 rads to the mediastinum in 5 to 6 weeks (with proper spinal cord shielding) is the current recommended treatment for carcinomas. Lower radiation doses (3000–4000 rads) are used for lymphomas. Bulky masses, however, may occasionally require a total dose of 5000 rads.

The higher initial daily radiation doses apparently produce more rapid regression than lower daily doses of 150–200 rads. The concomitant use of such diuretics as furosemide (20 to 80 mg daily in divided doses) or ethacrynic acid (50 to 200 mg daily in divided doses) is recommended during the first 2 to 5 days of treatment. If diuretics are used, the clinician should be alert to the possibility of inappropriate ADH secretion, since the use of potent diuretics may worsen the hyponatremia associated with this condition.

The emergency use of nitrogen mustard (0.4 mg/kg) during the initial radiotherapy course is no longer recommended. A prospective trial in patients with the SVC syndrome demonstrated that combining this agent with radiation therapy produced no quicker or more complete resolution of the SVC syndrome than radiation therapy alone. The routine early use of corticosteroids is controversial; however, they may be useful during initial treatment in dyspneic patients with severe SVC obstruction and markedly dilated veins.

Subjective improvement and/or decreased venous distention are usually noted within 72 hours of initiation of radiation therapy. Further diagnostic evaluations may be performed at this time, if a tissue diagnosis could not be made initially.

An objective response, with diminution in facial swelling, regression of the mediastinal mass, and decreased venous engorgement, was noted in 60% to 70% of patients with carcinomas and 80% of those with lymphomas within 14 days of initiation of radiation therapy in Perez's series. Actuarial survival in 67 patients with lung cancers of various histologies was approximately 20% at 1 year and less than 10% at 2 years. Approximately 50% of patients with lymphomas and the SVC syndrome were alive after 24 months.

D.G.

Davenport D, Ferree C, Blake D, Raben M: Radiation therapy in the treatment of superior vena caval obstruction. Cancer 42:2600–2603, 1978.
Thirty-five patients with SVC obstruction were treated with initially high daily radiation doses; there were no complications.

Fisherman W, Bradfield J: Superior vena caval syndrome: Response with initially high daily dose irradiation. South Med J 66:667–680, 1973.
Twelve patients with the syndrome are discussed. Good literature review.

Krishnamurthy G, Bland W, et al: Superior vena caval syndrome scintiphotographic evaluation of response to radiation therapy. Am J Roentgenol 117:609–614, 1973.
Serial scintigraphic studies are described and discussed.

Levitt S, Jones T, et al: Treatment of malignant superior vena caval obstruction. A randomized study. Cancer 24:447–451, 1969.
No differences were found when nitrogen mustard and XRT and XRT alone were compared in therapy of SVC obstruction.

Perez CA, Presant CA, Van Amburg AL III: Management of superior vena cava syndrome. Semin Oncol 5:123–134, 1978.
In this analysis of 84 patients with malignant SVC obstruction, the most common physical findings were: thoracic vein distention (67%), neck vein distention (59%), facial edema (56%), and tachypnea (40%). Diagnostic methods providing the diagnosis were: thoracotomy (100%), mediastinoscopy (81%), bronchoscopy (62%), lymph node biopsy—nonpalpable (50%), cytology (63%). Actuarial survival at 24 months was: <10% for carcinomas, 50% for lymphomas.

Rubin P, Green J, et al: Superior vena caval syndrome. Slow low dose versus rapid high dose schedules. Radiology 81:388–401, 1963.
Report shows effectiveness of initial high daily dose rate irradiation.

3. URETERAL OBSTRUCTION

Long-standing hydronephrosis can progressively destroy renal function. If infection does not occur, renal function may return after 50 to 70 days of obstruction, but this is the outside limit for restoration of useful kidney function. Obstructive uropathy impairs all functions of the kidney, including concentrating ability, but does not reduce the ability to produce a dilute urine. The most common causes of ureteral obstruction are renal calculi, injuries to the urinary tract, extrinsic compression by neoplastic diseases, and developmental abnormalities. The causes of ureteral obstruction may be divided into extrinsic and intrinsic.

Extrinsic obstruction may have vascular causes: aneurysms of the aorta or iliac vessels may compress the ureters, causing hydronephrosis; ovarian veins may create obstruction as they join the vena cava, especially in women who have had multiple pregnancies. Obstruction may arise from gastrointestinal disorders: Crohn's disease of the colon may produce extensive retroperitoneal inflammation and ureteral entrapment; appendicitis and diverticulitis with perforation may produce abscesses and resultant ureteral obstruction. Conditions of female pelvic organs, such as pregnancy, endometriosis, uterine prolapse, and tubo-ovarian abscesses, may all lead to ureteral obstruction and hydronephrosis. Retroperitoneal fibrosis may be idiopathic, may be related to drug ingestion (Sansert) or may follow high-dose abdominal irradiation. Retroperitoneal masses—benign processes such as hemorrhage, pus collections, cysts, and postoperative lymphoceles—may all compress the ureters. In neoplastic diseases lymphomas and sarcomas may produce ureteral obstruction, usually involving a single ureter. Both ureters may be obstructed by carcinomas of the bladder, prostate, and such gynecologic malignancies as ovarian and cervical carcinomas. The ureters may also be included in a ligature during pelvic operations, especially for cervical carcinoma.

Intrinsic causes of ureteral obstruction may be secondary to trauma or congenital abnormalities of the renal pelves, ureters, bladder, or urethra. Ureteral or bladder carcinomas may obstruct the ureter. Other, more inferiorly located, causes of ureteral obstruction are benign prostatic hypertrophy or carcinoma, tumors of the urethra or bladder neck, strictures of these structures, and congenital abnormalities.

Ureteral obstruction may have an insidious onset, and the first apparent sign may be renal failure. Symptoms of ureteral obstruction may be those of the underlying disorder, such as fever (infectious processes), flank pain and gastrointestinal disturbances (stone), and anorexia and associated weight loss (neoplasms). Hypertension from increased renin release may also be noted. In the acute postoperative period, ureteral obstruction may produce prolongation of ileus, abdominal pain, and fever.

Evaluation should include a careful history and physical examination. The ureteral obstruction may be caused by a primary malignancy, which should be searched for. An underlying inflammatory gastrointestinal lesion or pelvic abnormality may be discovered. The abrupt onset of severe back pain associated with a dissecting aneurysm of the abdominal aorta is characteristic and may lead to the diagnosis. The use of such drugs as Sansert should be ascertained. Physical examination may reveal an abdominal mass or bruit, abdominal tenderness, or lymphadenopathy, all of which may suggest the correct diagnosis. A complete blood count, electrolytes, BUN, creatinine, and creatinine clearance should all be performed. If urinalysis reveals microscopic hematuria, a urinary calculus should be suspected. A urine culture and sensitivity test should also be performed. Intravenous pyelography, with consideration of an infusion study if there is no initial renal function, may show delayed function or a nephrogram. A retrograde ureterogram may be necessary to localize the point of ureteral occlusion. Barium gastrointestinal studies may reveal either displacement of bowel by a mass or a primary gastrointestinal lesion. Ultrasound examination and computerized tomography may demonstrate hydronephrosis and extrinsic masses in the pelvis or retroperitoneum.

Arteriography or abdominal-pelvic venography may be indicated if either aneurysms or venous ureteral compression is suspected. A lymphangiogram is indicated for pelvic malignancies or for lymphomas. Cystoscopy will not only allow inspection of the urethra, bladder and ureteral orifices but will also enable a retrograde ureteral study to be performed.

Oliguria secondary to acute tubular necrosis and prerenal causes of oliguria such as hypovolemia or shock must be ruled out. However, it is rare for any of these to result in the complete anuria characteristic of total bilateral ureteral obstruction. If the history, physical examination, and laboratory studies reveal extrinsic compression of the ureters, the underlying disease process must be treated, if possible. If a malignant process is causing ureteral obstruction, a decision whether to treat the obstruction must be made. If no therapy is available for the underlying malignancy, a conservative approach is not to treat the urinary obstruction, allowing the patient to succumb to uremia rather than to painful distant metastases or to suffocation from pulmonary spread.

If the ureteral obstruction is to be treated, a temporary nephrostomy may be needed to restore renal function until the block is relieved. Allupurinol, 200 mg tid, may be necessary to prevent hyperuricemia in patients with non-Hodgkin's lymphomas and massive lymph node involvement. If feasible, radiotherapy should be used initially to treat malignant external ureteral obstruction, but if the tumor is sensitive to chemotherapy or if radiotherapy cannot be used, chemotherapy should be considered. Rarely, if renal function cannot be restored rapidly by nephrostomies, acute hemodialysis may be necessary until the obstruction can be relieved by radiotherapy-chemotherapy approaches. Until appropriate renal function is restored, fluid and electrolyte balance should be carefully monitored to prevent fluid overload, hyperkalemia, and hyponatremia.

D.G.

Persky L, Kursh E, Feldman S: Extrinsic obstruction of the ureter. *In* MF Campbell and JH Harrison (Eds), Urology. Philadelphia, W.B. Saunders, 1978. Pp. 415–447.
Differential diagnosis well detailed.
Rosenberg S: Ureteral Obstruction. *In* E Rubinstein and DD Federman (Eds), Scientific American Medicine. New York, Scientific American, 1978. Part 12, pp. VI–9.
Brief description of treatment of malignant causes of obstruction.
Sise JG, Crichlow RW: Obstruction due to malignant tumors. Semin Oncol 5:213–224, 1978.
Discusses ureteral obstruction due to malignant tumors.

---

4. MASS LESION IN THE BRAIN

Expanding intracranial mass lesions produce either insidious or rapid loss of neurologic function. Symptoms of increased intracranial pressure, such as headache, vomiting, and lethargy, develop rapidly if tumors or masses block the cerebral aqueduct or ventricular system. However, masses often initially produce progressive focal (and localizing) symptoms and signs. Brain tumors in adults are most commonly located supratentorially. Masses in the precentral area may produce weakness (and aphasia if located in a dominant hemisphere), spastic hemiparesis, or Jacksonian convulsions, while frontal lobe tumors may result in affect changes, anosmia, or dementia. Temporal lobe masses can cause hallucinations or aphasia (left lobe). Parietal lesions may result in cortical sensory changes, while visual abnormalities occur with occipital tumors or masses. Lesions of the pituitary, pineal gland, or posterior fossa (brain stem or cerebellum) may produce, respectively, visual field defects, acromegaly, or Cushing's disease; fixed pupils and paralysis of upward gaze; and cranial nerve palsies or station, gait, and coordination abnormalities.

Such cerebrovascular events as thrombosis or intracerebral hemorrhage may be mistaken for brain tumors. Other benign conditions that may be confused with cerebral neoplasms are postirradiation brain necrosis, pseudotumor cerebri, subdural hematomas, encephalitis, and arachnoiditis. Abscesses may occur secondary to fungal or bacterial infections, especially in such compromised hosts as patients receiving cancer chemotherapy or prolonged corticosteroid administration or those who have had organ transplantation.

Primary brain tumors are most common in the fifth and sixth decades and make up 5% of all neoplasms. In adults, gliomas make up one-half of all primary brain tumors, the majority being glioblastomas. Other primary brain tumors such as meningiomas (13% of all brain tumors), pineal tumors (<1%), pituitary adenomas (10% to 15%), acoustic neuromas (5%) and miscellaneous neoplasms make up the remainder. Approximately 15% to 25% of all brain tumors are metastases from such primary sites as lung, breast, kidney, and skin (melanoma).

A careful history and physical examination, including a detailed neurologic evaluation, should be performed. Chest radiographs may reveal a primary lung carcinoma. Skull radiographs may demonstrate a pineal shift intracranial calcification in a meningioma or craniopharyngioma, or osseous metastases. When an intracranial mass is suspected, a CT scan, which approaches 90% accuracy in detecting intracranial abnormalities, is indicated. Such scans may also be helpful in differentiating between intracranial hemorrhage, solid tumors with edema, and cystic masses. CT scans are probably more sensitive and accurate than radionuclide studies in evaluating mass lesions of the brain. The use of contrast-enhanced CT scans has also reduced the need for performing cerebral arteriography and pneumoencephalography.

If a cerebrovascular accident or other benign cause of increased intracranial pressure has been eliminated, a single, accessible intracerebral mass is preferably resected. If there is hydrocephalus, a shunt may be inserted to reduce elevated intracranial pressure. Dexamethasone, 16 mg daily in divided doses, is begun when the diagnosis of increased intracranial pressure is made. When primary brain tumors are incompletely excised or are malignant, postoperative radiation therapy is recommended.

Metastatic brain lesions are multiple in 40% to 60% of cases. Surgery should be considered for patients with solitary metastases and a free interval of 12 months or more since the treatment of the primary neoplasm. Surgical exploration should also be considered when the etiology of a lesion is uncertain or if rapidly increasing intracranial pressure persists despite the use of a shunt procedure or high-dose corticosteroids. Radiotherapy is used when multiple brain metastases are present. In irradiating brain metastases, the whole brain is treated. Radiation fractionations of 2000 rads in a week, 3000 rads in 2 weeks, or 4000 rads in 3 weeks to the whole brain are all equally effective. More rapid courses have been used but have resulted in an increased early mortality and decreased survival. The mean postirradiation survival time for patients with brain metastases averages only 5 months, but neurologic improvement may be noted in 60% of the patients and major functional improvement in approximately 40%.

D.G.

Abrams H, McNeil B: Medical implications of computed tomography. N Engl J Med 298:255–261, 1978.
Article discusses CT scanning of the brain.
Ashworth B: The early diagnosis of cerebral tumor. Practitioner 221:59–65, 1978.
Clear discussion of tumor evaluation, including history and physical examination, tests, and differential diagnosis.
Berry H, Parker R, Gerdes A: Irradiation of brain metastases. Acta Radiol 13:535–544, 1974.
In the 124 patients discussed, the main primary sites were lung, breast, and

unknown; 44% were multiple. Mean survival was 4.7 months; 41% showed functional improvement.

Brismar J, Roberson G, Davis K: Radiation necrosis of the brain. Neuroradiological consideration with computed tomography. Neuroradiology 12:109–113, 1976.

CT scans are shown to be important in making the diagnosis of radiation necrosis of the brain.

Butler AR, Passalaqua AM, Bernstein A, Kricheff II: Contrast enhanced CT scan and radionuclide brain scan in supratentorial gliomas. Am J Roentgenol 132:607–611, 1979.

Contrast-enhanced CT examination is the best single examination for a suspected brain tumor.

Coleman RE, Cooper MD: Conventional methods of diagnosis using nuclear scan and recent progress with radionuclide transaxial tomography. NCI Monograph No. 46:97–108, Dec. 1977.

CT scans are compared to radionuclide imaging, EEG's, and invasive studies.

Deutsch M, Parsons J, Mercado R: Radiotherapy for intracranial metastases. Cancer 34:1607–1611, 1974.

In this retrospective study 65 patients were given 3000 rads in 2 weeks to the whole brain with a 900 rad boost to the area of involvement. There was no evidence that prior craniotomy improved radiotherapy results.

Fager C: Indications for neurosurgical intervention in metastatic lesions of the central nervous system. Med Clin North Am 59:487–494, 1975.

Article discusses management of brain and spinal cord metastases. Recommends surgical intervention in patients with breast or renal primary sites with long free interval and for those with single metastases with long free interval.

Fishman R: Brain edema. N Engl J Med 293:706–711, 1975.

Excellent review of pathophysiology of brain edema.

Gercovich F, Luna M, Gottlieb J: Increased incidence of cerebral metastases in sarcoma patients with prolonged survival from chemotherapy. Cancer 36:1843–1851, 1975.

Of 456 patients with sarcomas at the M. D. Anderson Hospital who relapsed, only 6 had relapses in the central nervous system; however, when chemotherapy prolonged survival, 5 of 14 who had relapses had them in the CNS.

Hindo W, DeTrana F, Lee M, Hendrickson F: Large dose increment irradiation in treatment of cerebral metastases. Cancer 26:138–141, 1970.

Over 50 patients received 1000 rads in a single dose; improvement was noted in 65%, but there were 3 early deaths.

Kramer R, Janetos G, Perlstein G: An approach to contrast enhancement in computed tomography of the brain. Radiology 116:641–647, 1975.

Reviews the accuracy of CT scanning.

Lang E, Slater J: Metastatic brain tumors—Results of surgical and nonsurgical management. Surg Clin North Am 44:865–872, 1964.

Survival was poor in patients with lung cancer, but there was long postcraniotomy survival in some patients with melanoma and the breast as primary sites.

Posner JB, Chernik NL: Intracranial metastases from systemic cancer. *In* BS Schoenberg (Ed), Advances in Neurology. New York, Raven Press, 1978. Vol. 19, pp. 579–592.

Article discusses both frequency of metastases and distribution of primary sites.

Simionescu MA: Metastatic tumors of the brain. J Neurosurg 17:861–873, 1960.

In 195 patients with such tumors, 56% were solitary, 18% showed sudden symptoms, and in 43% onset was more insidious over 1 to 3 months. Postoperative mortality was 38%.

Vick NA: Intracranial tumors. *In* Grinker's Neurology. Springfield, Ill., Charles C Thomas, 1976. Pp. 392–470.
Detailed review of intracranial tumors.

Wilson CB: Clinical manifestations of intracranial tumors. Semin Oncol 2:5–10, 1975.
Gives short description of clinical sequelae of increased intracranial pressure.

Young D, Posner J, Chu F, Neisce F: Rapid course radiation therapy of cerebral metastases: Results and complications. Cancer 34:1069–1076, 1974.
Therapy of 750 rads twice in three days was compared retrospectively to 3000 rads in 3 weeks. Neurological improvement was similar in the two groups. There was an increase in complications (with five deaths) in patients with increased intracranial pressure who were in the rapid fractionation group. There was also decreased survival (59 days versus 116 days) in this group.

5. SPINAL CORD AND NERVE ROOT COMPRESSION

Almost two-thirds of patients with rapidly evolving spinal cord compression (SCC) have neoplastic encroachment upon the spinal cord as its cause. Approximately 5% of patients with systemic cancers develop this complication. Primary tumors resulting in spinal cord compression may be intramedullary (within the spinal cord), extramedullary (within the dura mater), or extradural. Ependymomas, astrocytomas, and benign cystic lesions are the most common intramedullary neoplastic causes of spinal cord compression. Extramedullary tumors that may cause this syndrome are neurofibromas and meningiomas. Extradural lesions within the spinal canal but outside the dura mater which may produce cord compression are meningiomas, angiomas, and chordomas. Neurofibromas may also protrude through an intervertebral foramen and compress the spinal cord.

Metastases from lung, breast, prostate, and renal carcinomas are common causes of spinal cord compression. Metastatic lesions usually compress the spinal cord anteriorly by direct extension from a vertebral body, less frequently by growth through an intervertebral foramen or from metastases to the extradural fat. Lymphoma and multiple myeloma may also produce spinal cord or nerve root compression; however, only 6% to 10% of patients with lymphomas develop this complication. Since anterior compression is common, the usual posterior laminectomy may not completely relieve the pressure upon the spinal cord, a possible explanation for the relative ineffectiveness of surgery alone in the treatment of SCC.

Rare, nonneoplastic causes of spinal cord compression are extradural abscesses, with or without adjacent osteomyelitis and spinal tuberculosis (Pott's disease). Rheumatoid arthritis, cervical spondylosis, and herniated thoracolumbar intervertebral discs may all result in SCC. Paraplegia may also result from the Guillain-Barré syndrome, multiple sclerosis, radiation myelitis, and spinal artery thrombosis. Other than herniated discs, however, all these benign causes of spinal cord compression are quite rare.

If neoplastic spinal cord compression progresses, it will ultimately result in paralysis. Earlier symptoms usually precede paralysis, however. The first symptom in 96% of patients is *pain*, either localized to the back, radiating in a belt-like distribution through the thoracolumbar regions, or extending to the groin or lower extremities. Pain is often present for weeks or months before the diagnosis of SCC is made. Weakness, sensory changes, bladder dysfunction, and ataxia are rarely initial symptoms of SCC (<2%); however, the first three *are noted* in 76%, 57%, and 51% of patients, respectively, at the time of diagnosis. The onset of all these symptoms may be insidious, as is the case with most primary tumors of the spinal cord and meninges, or may occur rapidly, in a matter of days to weeks, as is common with metastatic lesions.

The diagnosis of SCC must be made early so that treatment to restore sensory and motor function can be carried out before the damage is irreversible. A careful history may reveal evidence of a prior or coexisting malignancy. A detailed neurologic examination is also essential in both diagnosing and localizing the level of spinal cord impairment. Appropriate radiographs may reveal the presence of a paravertebral mass, bone destruction, or collapse. CSF protein elevations higher than 100 mg/ml are noted in the majority of patients with SCC, but cytologic findings are almost always negative. Rare reports have described progression of SCC symptomatology after a lumbar puncture, so caution is indicated in the case of a patient with rapidly progressing signs. If a myelogram is indicated, lumbar myelography is ordinarily performed. Cisternal myelography should also be carried out to localize the superior level of the block and to aid in planning the extent of the radiation therapy treatment volume. If a well-defined single thoracic or lumbar spine abnormality seen on x-ray or bone scan is likely to be a solitary metastasis, however, the cisternal myelogram may be occasionally omitted.

If an intrinsic neuropathy such as radiation-induced transverse myelitis or Guillain-Barré syndrome has been ruled out and neoplastic involvement is suspected, therapy should begin immediately. Historically the most commonly used initial treatment was decompressive laminectomy, with or without the use of concomitant corticosteroids and postoperative radiation therapy. However, in a recent nonrandomized study of 235 patients in which 170 were treated by radiation therapy alone and 65 by decompressive laminectomy followed by irradiation, no differences in outcome were noted between the two groups. The policy of the Stanford Medical Center at present is to begin corticosteroids (Decadron, 10 mg IV) when the diagnosis of neoplastic spinal cord compression is made and to continue their use (80 to 100 mg daily in divided doses) for three days, while high-dose irradiation is being delivered. The corticosteroids are then rapidly tapered as tolerated. Patients are initially managed nonsurgically with three exceptions: 1. Patients who have received prior high-dose irradiation to the site of block, which precludes further adequate radiation therapy, receive decompressive laminectomy. 2. Patients with no known primary malignancy or those in whom a neoplastic cause of SCC is questionable are also treated surgically. 3. Patients whose neurologic condition deteriorates while being irradiated receive decompressive laminectomy. All others, even those patients with rapid onset of neurologic impairment, are initially irradiated.

After the institution of Decadron, 400 rads daily for 3 days are delivered to the involved spinal cord segments. After these three initial high-dose fractions, conventional radiotherapy treatment is then given to the area of the block (with generous margins) for a total dose of 3500–4000 rads in 4 to 5 weeks. Outpatients should be hospitalized during the initial high-dose radiation course and thereafter depending upon their clinical status. Neurologic checks are made every 2 hours during the first 3 days to judge the patient's response to radiation therapy, so that decompressive laminectomy may be performed if further deterioration occurs.

The completeness of response to therapy depends on the rapidity of onset of spinal cord compression, whether or not a complete block is present and if paraplegia or quadriplegia has occurred, and the length of time that these complications have existed. Patients who are ambulatory at the start of therapy have the best prognosis (60% to 80% chance of continued ambulation for carcinomas and lymphomas, respectively), but only 0% to 10% of paraplegic patients can be expected to become ambulatory. Those with lymphomas have the best chance for long-term improvement in neurologic status after treatment.

D.G.

Bruckman JE, Bloomer WD: Management of spinal cord compression. Semin Oncol 5:135–140, 1978.
  Review details diagnostic methods, treatment, and outcome.
Friedman M, Kim T, Panahon A: Spinal cord compression of malignant lymphoma. Cancer 37:1485–1491, 1976.
  In 73 patients with spinal cord compression, 75% of unirradiated patients responded, and 46% of those who had received prior irradiation responded to additional radiation. Good literature review.
Gilbert R, Kim J, Posner J: Epidural spinal cord compression from metastatic tumor: Diagnosis and treatment. Ann Neurol 3:40–51, 1978.
  In a series of 235 patients, 170 were treated with radiotherapy alone and 65 with surgery and radiotherapy. The authors concluded that radiation therapy alone was as effective as decompressive laminectomy plus irradiation in treating epidural cord compression from metastatic cancer.
Harries B: Spinal cord compression. Br Med J 1:611–614, 1970.
  Excellent discussion of differential diagnosis, types of paralysis that occur, and treatment.
Kramer S: Complications of radiation therapy: The central nervous system. Semin Roentgenol 9:75–83, 1974.
  Good description of clinical radiation spinal cord injury.
Posner J, Howieson J, Cvitovic E: Disappearing spinal cord compression: Oncolytic effect of glucocorticoids (and other chemotherapeutic agents) on epidural metastases. Ann Neurol 2:409–413, 1977.
  Case reports show effectiveness of corticosteroids in reducing symptoms and signs of spinal cord compression.
White W, Patterson R, Bergland R: Role of surgery in the treatment of spinal cord compression by metastatic neoplasm. Cancer 27:558–561, 1971.
  In a large series, 226 patients were treated by decompressive laminectomy. Over half of the patients also received radiation therapy and 36% of the total became ambulatory.

6. MENINGEAL TUMOR INFILTRATION

Infiltration of the meninges by malignant tumor cells is being recognized in cancer patients with increasing frequency as their overall survival increases. This phenomenon was first reported in acute leukemia of childhood, where a tenfold increase in the incidence of meningeal leukemia was noted with the advent of chemotherapy. The incidence was so high (approximately 50%) in patients with relapsing acute lymphoblastic leukemia (ALL) that effective prophylactic treatment to the central nervous system (CNS) has become a pivotal part of initial management. In other malignancies as well, meningeal disease may be the first site of relapse and is frequently associated with bone marrow involvement, but the role of prophylactic CNS therapy is not well established. Leptomeningeal metastases are found in about 4% of cancer patients at autopsy, with metastatic adenocarcinoma of the breast or lung accounting for the majority of cases. In spite of effective systemic chemotherapy, malignant cells in the meninges may continue to proliferate, causing widespread multifocal seeding and sheet-like tumor cell growth along the surfaces of the brain and spinal cord. This lack of meningeal tumor control, in the face of systemic control, is thought to be due to the blood-brain barrier and consequent ineffective antitumor drug concentration in the CNS.

The symptoms of meningeal tumor involvement may include headache (usually diffuse and severe), nausea, vomiting, lethargy, confusion or changes in memory, leg or low back pain, unsteady gait, paresthesias, double vision, neck pain or stiffness, and seizures. Symptoms are usually present for less than 3 weeks but sometimes for as long as 3 to 6 months. Because many complaints are vague and not specific or focal, the clinical diagnosis may be elusive. Common admitting diagnoses other than meningeal tumor include infectious meningitis (tuberculous, fungal), parenchymal central nervous system or extradural metastases, metabolic or drug encephalopathy, viral encephalitis, multifocal leukoencephalopathy, subdural hematoma, and even herniated disc.

Meningeal disease may be suspected when there are symptoms and/or signs of structural disease involving the neuraxis at more than one anatomic site. In general the neurologic examination will uncover more widespread dysfunction than the patient's symptoms would suggest: in particular, abnormalities of cognitive function, cranial nerves, and/or spinal roots. In all instances the diagnosis is established by cerebrospinal fluid (CSF) examination, in which findings of increased pressure, increased white blood cell count, and protein with decreased glucose are typical. In no case is the CSF exam entirely normal, although an elevated pressure may be the only abnormality. Multiple taps may be required to obtain malignant CSF cytologic findings, since the first CSF examination is positive in less than half the patients. At least three taps may be necessary, and even though there may be fewer than 4 cells seen on routine cell count, the cytology can still be positive. Other laboratory examinations are less helpful in making the specific diagnosis of meningeal tumor but may aid in ruling out other neuropathologic conditions. A myelogram will sometimes demonstrate multiple, nodular, meningeal lesions and can rule out extradural compression. Computed tomography of the brain can demonstrate retro-orbital masses, parenchymal metastases, hydrocephalus, and sometimes even meningeal deposits. Diffuse slowing and occasional asymmetry may be seen on EEG. Skull x-rays, brain scan, arteriography, and pneumoencephalography are of little additional value.

Since the entire neuraxis is invaded by tumor, the therapy of meningeal disease must encompass not only the symptomatic site but all areas at risk. Without treatment the patient with meningeal tumor has a survival time of less than 6 weeks; with treatment, survival may be prolonged by 4 to 5 months for patients with carcinomatous meningitis and even longer (>12 months) for those with leukemic infiltration. There are several methods of treating meningeal disease: craniospinal irradiation and intrathecal (IT) or intraventricular chemotherapy with or without local irradiation to the symptomatic site. Since craniospinal irradiation causes severe bone marrow depression and patients frequently require concurrent systemic chemotherapy, this extent of irradiation has been supplanted by involved field treatment, usually to the whole brain, plus CSF chemotherapy.

Methotrexate is the drug most commonly used for the treatment of meningeal disease, although cytosine arabinoside also appears to be effective. Methotrexate can be administered by lumbar puncture into the intrathecal space or via an Ommaya reservoir into the intraventricular space. The distribution of methotrexate within the CSF is more reproducible with Ommaya reservoir administration, and it has been demonstrated recently that this is probably a more effective means of meningeal tumor therapy. On the other hand, intraventricular chemotherapy via an Ommaya reservoir may be complicated by infection or incorrect placement. The dose of methotrexate given by either route is 6 to 12 mg/M² (15 mg maximum) two times a week until the CSF clears; the schedule is then lengthened to monthly maintenance therapy. The drug should be diluted in sterile nonbacteriostatic saline, water, or Eliot's B solution.

Blood count depression is a common side-effect of CSF methotrexate therapy and can be ameliorated by the use of leucovorin rescue. Because leucovorin rapidly enters the CSF, its use must be delayed for 12 to 24 hours following intrathecal or intraventricular methotrexate to avoid reversing methotrexate's antitumor activity. The usual dose of leucovorin is 3 to 6 mg po every 6 hours for 4 or more doses.

Other toxicities of CSF methotrexate administration include fever, headache, aseptic meningitis, lumbar arachnoiditis, paraparesis, paraplegia, and sensory loss. In addition, a necrotizing leukoencephalopathy has been described in patients receiving both whole brain irradiation and intrathecal or systemic methotrexate. The neurotoxicities of CSF methotrexate therapy appear to correlate with the cumulative total of drug administered as well as with high local concentration and prolonged exposure.

C.P.

Band PR, Holland JF, Bernard J, et al: Treatment of central nervous system leukemia with intrathecal cytosine arabinoside. Cancer 32:744–748, 1973.
Intrathecal cytosine arabinoside was shown to be transiently effective. No hematological toxicity was noted.

Bleyer WA, Drake JC, Chabner BA: Neurotoxicity and elevated cerebrospinal-fluid methotrexate concentration in meningeal leukemia. N Engl J Med 289:770–773, 1973.
Neurotoxicity developed in 5 of 25 patients receiving intrathecal methotrexate; it was related to prolonged exposure to elevated concentrations of methotrexate.

Bleyer WA, Pizzo PA, Spence AM, et al: The Ommaya reservoir: Newly recognized complications and recommendations for insertion and use. Cancer 41:2431–2437, 1978.
A useful guide.

Bleyer WA, Poplack DG: Intraventricular versus intralumbar methotrexate for central-nervous-system leukemia: Prolonged remission with the Ommaya reservoir. Med Pediatr Oncol 6:207–213, 1979.
Reinduction of CNS remission was accomplished with Ommaya reservoir administration in spite of prior intralumbar failure.

Duttera MJ, Bleyer WA, Pomeroy TC, et al: Irradiation, methotrexate toxicity, and the treatment of meningeal leukemia. Lancet 2:703–707, 1973.
This prospective randomized study of 31 patients with meningeal leukemia compared intrathecal methotrexate alone vs. IT methotrexate plus 2400 rads to the cranium.

Glass JP, Melamed M, Chernik NL, Posner JB: Malignant cells in cerebrospinal fluid (CSF): The meaning of a positive CSF cytology. Neurology 29:1369–1375, 1979.
Of 51 patients with autopsy evidence of meningeal disease, 41% had a negative CSF cytology premortum.

Griffin JW, Thompson RW, Mitchinson MJ, et al: Lymphomatous leptomeningitis. Am J Med 51:200–208, 1971.
Lymphomatous leptomeningitis is seen most commonly in diffuse histiocytic lymphoma; median survival of 20 patients was 3 months.

Hustu HO, Aur RJA, Verzosa MS, et al: Prevention of central nervous system leukemia by irradiation. Cancer 32:585–597, 1973.
Excellent review of the St. Jude's experience of CNS prophylaxis using 2400 rads craniospinal irradiation or 2400 rads cranial irradiation plus intrathecal methotrexate.

Little JR, Dale AJD, Okazaki H: Meningeal carcinomatosis: Clinical manifestations. Arch Neurol 30:138–143, 1974.
Meningeal carcinomatosis was seen most commonly in patients with adenocarcinoma of the breast and lung.

Olson ME, Chernik NL, Posner JB: Infiltration of the leptomeninges by systemic cancer: A clinical and pathologic study. Arch Neurol 30:122, 1974.
An excellent clinicopathological analysis of 50 patients with meningeal cancer.

Posner JB: Management of central nervous system metastases. Semin Oncol 4:81, 1977.
Excellent review of the management of intracranial, spinal, and leptomeningeal metastases.

Price RA, Jamieson PA: The central nervous system in childhood leukemia: II. Subacute leukoencephalopathy. Cancer 35:306–318, 1975.
Leukoencephalopathy occurred in patients who had received greater than 2000 rads whole brain irradiation and systemic methotrexate. Intrathecal therapy alone did not appear to contribute to the development of leukoencephalopathy.

Rubinstein LJ, Herman MM, Long TF, Wilbur JR: Disseminated necrotizing leukoencephalopathy: A complication of treated central nervous system leukemia and lymphoma. Cancer 35:291–305, 1975.
Describes clinicopathological features of leukoencephalopathy in 5 patients following whole brain irradiation and intrathecal chemotherapy.

Shapiro WR, Young DF, Mehta BM: Methotrexate: Distribution in cerebrospinal fluid after intravenous, ventricular, and lumbar injections. N Engl J Med 293:161–166, 1975.
Distribution of methotrexate within the CSF was most reproducible with Ommaya reservoir administration.

Simone JV, Aur RJA, Hustu HO, Verzosa M: Acute lymphocytic leukemia in children. Cancer 36:770–774, 1975.
Excellent review of systemic therapy and the role of CNS prophylaxis. Article also discusses the development of leukoencephalopathy in patients receiving weekly systemic methotrexate (<50 mg/m²) maintenance for at least 6 months.

Young RC, Howser DM, Anderson T, et al: Central nervous system complications of non-Hodgkin's lymphoma—the potential role for prophylactic therapy. Am J Med 66:435–442, 1979.
A retrospective study of 38 patients: Aggressive histologies and bone marrow or bone involvement correlated with the development of lymphomatous meningitis.

7. FEVER AND NEUTROPENIA

Infection is the cause of death in almost half of all patients with malignant disease; and as surgery, radiation therapy, and chemotherapy are employed more frequently, the risk of subsequent infection increases. Normal host defenses to infection may be altered by the malignancy itself, by its treatment, or by other factors such as malnutrition or advanced age. The mechanical barriers of the skin and mucous membranes may be disrupted by indwelling catheters, surgical procedures, drug- or radiation-induced mucositis, decubitus ulceration, or tumor infiltration. Phagocytic defenses may be seriously compromised by neutropenia (drug- or radiation-induced, or secondary to tumor infiltration of bone marrow or hypersplenism) and/or granulocytic dysfunction. Cell-mediated immunity is frequently abnormal in patients with lymphomas or metastatic solid tumors; and corticosteroids impair cutaneous delayed hypersensitivity as well as in vitro lymphocyte responsiveness. Hypogammaglobulinemia and/or diminished antibody responses may be seen in chronic lymphocytic leukemia, multiple myeloma, and lymphomas. Moreover, chemotherapy impairs primary antibody responses, and splenectomy (as performed for lymphoma staging) reduces opsonic activity.

More than 60% of febrile episodes in cancer patients are due to proved or presumptive infection, in most instances in the setting of neutropenia. With a fall in the number of granulocytes to below 1500/mm^3, the risk of infection is approximately 12%, and below 100/mm^3 the risk increases to nearly 100%. In addition the severity of infection and its associated mortality rate correlate not only with the level of granulocytopenia but with its duration. In the neutropenic patient, bacteremia with an indeterminate source and pneumonia are the most common infectious complications. Gram-negative bacteria are isolated from the blood in over half the cases, in particular *Escherichia coli, Pseudomonas aeruginosa*, and *Klebsiella pneumoniae. Staphylococcus aureus, Bacteroides* sp., and multiple bacterial species are also commonly identified. Candidemia accounts for less than 8% of positive blood cultures, and other fungal infections are identified even less often, although fungal superinfections are documented at autopsy in up to 50% of patients with leukemia or lymphoma (but in <10% of those with solid tumors).

The prognosis of the cancer patient with sepsis depends upon multiple factors, including causative organism (*Ps. aeruginosa, Klebsiella* sp., polymicrobic, and *Candida* sp. infections are associated with >50% mortality); source of infection (>70% mortality with pulmonary infections); degree and duration of neutropenia (approximately 40% mortality with <500/mm^3, but increasing to >80% if granulocytopenia persists for more than 10 days); presence of shock (mortality of 70%); prompt and appropriate antibiotic therapy; and extent of underlying malignancy.

The febrile, neutropenic patient may present a difficult diagnostic problem, since the usual signs and symptoms (other than fever) of localized infection may be absent. A thorough physical examination should include particular attention to even minimal tenderness or erythema, since cellulitis may be subtle and abscesses rarely become fluctuant. Bacterial and fungal cultures of blood (both aerobic and anaerobic), sputum, and urine should be obtained, along with cultures from any other suspicious sites, including cerebrospinal fluid. Lung infections are often clinically occult, and a chest x-ray can detect "silent" pulmonary infiltrates. Serologic tests for viral, fungal, or protozoan infections may be useful. The nitrobluetetrazolium (NBT) test and limulus assay should not be relied upon to exclude infection.

Since the relationship of granulocytopenia with infection is well established, prompt antimicrobial therapy is indicated in the febrile, neutropenic patient, unless a bacterial etiology can be categorically excluded. Antibiotics should be bactericidal rather than bacteriostatic, administered intravenously, and have a broad spectrum of activity covering both gram-negative and gram-positive organisms. Rather than awaiting documentation of bacteremia (which may take several days), treatment should be initiated immediately after appropriate cultures, on the presumption that bacteremia exists. Typical drug combinations utilized in this setting include a cephalosporin (cephalothin or cephazolin) plus carbenicillin or gentamicin, or carbenicillin plus gentamicin, or all three drugs. In one study, cephalothin plus gentamicin was found to be more nephrotoxic

(12% incidence) than the other two regimens (<4%). Once the causative organism is identified, antibiotic therapy can be adjusted according to drug susceptibility and kind of infection. In spite of rapid defervescence, antibiotics should be continued for at least 7 days, since earlier discontinuation may result in relapse of infection. If a patient has persistent neutropenia and fever on antibiotics, a third antibiotic should be added, and thorough search for the cause of infection should be continued. Granulocyte transfusions may be of value, since they can improve survival significantly in septic patients with prolonged neutropenia. In general, treatment with antifungal, antituberculous, and antiprotozoal agents should require identification of the causative organism and not be used empirically.

At least 20% of patients with bacteremia will develop circulatory shock, usually associated with gram-negative organisms, and this complication is frequently fatal (>70% mortality). Shock is probably secondary to the release of endotoxin (a cell-wall lipopolysaccharide) and the resultant generation of vasoactive kinins. Clinical manifestations include chills, fever, hypotension, hyperpnea, tachypnea, oliguria or anuria, and changes in mentation. Metabolic acidosis, hepatocellular dysfunction, and thrombocytopenia are commonly documented. Besides appropriate antibiotic therapy, treatment of circulatory shock requires rapid correction of the effective blood volume with fluids (monitoring central venous or pulmonary artery pressure), oxygen, correction of acidosis, and sometimes the addition of vasoactive drugs (such as dopamine, isoproterenol, or digitalis). The use of high-dose corticosteroids remains controversial but is probably of value.

C.P.

Bloomfield CD, Kennedy BJ: Cephalothin, carbenicillin, and gentamicin combination therapy for febrile patients with acute nonlymphocytic leukemia. Cancer 34:431–437, 1974.
This drug combination is an effective antibiotic regimen for empiric therapy of febrile, neutropenic patients.
Bodey GP, Buckley M, Sathe YS, Freireich EJ: Quantitative relationships between circulating leukocytes and infection in patients with acute leukemia. Ann Intern Med 64:328–340, 1966.
The incidence and severity of infection increases with the degree and duration of granulocytopenia (<1500/mm³).
Bodey GP, Rodriguez V, Cabanillas F, Freireich EJ: Protected environment-prophylactic antibiotic program for malignant lymphoma: Randomized trial during chemotherapy to induce remission. Am J Med 66:74–81, 1979.
Frequency of infection was significantly less for patients in the PEPA program.
Gill FA, Robinson R, Maclowry JD, Levine AS: The relationship of fever, granulocytopenia and antimicrobial therapy to bacteremia in cancer patients. Cancer 39:1704–1709, 1977.
This retrospective study shows that the discontinuance of antimicrobial therapy in the presence of persistent granulocytopenia and fever was associated with subsequent bacteremia within 4 days in 47% of episodes.
Herzig RH, Herzig GP, Graw RG, et al: Successful granulocyte transfusion therapy of gram-negative septicemia: A prospectively randomized controlled study. N Engl J Med 296:701–705, 1977.
The addition of granulocyte transfusions to appropriate antibiotic therapy in 16 neutropenic patients with gram-negative sepsis significantly improved survival for those with prolonged granulocytopenia (>10 days).
Higby DJ, Burnett D: Granulocyte transfusions: Current status. Blood 55:2–8, 1980.

An excellent summary of the indications for granulocyte transfusion, methods of granulocyte harvesting, and assessment of response to therapy.

Ketchel SJ, Rodriguez V: Acute infections in cancer patients. Semin Oncol 5:167–179, 1978.
Includes a good review of antibacterial therapy.

Pizzo PA, Robichaud KJ, Gill FA, et al: Duration of empiric antibiotic therapy in granulocytopenic patients with cancer. Am J Med 67:194–200, 1979.
Of 33 patients who defervesced on prophylactic antibiotics, none of 16 had infectious sequelae with continued therapy until granulocytopenia resolved, whereas 7 of 17 developed infectious sequelae when the antibiotics were discontinued while the patients were still granulocytopenic.

Rodriguez V, Burgess M, Bodey GP: Management of fever of unknown origin in patients with neoplasms and neutropenia. Cancer 32:1007–1012, 1973.
During 81 febrile episodes in 76 neutropenic patients, the cause of fever could not be identified in 72% of the episodes.

Schimpff SC, Aisner J: Empiric antibiotic therapy. Cancer Treat Rep 62:673–680, 1978.
An excellent review with pragmatic management recommendations.

Schumer W: Steroids in the treatment of clinical septic shock. Ann Surg 184:333–341, 1976.
This prospective randomized trial comparing steroids to placebos demonstrates a significant decrease in mortality for those surgical patients in septic shock who received corticosteroids.

Singer C, Kaplan MH, Armstrong D: Bacteremia and fungemia complicating neoplastic disease: A study of 364 cases. Am J Med 62:731–742, 1977.
An excellent analysis of the clinical features, diagnoses, and prognostic factors of bacteremia and fungemia.

The EROTC International Antimicrobial Therapy Project Group: Three antibiotic regimens in treatment of infection in febrile granulocytopenic patients with cancer. J Infect Dis 137:14–29, 1978.
Although equally effective antimicrobial regimens, cephalothin plus gentamicin was more nephrotoxic (12% incidence) than carbenicillin plus cephalothin (4%) or carbenicillin plus gentamicin (2%).

Young LS, Martin WJ, Meyer RD, et al: Gram-negative rod bacteremia: Microbiologic, immunologic, and therapeutic considerations. Ann Intern Med 86:456–471, 1977.
A good review.

8. DISSEMINATED INTRAVASCULAR COAGULATION

Laboratory evidence of coagulation abnormalities in cancer patients is found frequently. Often these abnormalities are attributable to intravascular coagulation and associated fibrinolysis. The syndrome of disseminated intravascular coagulation (DIC) may be triggered by the release of thromboplastic material into the circulation, the activation of factor XII by epinephrine, or shock with the development of lactic acidosis. Fibrinolysis usually accompanies intravascular coagulation, and the resultant laboratory and clinical findings reflect the dynamic balance between these two processes. Because the rates of intravascular coagulation, fibrinolysis, and the production of clotting factors and platelets vary during DIC, laboratory measurements (other than the presence of fibrinogen-fibrin degradation products) may be normal or abnormal. There may be compensated DIC, in which the consumption of coagulation factors and platelets is balanced by their production in the liver and bone marrow; decompensated DIC, in which consumption outstrips production; or overcompensated DIC, in which production surpasses consumption. The laboratory states of coagulopathy do not necessarily have a correlation with the clinical syndromes of subclinical chronic DIC, acute hemorrhagic DIC, or thrombotic DIC. In fact all three clinical syndromes can be seen with any of the three laboratory settings.

The hemorrhagic and/or thrombotic, as well as asymptomatic, forms of DIC have all been documented in association with malignancy, and their common pathophysiologic mechanism is thought to be the release of thromboplastin-like material from the tumor itself (such as cellular secretions, enzymes, cell membrane or cytoplasmic components). Subclinical DIC (defined as the laboratory presence of fibrinolysis, i.e., the presence of fibrinogen-fibrin degradation products, in the asymptomatic patient) represents the most common form of the syndrome, and although its true incidence is unknown, it has been identified in as many as 86% of patients with lung cancer. Moreover, fibrinogen and platelet turnover studies by one group showed that in 13 of 13 cancer patients studied, these measurements were 3 times greater than normal in the face of normal platelet counts and fibrinogen concentrations. Chronic subclinical DIC is more frequently documented in patients with metastatic disease and, in particular, those with cancers of the prostate, lung, breast, and pancreas.

The hypercoagulable form of DIC is associated with thrombophlebitis (Trousseau's syndrome), nonbacterial thrombotic endocarditis, and small vessel occlusions with microinfarcts (e.g., in kidneys or brain). Migratory thrombophlebitis is seen classically in patients with cancer of the body or tail of the pancreas. Thrombotic complications are also common in lung, stomach, and ovarian cancer.

The hemorrhagic form of DIC is seen in approximately 10% of patients with cancer and in almost all patients with acute promyelocytic leukemia. It is associated with sepsis, liver dysfunction, or surgical procedures; and in patients with acute leukemia it may be seen in association with very high white blood cell counts and/or with therapy. Prognosis is poor in cancer patients with hemorrhagic DIC: in one series, 75% died within 30 days of its diagnosis.

Typical laboratory findings in patients with DIC include the presence of fibrinogen-fibrin degradation products (FDP); hypofibrinogenemia; thrombocytopenia; prolonged prothrombin, partial thromboplastin, and thrombin times; decreased factors V, VIII, and X; poor clot formation; and the presence of microangiopathic hemolytic anemia and cryoproteins. The most sensitive test, particularly in chronic subclinical DIC, is that for FDP, since fibrinolysis is almost always present with intravascular coagulation. Other laboratory findings may be low (decompensated), high (overcompensated), or normal (compensated), depending upon the dynamic balance of consumption and production.

Causes of acute hemorrhagic DIC, other than malignancy, include obstetric complications, infections, surgical procedures, trauma, heat stroke, shock, incompatible blood transfusions; while giant hemangioma, collagen vascular diseases, aortic aneurysm, sarcoidosis, and amyloidosis have been documented in association with chronic DIC. Any of the above conditions may exacerbate the subclinical DIC of malignancy, as illustrated by the common problem of postoperative hemorrhage in the patient with prostate cancer.

Since DIC is usually secondary to some underlying condition, the most effective therapy is to treat the primary disease process. Chronic DIC rarely requires therapy, since patients are often asymptomatic. Thrombotic complications can be treated appropriately with heparin and then chronically with warfarin, although some patients may require long-term heparin to control recurrent thrombophlebitis.

Acute hemorrhagic DIC should be anticipated in patients with acute promyelocytic leukemia or those with chronic DIC and sepsis, for example. Heparin therapy can be very hazardous in the setting of thrombocytopenia and hemorrhage and should be reserved for those patients with severe clinical bleeding. Often hemorrhagic DIC is acute but self-limited and in these circumstances, may call for replacement of coagulation factors (with cryoprecipitate and fresh frozen plasma) and platelets. Antifibrinolytic agents (E-aminocaproic acid, EACA) are generally contraindicated.

C.P.

Alving BM, Abeloff MD, Bell W: Spontaneous remission of recurring disseminated intravascular coagulation associated with prostatic carcinoma. Cancer 37:928–930, 1976.
This case report emphasizes the clinical and subclinical aspects of chronic DIC.

Bowie EJW, Owen CA Jr: Hemostatic failure in clinical medicine. Semin Hematol 14:341–364, 1977.
A good review of intravascular coagulation and fibrinolysis (DIC), both acute and chronic.

Collins RC, Al-Mondhiry H, Chernik NL, Posner JB: Neurologic manifestations of intravascular coagulation in patients with cancer: A clinicopathologic analysis of 12 cases. Neurology (Minneap) 25:795–806, 1975.
Generalized brain dysfunction associated with coagulation abnormalities and the presence of multifocal brain infarcts at autopsy were documented in 12 of 1,459 patients with cancer.

Cooper HA, Bowie EJW, Owen CA: Evaluation of patients with increased fibrinolytic split products (FSP) in their serum. Mayo Clin Proc 49:654–657, 1974.
Article illustrates "compensated," "decompensated," and "overcompensated" patterns of laboratory values in DIC.

Davis RB, Theologides A, Kennedy BJ: Comparative studies of blood coagulation and platelet aggregation in patients with cancer and nonmalignant diseases. Ann Intern Med 71:67–80, 1969.
Thrombocytosis prior to therapy and the presence of fibrin split products were only detected in patients with cancer.

Gralnick HR, Marchesi S, Givelber H: Intravascular coagulation in acute leukemia: Clinical and subclinical abnormalities. Blood 40:709–718, 1972.
Laboratory evidence of intravascular coagulation is commonly seen in acute leukemia and may be entirely asymptomatic.

Gralnick HR, Tan HK: Acute promyelocytic leukemia: A model for understanding the role of the malignant cell in hemostasis. Hum Pathol 5:661–673, 1974.
Excellent review of intravascular coagulation in association with acute promyelocytic leukemia.

Hagedorn AB, Borie EJW, Elveback LR, Owen CA: Coagulation abnormalities in patients with inoperable lung cancer. Mayo Clin Proc 49:647–653, 1974.
Tests for soluble fibrin and fibrinolysis were positive in 37 of 43 (86%) lung cancer patients studied prospectively and none had symptomatic DIC.

Harker LA, Slichter SJ: Platelet and fibrinogen consumption in man. N Engl J Med 287:999–1005, 1972.
Platelet and fibrinogen turnover was three times normal in 13 cancer patients although platelet counts and fibrinogen concentrations were normal.

Kazmier FJ, Bowie EJW, Hagedorn AB, Owen CA: Treatment of intravascular coagulation and fibrinolysis (ICF) syndromes. Mayo Clin Proc 49:665–672, 1974.
A good review.

Sack GH, Levin J, Bell WR: Trousseau's syndrome and other manifestations of chronic disseminated coagulopathy in patients with neoplasms: Clinical, pathophysiologic and therapeutic features. Medicine 56:1–37, 1977.
This article provides a comprehensive analysis of 182 patients with migratory thrombophlebitis (96), hemorrhagic phenomena (75), arterial emboli (45), or all three manifestations of DIC (12).

Weick JK: Intravascular coagulation in cancer. Semin Oncol 5:203–211, 1978.
A brief review of the physiology of intravascular coagulation, clinical problems seen in cancer patients, and treatment.

9. HYPERVISCOSITY

The viscosity of whole blood is dependent upon the interaction of blood cells and plasma proteins. Hyperviscosity, therefore, may be due to an elevated serum viscosity, an increased number of blood cells (polycythemia, leukemia), the aggregation of erythrocytes by paraproteins, or an increased resistance of cells to deformation (sickle cells, spherocytes). In patients with malignant disease, the syndromes of hyperviscosity are associated with the first three mechanisms.

Serum hyperviscosity is seen most commonly in Waldenström's macroglobulinemia and multiple myeloma. The resistance to flow (viscosity) of a protein fluid such as serum depends on both the concentrations and the intrinsic viscosity of the individual proteins in solution. The IgM molecule of macroglobulinemia has a high molecular weight (1×10^6) as well as an unusual shape (five projections from a central core) and a large size. These characteristics contrast with the relatively small size (molecular weight of 160,000) and usually symmetric shape of the myeloma IgG and IgA paraproteins. It is not surprising, then, that the serum viscosity of the dysproteinemias and the syndrome of hyperviscosity have a correlation not only with the protein concentration but, more importantly, with the nature, state, and special characteristics of the individual paraproteins. Consequently, for a given concentration of paraprotein, the mean serum viscosity is highest for IgM and significantly less for IgG and IgA. Although almost 80% of patients with myeloma have an abnormally elevated serum viscosity (normal = 1.4 to 1.8), fewer than 5% have a relative serum viscosity of more than 4.0, and rarely are patients symptomatic. On the other hand, up to 40% of the patients with macroglobulinemia have a relative serum viscosity of more than 5.0, and many of these patients are symptomatic. The postulated molecular mechanisms responsible for the development of serum hyperviscosity include high concentrations of monomeric proteins; molecular asymmetry (IgM); stable protein aggregation (IgG_3); unstable protein aggregation (IgG_3); and reversible polymerization (IgA).

In general, the relative viscosity of serum as measured in an Ostwald viscometer correlates with the viscosity of whole blood in the dysproteinemias.

Occasionally, however, the whole blood viscosity is elevated while the serum viscosity is low, probably indicating extensive erythrocyte-paraprotein interaction. In either case the development of symptoms and signs of hyperviscosity are dependent upon many factors, including the degree of serum and whole blood viscosity, the hematocrit, the presence of microvascular disease or cardiac insufficiency, and local pH and ionic strength. With a relative serum viscosity of 5 to 10, most patients are symptomatic, while all have symptoms with a viscosity of ⩾10. Symptoms and signs of serum hyperviscosity include hemorrhagic diathesis (epistaxis, gingival, and mucous membrane bleeding; retinal hemorrhage; purpura); neurologic disorders (acute and chronic encephalopathy, peripheral neuropathy, strokes, seizures, subarachnoid hemorrhage); ocular manifestations (retinopathy, venous distention, hemorrhage with impaired vision); and cardiovascular abnormalities (congestive heart failure, expanded plasma volume with anemia).

Plasmapheresis can effectively treat the symptoms and signs of serum hyperviscosity, as it removes intravascular paraprotein. Since there is a nonlinear relationship between serum viscosity and IgM concentration, relatively small reductions in paraprotein concentrations may greatly reduce the serum viscosity. However, because plasmapheresis has no effect on the basic disease process, discontinuance will result in recurrence of the syndrome in 2 to 3 weeks. Therefore it is recommended that plasmapheresis be performed every 1 to 2 weeks.

Hyperviscosity of whole blood may be caused by increased numbers of cells, as in leukemia or polycythemia. Although the major determinant of viscosity in this instance is the number of cells, other factors may include the rate of shear in blood vessels, the plasma viscosity, the plasma protein morphology and concentration, the blood cell morphology and membrane characteristics, and the blood cell deformability. Leukostasis with intravascular leukemic aggregates or thrombi is usually associated with very high leukocyte counts (> 100,000/mm^3) and symptoms or signs referable to the cardiopulmonary or central nervous systems. Interestingly, it is rarely seen in lymphocytic leukemias (acute or chronic) but may contribute to death in up to 25% of patients with myelogenous leukemias (acute or chronic). The difference between the effects of leukemic lymphoid and of myeloid cells on blood viscosity has been attributed to the relatively larger size and rigidity of myeloblasts as compared to lymphoblasts.

Polycythemia (as in polycythemia vera, or as occasionally associated with renal cell carcinoma, hepatocellular carcinoma, lung or prostate cancer, or uterine fibromata) may also cause whole blood hyperviscosity with increased viscous resistance to flow in the microcirculation and decreased effective tissue perfusion. Correlation of hematocrit level and blood viscosity depends upon the rate of shear, so that for a given hematocrit, viscosity is greater in capillaries than in large vessels. Here the syndrome of hyperviscosity is one of retarded blood flow with organ congestion, reduced capillary perfusion, and increased cardiac work. Treatment of either white cell or red cell hyperviscosity requires a reduction in the number of circulating cells, either by removing the cells with leukopheresis or phlebotomy or by treating the basic disease process.

C.P.

Alexanian R: Blood volume in monoclonal gammopathy. Blood 49:301–307, 1977.
The plasma volume was significantly increased for the hematocrit in 30% of patients, and the total blood volume was elevated in 45%.

Bloch KJ, Maki DG: Hyperviscosity syndromes associated with immunoglobulin abnormalities. Semin Hematol 10:113–124, 1973.
An excellent review of the clinical presentation, diagnosis, and therapy of the hyperviscosity syndrome.

Capra JD, Kunkel HG: Aggregation of γG3 proteins: Relevance to the hyperviscosity syndrome. J Clin Invest 49:610–621, 1970.
Article demonstrates concentration and temperature dependent aggregation of γG3 myeloma proteins that were associated with the clinical findings of the hyperviscosity syndrome.

MacKenzie MR, Babcock J: Studies of the hyperviscosity syndrome: II. Macroglobulinemia. J Lab Clin Med 85:227–234, 1975.
Relative serum viscosity of levels of ≥ 6.0 were found to correlate with IgM protein concentrations of ≥ 5.0 gm/100 ml or with molecular asymmetry.

MacKenzie MR, Brown E, Fudenberg HH, Goodenay L: Waldenström's macroglobulinemia: Correlation between expanded plasma volume and increased serum viscosity. Blood 35:394–408, 1970.
An expanded plasma volume was documented in 17 patients, and its extent correlated with the degree of increase in the relative serum viscosity.

MacKenzie MR, Fudenberg HH, O'Reilly RA: The hyperviscosity syndrome: I. In IgG myeloma. The role of protein concentration and molecular shape. J Clin Invest 49:15–20, 1970.
Demonstrates the role of protein concentration and molecular asymmetry in the development of an increased relative serum viscosity.

MacKenzie MR, Lee TK: Blood viscosity in Waldenström macroglobulinemia. Blood 49:507–510, 1977.
Whole blood viscosity was found to correlate with relative serum viscosity, and symptomatic patients usually had whole blood viscosity values of ≥ 8.0 centipoises.

Mannik M: Blood viscosity in Waldenström's macroglobulinemia. Blood 44:87–98, 1974.
Blood viscosity is dependent upon both hematocrit and macroglobulin concentration.

McKee LC Jr, Collins RD: Intravascular leukocyte thrombi and aggregates as a cause of morbidity and mortality in leukemia. Medicine 53:463–478, 1974.
This autopsy study of 201 patients with leukemia correlated pathological findings with peripheral leukocyte counts.

Solomon A, Fahey JL: Plasmapheresis therapy in macroglobulinemia. Ann Intern Med 58:789–800, 1963.
Plasmapheresis in 10 patients effectively reduced serum macroglobulin level and relative serum viscosity, and improved symptoms of hyperviscosity.

Wells R: Syndromes of hyperviscosity. N Engl J Med 283:183–186, 1970.
A good review of blood hyperviscosity and its etiology (secondary to dysproteinemias, increased cell numbers, or diminished red cell deformability).

10. HYPERCALCEMIA

Hypercalcemia is a common metabolic complication of malignancy, developing in as many as 25% of patients with metastatic breast cancer or squamous carcinoma of the lung. It is also frequently associated with tumors of the kidney, head and neck, cervix, and prostate, and with neuroblastoma and melanoma, as well as with many hematologic malignancies (myeloma, lymphoma, leukemia). Causes of hypercalcemia, other than malignancy, that may coexist in the patient with cancer include hyperparathyroidism, sarcoidosis, vitamin D intoxication, and thiazide administration.

At least three humoral mechanisms have been postulated by which malignancy causes enhanced resorption of bone and subsequent hypercalcemia. The first and most common is direct invasion of bone, thought to be mediated initially by the tumor cell release of prostaglandins. Organ culture studies have demonstrated enhanced bone resorption by prostaglandins E_1 and E_2 derived from animal tumors. In addition, inhibitors of prostaglandin synthesis (indomethacin) have been shown to reverse the tumor-induced hypercalcemia in such animals. Similar studies are becoming available in humans: high levels of prostaglandin metabolites have been found in the urine of cancer patients with hypercalcemia, and in those patients without demonstrable bony metastases, indomethacin has reversed the hypercalcemia. This mode of treatment has little practical utility, however, since more than 80% of cancer patients with hypercalcemia will have demonstrable bony metastases by x-ray or scan. Ectopic production of parathyroid hormone (PTH) by malignant tumors probably accounts for most instances of hypercalcemia without demonstrable bone metastases. Increased levels of immunoreactive PTH may be found in tumor tissue or blood; and with removal of the nonparathyroid cancer, there is resolution of the hypercalcemia. Squamous cell carcinomas of the lung or head and neck as well as renal cell carcinoma are most commonly associated with this syndrome. Ectopic production can usually be differentiated from primary hyperparathyroidism by the serum level of immunoreactive parathormone (iPTH) relative to the serum calcium, with iPTH being higher in the primary disorder. In hematologic malignancies the osteoclastic resorption of bone may be mediated by a soluble polypeptide, osteoclast activating factor (OAF), elaborated by the tumor.

The clinical syndrome of hypercalcemia is usually manifested by anorexia, nausea, constipation, polydipsia, and polyuria. The spectrum of symptoms will depend in part on the rapidity of onset, the patient's prior general condition, and the presence or absence of other underlying diseases (such as renal or CNS). In addition hypercalcemia may be exacerbated by immobilization or by estrogens, androgens, or progestins in the treatment of breast cancer.

Diagnostic studies in the evaluation of hypercalcemia may include serum calcium (two determinations to check for accuracy), phosphate, alkaline phosphatase, BUN, creatinine, electrolytes, serum iPTH, and urinary calcium. Since calcium is 50% protein-bound, a total serum protein aids in determining the ionized fraction, which probably accounts for symptomatic hypercalcemia. The electrocardiogram may show tachycardia, a shortened Q-T interval, and a cove-like broadening of the T wave. X-rays of the chest may suggest tumor, sarcoidosis, or even bony changes of hyperparathyroidism. Abdominal flat plate may show bone metastases.

Hypercalcemia may be treated in a variety of ways, with the choice of therapy dictated by the clinical condition of the patient and the degree of calcium elevation. Hydration with sodium chloride is usually all that is necessary for patients with a calcium value of <13 mg/100 ml. For those with levels of 13 to 15 mg/100 ml, vigorous saline hydration and intermittent intravenous furosemide may result in a prompt calcium diuresis. Close attention must be paid to the patient's cardiovascular status, and thiazide diuretics should not be used, since they depress urinary calcium excretion. Corticosteroids may be added and are most effective in hypercalcemia secondary to myeloma, breast cancer, and lymphomas. Oral phosphates are of little value: they act slowly, cannot be used in renal failure, and cause metastatic soft tissue calcification. When there are unresponsive calcium levels of 13 to 15 mg/100 ml or levels greater than 15 mg/100 ml, a single intravenous dose of mithramycin (25 μg/kg) will usually reverse the hypercalcemia within 24 to 48 hours. Because of its toxicity (thrombocytopenia, coagulopathy, renal and hepatic dysfunction) and potential hypocalcemic effects, mithramycin should not be repeated more frequently than every 48 hours. Other drugs that have been used in hypercalcemia include actinomycin D, porcine calcitonin, and indomethacin.

Since the cause of hypercalcemia in cancer patients is usually the malignancy, control of the metabolic disorder rests with control of the tumor. Therapy directed toward the malignancy should follow once the hypercalcemia is medically treated.

C.P.

Bender RA, Hansen H: Hypercalcemia in bronchogenic carcinoma: A prospective study of 200 patients. Ann Intern Med 80:205–208, 1974.
  Hypercalcemia was seen in 23% of patients with epidermoid, in 12.7% with large cell undifferentiated, in 2.5% with adenocarcinoma, and in none with small cell carcinoma.
Benson RC, Riggs BL, Pickard BM, Arnaud CD: Radioimmunoassay of parathyroid hormone in hypercalcemic patients with malignant disease. Am J Med 56:821–826, 1974.
  Of 108 patients with hypercalcemia, 103 (95.3%) had elevated serum iPTH relative to serum calcium. Primary hyperparathyroidism could be differentiated from ectopic PTH production by a higher iPTH value in the primary disorder.
Kennedy BJ: Metabolic and toxic effects of mithramycin during tumor therapy. Am J Med 49:494–503, 1970.
  Hypocalcemia and hypophosphatemia were seen in 93% of normocalcemic patients treated with mithramycin; hypercalcemia was effectively controlled with small intermittent dosage of this drug.
Mundy GR, Raisz LG, Cooper RA, et al: Evidence for the secretion of an osteoclast stimulating factor in myeloma. N Engl J Med 291:1041–1046, 1974.
  This article describes the secretion of a soluble factor (OAF) produced by myeloma cells that stimulates osteoclastic activity in adjacent bone.
Muggia FM, Heinemann HO: Hypercalcemia associated with neoplastic disease. Ann Intern Med 73:281–290, 1970.
  A good review.
Myers WPL: Hypercalcemia in neoplastic disease. Arch Surg 80:308–318, 1960.
  In this retrospective study of 430 patients with hypercalcemia and malignancy, breast and lung cancer were most commonly associated with hypercalcemia.
Myers WPL: Differential diagnosis of hypercalcemia and cancer. CA 27:258–272, 1977.
  Excellent review of the differential diagnosis, pathogenesis, and therapy of cancer-induced hypercalcemia.
Seyberth HW, Segre GV, Morgan JL, et al: Prostaglandins as mediators of hypercalcemia associated with certain types of cancer. N Engl J Med 293:1278–1283, 1975.
  Aspirin and indomethacin were used successfully in some patients with hypercalcemia and increased urinary levels of E-prostaglandin metabolites.
Vaughn CB, Vaitkevicius VK: The effects of calcitonin in hypercalcemia in patients with malignancy. Cancer 34:1268–1271, 1974.
  Porcine calcitonin is effective in hypercalcemia and is not toxic.

11. ADRENAL INSUFFICIENCY AND PITUITARY INSUFFICIENCY

Metastatic tumor involvement of the adrenals is commonly found in cancer patients at autopsy, while clinical symptoms and signs of adrenal insufficiency are rare. At autopsy the adrenals contain metastatic disease in approximately 10% of cancer patients, with the breast and lung the most common primary sites. In spite of this frequency there have been few case reports describing the development of adrenal insufficiency as a result of metastatic tumor. The apparent rarity of this clinical syndrome secondary to adrenal metastases may be due to multiple factors: inaccurate diagnosis, since the symptoms of metastatic disease may mimic adrenal insufficiency; treatment of metastatic cancer with corticosteroids, masking adrenal insufficiency; and nonperformance of diagnostic tests, since patients are otherwise terminally ill.

In the cancer patient the most common causes of adrenal insufficiency are bilateral adrenalectomy (as for palliative therapy of metastatic breast or prostate cancer), with inadequate steroid replacement, and chronic corticosteroid therapy with rapid withdrawal or inadequate replacement.

Causes of adrenal insufficiency other than cancer include destruction of the adrenals by an autoimmune process, tuberculosis, fungal infection, amyloidosis, and hemorrhage. In addition adrenal atrophy can result from drug therapy with mitotane (o,p'-DDD) when used as adrenocortical carcinoma or aminoglutethimide when used for a "medical adrenalectomy" in metastatic breast cancer.

In cancer patients with adrenal insufficiency, the development of an addisonian crisis results from a relative cortisol deficiency, aldosterone deficiency, extracellular volume deficiency, and the addition of some precipitating stress. The symptoms of adrenal insufficiency may include nausea, vomiting, apathy, weakness, anorexia, abdominal pain, postural syncope, and hyperthermia. Because these symptoms are relatively nonspecific, particularly in the patient with metastatic cancer, the diagnosis should be entertained whenever there is a rapidly deteriorating clinical situation without obvious cause. Laboratory studies may reveal hyponatremia, hyperkalemia, hypoglycemia, prerenal azotemia, and hemoconcentration. A serum cortisol value may add little information, since it may be within normal range but inappropriately low for the clinical stress. An ACTH stimulation test may be diagnostically useful.

The management of acute adrenal insufficiency includes adequate corticosteroid replacement (at least 300 mg of hydrocortisone daily in divided doses) and hydration with glucose and saline. The intravenous route of administration is preferable for all patients initially, since intramuscular or oral routes may not provide adequate absorption. Mineralocorticoid replacement is not necessary initially, since large doses of hydrocortisone have adequate mineralocorticoid effect.

A search for infection should be undertaken in all patients with acute adrenal insufficiency, and prophylactic antibiotic therapy should be considered for patients who are leukopenic.

Like adrenal metastases, metastatic involvement of the pituitary is frequently seen at autopsy, while clinical findings of hypopituitarism are rare. When clinically apparent, metastatic disease in the pituitary may present as diabetes insipidus and may be seen in as many as 1% of women with metastatic breast cancer. Abnormalities of anterior pituitary function are more commonly associated with primary pituitary tumors, pituitary infarction, infections, granulomatous diseases (sarcoidosis or histiocytosis), radiation therapy, and disease processes involving the hypothalamus.

Patients with anterior pituitary dysfunction or ablation may develop symptoms or signs of adrenal insufficiency, with inadequate steroid replacement, but unlike those with the primary disorder, they possess an intact renin-angiotensin-aldosterone system and thus do not need mineralocorticoid replacement.

Gonadotropin and thyrotropin deficiencies occur early in patients with anterior pituitary dysfunction, and attention to sex hormone and thyroid replacement is important.

Following hypophysectomy (as for therapy of a pituitary tumor or for palliation of metastatic breast or prostate cancer), there is complete ablation of anterior pituitary function and variable preservation of antidiuretic hormone (ADH) release. Since ADH is synthesized in the hypothalamus and fibers ending in the median eminence can release ADH, removal of the posterior lobe of the pituitary usually results in only transient polyuria.

In many cases diabetes insipidus (DI) can be difficult to recognize in the patient with metastatic cancer, since the symptoms of polyuria may be secondary to many other factors (renal disease, psychogenic water intoxication, diabetes mellitus, hypercalcemia, or hypokalemia). Metastatic tumor is the cause of DI in approximately 20% of patients, however.

Whatever its cause, the syndrome of central diabetes insipidus results from inadequate vasopressin release in response to physiologic stimuli. Its diagnosis rests on demonstrating a plateau of urine osmolality after fluid deprivation that rises with exogenous administration of vasopressin. Other diagnostic studies, such as hypertonic saline infusion and measurements of ADH, are of less value.

The choice of therapy for DI depends on the clinical circumstance, but at all times, attention must be paid to urine volumes, specific gravity, body weight, and intake and output measurements. Aqueous vasopressin has a short duration of action (4 to 6 hours) and is most commonly used in acute DI. Therapy for chronic mild DI may include chlorpropamide, thiazides, clofibrate, or carbamazepine. For severe DI the most satisfactory long-acting therapy is 1-desamino-8-d-arginine vasopressin (DDAVP).

C.P.

Hill GJ, Wheeler HB: Adrenal insufficiency due to metastatic carcinoma of the lung. Cancer 18:1467–1473, 1965.
   A rare cause of clinically apparent adrenal insufficiency is discussed.
Himathongkam T, Newmark SR, Greenfield M, Dluhy RG: Acute adrenal insufficiency. JAMA 230:1317–1318, 1974.
   Brief review of clinical manifestations and therapy.
Houck WA, Olson KB, Horton J: Clinical features of tumor metastasis to the pituitary. Cancer 26:656–659, 1970.
   In patients with diabetes insipidus, metastatic cancer is the cause of the disorder in 20%.
Miller M, Dalakos T, Moses AM, et al: Recognition of partial defects in antidiuretic hormone secretion. Ann Intern Med 73:721–729, 1970.
   This article describes the utility of the water deprivation test, with a subsequent test dose of aqueous vasopressin, in evaluating central diabetes insipidus.
Moses AM, Miller M, Streeten DPH: Pathophysiologic and pharmacologic alterations in the release and action of ADH. Metabolism 25:697–721, 1976.
   Discusses all aspects of ADH. An excellent review.
Robinson AG: DDAVP in the treatment of central diabetes insipidus. N Engl J Med 294:507–511, 1976.

*1-Desamino-8-d-arginine vasopressin is an effective synthetic analogue of va-
sopressin; it has a long duration of action (8 to 20 hours) and no apparent side
effects. It is administered by intranasal spray.*

Samaan NA, Bakdash MM, Caderao JB, et al: Hypopituitarism after external
irradiation: Evidence for both hypothalamic and pituitary origin. Ann Intern
Med 83:771–777, 1975.

*Radiation therapy portals that encompass the base of the skull may cause
hypothalamic and/or pituitary dysfunction.*

Shucart WA, Jackson I: Management of diabetes insipidus in neurosurgical
patients. J Neurosurg 44:65–71, 1976.

A good review.

Snyder PJ, Jacobs LS, Rabello MM, et al: Diagnostic value of thyrotrophin-
releasing hormone in pituitary and hypothalmic diseases: Assessment of
thyrotrophin and prolactin secretion in 100 patients. Ann Intern Med
81:751–757, 1974.

*Subtle abnormalities of pituitary and hypothalamic function can be detected
by TSH and prolactin responses to TRH.*

Yap H-Y, Tashima CK, Blumenschein GR, Eckles N: Diabetes insipidus and
breast cancer. Arch Intern Med 139:1009–1011, 1979.

*This report covers 39 patients with metastatic involvement of the neuro-
hypophysial system.*

12. SYNDROME OF INAPPROPRIATE ANTIDIURETIC HORMONE SECRETION

The syndrome of inappropriate antidiuretic hormone secretion (SIADH) is a
common problem in the patient with cancer. At least 50% of patients with small
cell carcinoma of the lung have impaired water excretion when challenged with
a water load; and of those patients with documented SIADH, approximately
two-thirds are found to have malignant disease. Lung cancer is most frequently
diagnosed and in the majority (87%) of cases is small cell carcinoma, while
epidermoid and adenocarcinoma are rarely seen. Other malignancies reported
to occur in association with SIADH include pancreatic carcinoma, lymphoma,
and thymoma.

The clinical syndrome of inappropriate ADH secretion results in excessive
retention of water, which persists in spite of a concomitant reduction in the
osmolality of the serum and extracellular fluid. Since patients are unable to
excrete a dilute urine, the extracellular fluid volume expands and hyponatremia develops. Typical symptoms include anorexia, nausea, vomiting, weight
gain, weakness, irritability, personality changes, mental confusion, seizures,
and coma. The extent of symptomatology usually relates to the degree of
hyponatremia and its duration.

SIADH may be diagnosed clinically when there is hyponatremia with hypo-
osmolality of the serum and extracellular fluid; continued renal excretion of
sodium; absence of fluid volume depletion; urine osmolality greater than that
appropriate for the plasma osmolality; and normal renal and adrenal function.
Diseases that may simulate the syndrome include adrenal insufficiency, hypothyroidism, dilutional hyponatremia (as seen in congestive heart failure, renal
failure, or liver disease with ascites), primary polydipsia, and hyponatremia
secondary to sodium depletion (as seen in renal disease, vomiting or diarrhea,
or diabetic acidosis).

The water-loading test is useful in diagnosis but is safe only when the serum sodium is greater than 125 mEq/liter and the patient is asymptomatic. Plasma and/or urinary ADH concentrations are inappropriately elevated, and in patients with malignancy, the ADH levels may be partially suppressible with water loading.

In the patient with cancer, SIADH is thought to be due to synthesis and secretion of antidiuretic hormone by tumor tissue. In vitro studies have demonstrated this capacity in small cell carcinoma of the lung and the ADH released appears to be identical with that produced by the normal neurohypophyseal system. In addition neurophysin (a carrier protein of the posterior pituitary) has been identified in blood and tumor tissue of patients with small cell carcinoma and SIADH.

However, there are other causes of SIADH that should be considered in the cancer patient. Pulmonary infections such as tuberculosis, lung abscess, and pneumonia (either viral or bacterial) have been reported to cause SIADH and may coexist in the cancer patient. Many central nervous system disorders have been associated with the syndrome, including skull fracture, subdural hematoma, cerebrovascular accident, hydrocephalus, cerebral atrophy, meningitis, encephalitis, and metastic tumor. Several drugs have been reported to cause SIADH (chlorpropamide, carbamazepine, thiazide diuretics, oxytocin, and in particular the antineoplastic agents vincristine and cyclophosphamide). Such drug-induced hyponatremia can be aggravated further by encouraging water intake, as is often done to prevent cyclophosphamide-induced cystitis.

The hyponatremia of SIADH can usually be corrected by restriction of fluid intake. If there are symptoms of severe water intoxication, however, then hypertonic saline alone or with furosemide may be administered intravenously. In either case electrolytes must be monitored closely. All drugs that might produce or exacerbate the syndrome should be discontinued, and other causes of SIADH should be identified and treated, if possible. It is well known that effective tumor treatment results in resolution of the syndrome.

There are no drugs available that simply suppress the synthesis or release of ADH from tumor tissue. Both lithium carbonate and demethylchlortetracycline have been reported to induce polyuria by interfering with the renal action of ADH, and thus they may be useful in improving hyponatremia and the symptoms of SIADH. These drugs may be of particular benefit to the cancer patient receiving palliative treatment, when fluid restriction may be difficult.

C.P.

Bartter FC, Schwartz WB: The syndrome of inappropriate secretion of antidiuretic hormone. Am J Med 42:790–806, 1967.
An excellent review of the clinical features, pathophysiology, etiology, and therapy of SIADH.
Baumann G, Lopez-Amor E, Dingman JF: Plasma arginine vasopressin in the syndrome of inappropriate antidiuretic hormone secretion. Am J Med 52:19–24, 1972.
Plasma vasopressin levels (in 7 patients) were inappropriately high for the concurrent blood osmolality, and abnormal vasopressin concentrations could not be completely suppressed with hydration.
Cheng KW, Friesen HG: Studies of human neurophysin by radioimmunoassay. J Clin Endocrinol Metab 36:553–560, 1973.
Elevated serum levels of neurophysin were detected in patients with SIADH. Tumor tissue was found to contain both neurophysin and vasopressin.
Cherrill DA, Stote RM, Birge JR, Singer I: Demeclocycline treatment in the syndrome of inappropriate antidiuretic hormone secretion. Ann Intern Med 83:654–656, 1975.

This case report describes demeclocycline therapy of chronic SIADH in a patient with small cell carcinoma.

Cutting HO: Inappropriate secretion of antidiuretic hormone secondary to vincristine therapy. Am J Med 51:269–271, 1971.

A case report describing the transient development of inappropriate ADH following vincristine administration.

DeFronzo RA, Braine H, Colvin OM, Davis PJ: Water intoxication in man after cyclophosphamide therapy: Time course and relation to drug activation. Ann Intern Med 78:861–869, 1973.

Intravenous cyclophosphamide (>50 mg/kg) induced impaired water excretion in 17 of 19 cancer patients 4 to 12 hours after administration.

George JM, Capen CC, Phillips AS: Biosynthesis of vasopressin in vitro and ultrastructure of a bronchogenic carcinoma: Patient with the syndrome of inappropriate secretion of antidiuretic hormone. J Clin Invest 51:141–148, 1972.

In vitro synthesis of vasopressin by tumor tissue (small cell carcinoma of the lung) was demonstrated in a patient with SIADH.

Hantman D, Rossier B, Zohlman R, Schrier R: Rapid correction of hyponatremia in the syndrome of inappropriate secretion of antidiuretic hormone: An alternative treatment to hypertonic saline. Ann Intern Med 78:870–875, 1973.

SIADH-induced symptomatic hyponatremia was corrected within 6 to 8 hours, utilizing furosemide diuresis and hypertonic saline with supplemental potassium to replace urinary electrolyte losses.

Miller M, Moses AM: Urinary antidiuretic hormone in polyuric disorders and in inappropriate ADH syndrome. Ann Intern Med 77:715–721, 1972.

Baseline ADH levels were normal in SIADH but inappropriately elevated after water loading.

White MG, Fetner CD: Treatment of the syndrome of inappropriate secretion of antidiuretic hormone with lithium carbonate. N Engl J Med 292:390–392, 1975.

This case report suggests lithium carbonate as chronic therapy for SIADH, but it also emphasizes the risks of lithium intoxication.

13. HYPOGLYCEMIA

Although fasting hypoglycemia is an uncommon problem in the clinic, it can be incapacitating and even life-threatening to patients with islet cell tumors, patients with large retroperitoneal or intrathoracic mesenchymal tumors, and occasionally patients with massive hepatic metastases. In many instances the symptoms of fasting hypoglycemia are insidious in onset, mimicking psychiatric or neurologic disorders, and they may be present for several years before the correct diagnosis is made (particularly with islet cell tumors, in which case a patient may have symptoms for as long as 10 to 20 years). Symptoms of reactive hypoglycemia (tremor, hunger, sweating) are relatively rare, while complaints of weakness, undue fatigue, dizziness, mental confusion, and somnolence are more typically seen in fasting hypoglycemia; and, if undetected, the symptoms of neuroglycopenia can progress to generalized seizures and/or coma. Hypoglycemic symptoms are usually apparent or exacerbated in early morning or late afternoon following a period of fasting and may be rapidly relieved by food.

Hypoglycemia may be iatrogenic (as with exogenous insulin), reactive, or spontaneous (and apparent during fasting). Causes of fasting hypoglycemia include islet cell tumors, extrapancreatic neoplasms, hepatocellular dysfunction, hypoadrenal and pituitary states, chronic starvation, alcohol-induced hypoglycemia, and idiopathic hypoglycemia of childhood. Making the diagnosis and identifying the cause of fasting hypoglycemia is frequently difficult. A blood glucose level of less than 40 mg/100 ml during fasting is commonly used to define hypoglycemia; however, normal women may have blood levels fall as low as 30 mg/100 ml. Marked fasting hypoglycemia is usually apparent within 12 to 18 hours but may require up to 72 hours of fasting to detect.

Whereas in general there is suppression of insulin with hypoglycemia, hypoglycemia due to islet cell tumors is associated with inappropriately elevated levels of insulin. Although the basal insulin level may be normal, with fasting, serial determinations of blood glucose and immunoreactive insulin (IRI) demonstrate an increasing ratio of IRI to blood glucose rather than the normal constant relationship. In addition the percentage of plasma proinsulin or C peptide is usually higher than normal. Provocative tests of insulin secretion are not of great value in the diagnosis of islet cell tumors and may risk severe hypoglycemia.

Unlike the case of islet cell tumors, which cause fasting hypoglycemia through excessive and/or inappropriate insulin secretion, the etiology of extrapancreatic tumor hypoglycemia is unknown. It is not likely to be caused by the same mechanism as islet cell tumors, since the relationship of IRI to blood glucose during fasting is normal. However, there is conflicting data regarding the presence of insulin-like material in extrapancreatic tumor tissue and/or in plasma of patients with fasting hypoglycemia. Other hypotheses for tumor hypoglycemia include inappropriately increased peripheral glucose utilization by the tumor itself and tumor secretion of specific inhibitors of hepatic gluconeogenesis.

Whatever its mechanism, the source of fasting hypoglycemia in these patients is the tumor itself. Extrapancreatic tumors are frequently large, clinically occult, and retroperitoneal. Although soft tissue sarcomas are most commonly associated with this syndrome, it has been documented in patients with benign mesenchymal tumors, adrenocortical carcinoma, hepatocellular carcinoma, melanoma, and even Hodgkin's disease. In contrast to the sometimes massive size (up to 20 kg) of extrapancreatic tumors associated with hypoglycemia, islet cell tumors are typically benign, single nodules within the pancreatic substance, and only 10% of patients present with overt malignant disease with metastases and are unresectable. Selective arteriography of the celiac and superior mesenteric arteries can aid in identifying the islet cell tumor nodule preoperatively. Its diagnostic accuracy depends on the tumor's size and vascularity.

Since the cause of tumor hypoglycemia is the tumor itself, effective treatment requires its removal. With islet cell tumors, surgery is usually all that is necessary, while large extrapancreatic tumors may not be amenable to any curative modality. Chemotherapy and/or radiation therapy may give transient benefit by reducing tumor bulk, and in particular streptozotocin is an effective palliative therapy for malignant insulinoma.

Palliation of hypoglycemic symptoms can sometimes be accomplished with diet alone but may require corticosteroids, growth hormone, or glucagon. Oral diazoxide, which inhibits insulin release, has been used effectively for palliation of islet cell tumor induced hypoglycemia.

C.P.

Abbasi A, Power L: Insulin and insulinlike activity in extracts of tumors associated with hypoglycemia. Diabetes 22:762–767, 1973.
Unlike 5 islet cell adenomas, 10 nonpancreatic tumors associated with hypoglycemia had no significant concentration of insulin or insulin-like activity in tumor extracts.

Broder LE, Carter SK: Pancreatic islet cell carcinoma: II. Results of therapy with streptozotocin in 52 patients. Ann Intern Med 79:108–118, 1973.
Objective tumor responses were seen in 50% of patients, with the median duration of response being approximately one year.

Fajans SS, Floyd JC: Fasting hypoglycemia in adults. N Engl J Med 294:766–772, 1976.
An excellent review of the physiology of euglycemia during fasting, the pathophysiology of hypoglycemia, and the differential diagnosis of fasting hypoglycemias.

Frerichs H, Track NS: Pharmacotherapy of hormone-secreting tumors. Clin Gastroenterol 3:721–732, 1974.
A comprehensive review of diazoxide therapy in islet cell tumor-induced hypoglycemia.

Marks V: Hypoglycaemia. 2. Other causes. Clin Endocrinol Metab 5:769–782, 1976.
An excellent review of hypoglycemia in association with extrapancreatic neoplasms.

Marks V, Samols E: Insulinoma: Natural history and diagnosis. Clin Gastroenterol 3:559–573, 1974.
An excellent review.

McFadzean AJS, Yeung RTT: Further observations on hypoglycaemia in hepatocellular carcinoma. Am J Med 47:220–235, 1969.
Hypoglycemia was documented in 38 of 142 patients (27%) with hepatocellular carcinoma.

Megyesi K, Kahn CR, Roth J, Gorden P: Hypoglycemia in association with extrapancreatic tumors: Demonstration of elevated plasma NSILA-S by a new radioreceptor assay. J Clin Endocrinol Metab 38:931–934, 1974.
Nonsuppressible insulin-like activity soluble in acid-ethanol (NSILA-S) was found to be elevated in plasma of 5 patients with hypoglycemia and non-islet cell tumors.

Rubenstein AH, Kuzuya H, Horwitz DL: Clinical significance of circulating C-peptide in diabetes mellitus and hypoglycemic disorders. Arch Intern Med 137:625–632, 1977.
Impaired suppression of serum C-peptide secretion was found in patients with insulinoma during porcine insulin-induced hypoglycemia.

Sherman BM, Pek S, Fajans SS, et al: Plasma proinsulin in patients with functioning pancreatic islet cell tumors. J Clin Endocrinol Metab 35:271–280, 1972.
An increased percentage of plasma proinsulin was detected in 21 patients with islet cell tumors (mean 37%) as compared to 10 normal controls (<20%).

Younus S, Soterakis J, Sossi AJ, et al: Hypoglycemia secondary to metastases to the liver: A case report and review of the literature. Gastroenterology 72:334–337, 1977.
Hypoglycemia improved after effective chemotherapy of massive metastic liver disease (adenocarcinoma of prostate).

PART II. DIAGNOSTIC PROBLEMS

Fever as a manifestation of malignant disease may present a difficult diagnostic problem for the clinician. While at least two-thirds of all cancer patients will have fever at some time during their illness, in most instances this symptom is attributable to infection. It is well recognized, however, that some neoplasms are associated with the development of fever in the absence of infection. Such tumor-associated fever has been documented in renal cell carcinoma (11% of patients); Wilms' tumor (20%); Ewing's tumor; carcinoma of the stomach, colon, and pancreas; leukemia; atrial myxoma; and primary and metastatic liver tumors (23%). In addition, fever is a common systemic symptom in Hodgkin's disease (27%) but is less frequently seen in the non-Hodgkin's lymphomas (3.5%). Although tumor-associated fever is found more frequently in advanced or metastatic disease, it can be seen in patients with localized disease as well.

The cause(s) of tumor-associated fever are unknown, although several mechanisms have been postulated, including (1) necrosis of rapidly growing lesions; (2) infiltration of the tumor by leukocytes in response to an inflammatory stimulus; (3) abnormal liver function with altered steroid conjugation; (4) undiagnosed infection or tumor-caused obstruction; and (5) release of pyrogen by tumor cells. Tumor cell production and releases of endogenous pyrogen has been reported in in vitro studies of renal cell carcinoma and Hodgkin's disease.

Many times a tumor-associated fever presents to the clinician as a fever of unknown origin (FUO). Classically such a fever is present for at least 3 weeks, rises to a temperature of at least 101°F, and has a still uncertain diagnosis after the patient has been hospitalized for a week. In most series of unselected patients, the etiology of FUO is infection in 30% to 40% of patients, malignancy in 20% to 30%, and collagen vascular disease in another 20%. As one might expect, at least half those patients with FUO and malignancy are found to have lymphomas. Similarly, if one looks at patients with FUO who undergo exploratory laparotomy for diagnosis, neoplasms account for 25% to 40% of positive findings, with lymphomas making up half the malignancies.

Since liver metastases and retroperitoneal tumors account for many of the neoplasms diagnosed at exploratory laparotomy in patients with FUO, it has been argued that liver biopsy and lymphography be performed prior to laparotomy. Unfortunately the diagnostic yield of these procedures appears to be relatively low. Lymphography, however, can direct the surgeon to suspicious nodal areas. In addition to lymph node sampling and open liver biopsy, splenectomy is sometimes performed on patients with FUO. Where it has been evaluated, the histopathology of the spleen has confirmed other laparotomy findings but has not identified the sole site of disease.

FUO is a rare problem in the patient with an already diagnosed malignancy. In one series only 47 of 6880 patients (0.7%) were found to have FUO. As in other FUO reports, the most common cause of unexplained fever was infection (57.4%), while 38.4% had tumor-associated fever.

Because tumor-associated fever is a rare cause of fever or FUO, its diagnosis must be one of exclusion. Although Pel-Epstein fever is said to be characteristic of Hodgkin's disease, the temperature pattern or height of fever cannot clearly distinguish between infection and tumor. Diagnostic evaluation should include a careful history and physical examination; laboratory, x-ray, and scan studies with attention to predisposing causes of infection; and appropriate cultures and serologies that include bacterial, acid-fast, and fungal organisms. In addition, the kind of malignancy, its disease extent, and the patient's prior therapy (particularly associated leukopenia) may help to direct the search for infection.

C.P.

Bernheim HA, Block LH, Atkins E: Fever—pathogenesis, pathophysiology, and purpose. Ann Intern Med 91:261–270, 1979.
A comprehensive review.

Bodel P: Tumors and fever. Ann NY Acad Sci 230:6–13, 1974.
Article provides description of in vitro studies of endogenous pyrogen production from human tumor cells.

Browder AA, Huff JW, Peterdorf RG: The significance of fever in neoplastic disease. Ann Intern Med 55:932–942, 1961.
An analysis of febrile episodes (not FUO) in 343 cancer patients, emphasizing the rarity of tumor-associated fever without infection (seen in 5.4%).

Dunnick NR, Castellino RA: Lymphography in patients with suspected malignancy or fever of unexplained origin. Radiology 125:107–111, 1977.
Of 44 patients studied, 13 had nonspecific benign reactive changes, and in the remainder studies were normal.

Geraci JE, Weed LA, Nichols DR: Fever of obscure origin—The value of abdominal exploration in diagnosis: Report of 70 cases. JAMA 169:1306–1315, 1959.
Of 70 patients with FUO, 21 (30%) were found to have malignancies at laparotomy, 10 of which were lymphomas.

Howard PH Jr, Hardin WJ: The role of surgery in fever of unknown origin. Surg Clin North Am 52:397–403, 1972.
Of 34 patients with FUO, 11 had exploratory laparotomy and 5 of the 11 were found to have neoplasms.

Jonsson K: The role of lymphography in the investigation of patients with fever of unknown origin. Acta Med Scand 198:135–136, 1975.
Of 21 patients with FUO who underwent lymphography, 8 had studies suggestive of lymphoma and 7 of these were histologically confirmed.

Klastersky J, Weerts D, Hensgens C, Debusscher L: Fever of unexplained origin in patients with cancer. Eur J Cancer 9:649–656, 1973.
FUO was identified in 47 of 6,880 patients (0.7%); the causes of FUO were infection (57.4%) and underlying neoplasm (38.4%).

Milton AS: Modern views of the pathogenesis of fever and the mode of action of antipyretic drugs. J Pharm Pharmacol 281:393–399, 1976.
An excellent review.

Mitchell DP, Hanes TE, Hoyumpa AM Jr, Schenker S: Fever of unknown origin: Assessment of the value of percutaneous liver biopsy. Arch Intern Med 137:1001–1004, 1977.
Diagnostic pathology was found in only 14% of patients with FUO; hepatomegaly and abnormal liver function tests were more common in those with positive biopsies.

Petersdorf RG, Beeson PB: Fever of unexplained origin: Report on 100 cases. Medicine 40:1–30, 1961.
A classic study that defines the criteria of FUO and emphasizes that most patients with FUO are suffering from unusual manifestations of common diseases.

15. LYMPHADENOPATHY

The human body contains more than 500 lymph nodes, any of which may become enlarged for a wide variety of reasons, including antigenic challenge, suppurative infection, granulomatous disease, primary lymph node disease, metastatic tumor (carcinoma, leukemia), drug effect, and congenital abnormality. Whenever lymph node enlargement is detected, its etiologic evaluation depends upon the location and distribution of adenopathy as well as such physical characteristics as size, shape, consistency, fixation to skin or underlying tissue, discrete or confluent nodal groups, superficial warmth or erythema, and sensitivity to palpation. The patient's history may reveal the duration of adenopathy, exposure to infections or drugs, known associated illnesses or family history, and possible systemic symptoms (fevers, sweats, weight loss). The physical examination may demonstrate other associated abnormalities in the regional drainage area of the enlarged lymph node (such as a breast mass in a patient with axillary adenopathy), or it may reveal more generalized lymphadenopathy. Since the most common cause of lymphadenopathy is infection, screening studies usually begin with cultures of the appropriate regional portals of entry and may subsequently include blood cultures, blood counts with white blood cell differential and review of peripheral smear, VDRL, mono spot test, febrile agglutinins, fungal serologies, skin tests, and chest x-ray.

The greatest challenge to the physician evaluating lymphadenopathy is when to do a lymph node biopsy. Various criteria apply, the first being documentation of nodal enlargement on two separate occasions. When localized adenopathy is present and the regional drainage area is unrevealing, a biopsy may reveal a metastatic tumor whose primary site is occult. On the other hand, the regional lymph node may be excised to document metastatic disease in the patient with an obvious primary tumor in that drainage area (such as a patient with supraclavicular adenopathy and a lung mass). When there is generalized lymphadenopathy, systemic infections or diseases should be excluded, if possible, prior to biopsy.

The diagnostic yield of a lymph node biopsy depends upon many factors in addition to patient selection. From the pathologist's viewpoint, it is important that the node be a representative sample; that it be excised completely with minimal trauma; that cytologic imprints, cultures, and special stains be anticipated at surgery; and that the histologic processing be done properly. From the surgeon's viewpoint, a peripheral lymph node biopsy is more likely to be diagnostic when it is removed from the supraclavicular or cervical region (70% to 80% of the time) than from the axilla or groin (40% to 50%). Approximately 75% of diagnostic peripheral lymph node biopsies (done in patients without other regional pathologic conditions) are malignant, and the majority of these are lymphomas (60%). Carcinomas may be diagnosed initially by lymph node biopsy, but it is unusual for the primary tumor to remain undetected. With axillary metastases, breast cancer is the most frequent occult primary tumor; and with cervical metastases, lung and head and neck cancer are the most common occult origins. More than one-third of patients who undergo peripheral lymph node biopsy have no specific diagnosis made. Within 12 months of the initial biopsy, however, up to 20% of these patients are found to have diseased lymph nodes, primarily due to lymphoma.

Lymphadenopathy in the chest or abdomen usually requires diagnostic biopsy if no associated peripheral or regional abnormalities are present. One possible exception to this may be the asymptomatic, characteristic, bilateral hilar adenopathy of sarcoidosis. In the abdomen, lymph node enlargement may be detected by physical examination, plain film of the abdomen, intravenous pyelogram, gastrointestinal x-rays, ultrasound, computed axial tomography, or lymphogram. None of these methods is diagnostic; however, they may assist the surgeon in identifying suspicious nodal groups. In the patient with already diagnosed malignancy or with probable metastatic disease from an identified primary site, lymph node aspiration with cytology may obviate the need for laparotomy and biopsy. The accuracy of this procedure is best for solid tumors and less so for lymphoma.

In order to increase the diagnostic yield of lymph node biopsy, a number of other tests may be applied to lymph node tissue. For example, a pathologic axillary or supraclavicular lymph node in a woman without a known primary tumor can be studied for estrogen-binding receptor protein. Electron micros-copy can be done on selected specimens to look for secretory granules (as in small cell carcinoma) or intercellular bridges (as in squamous carcinoma). A suspected lymphoma can be studied for the presence of a monoclonal population of B- or T-cells. Unfortunately, all these tests require freshly frozen specimens and thus require anticipatory planning prior to biopsy.

C.P.

Copeland EM, McBride CM: Axillary metastases from unknown primary sites. Ann Surg 178:25–27, 1973.
Breast carcinoma was the most frequent occult primary (30% of 60 patients).
Dorfman RF, Warnke R: Lymphadenopathy simulating the malignant lym-phomas. Hum Pathol 5:519–550, 1974.
An excellent discussion of the histopathological features in lymph nodes, analyzed according to the histological patterns observed in stimulated lymph nodes.
Murphy JF, Fred HL: Infectious lymphadenitis or lymphoma? Seven lessons. JAMA 235:742–743, 1976.
This article emphasizes that lymphoma may masquerade as infection with nodal pain, local inflammation, and fever.
Parker BR, Blank N, Castellino RA: Lymphographic appearance of benign conditions simulating lymphoma. Radiology 111:267–274, 1974.
Article discusses six patients with benign diseases and lymphograms consis-tent with lymphoma.
Ross GD: Identification of human lymphocyte subpopulations by surface marker analysis. Blood 53:799–811, 1979.
An excellent review of lymphocyte surface markers with extensive references.
Saltzstein SL: The fate of patients with nondiagnostic lymph node biopsies. Surgery 58:659–662, 1965.
Of 68 patients who had biopsies for peripheral lymphadenopathy, biopsies in 33 (48%) were diagnostic; an additional 6 (17%) later had a second biopsy, which revealed lymphoma.
Schroer KR, Franssila KO: Atypical hyperplasia of lymph nodes: A follow-up study. Cancer 44:1155–1163, 1979.
Within a median of 7 months following the original biopsy, 11 of 35 patients were found to have lymphoma.
Sinclair S, Beckman E, Ellman L: Biopsy of enlarged superficial lymph nodes. JAMA 228:602–603, 1974.
In a retrospective study of 135 patients who underwent superficial lymph node biopsy, 63% of biopsies were diagnostic (50% were lymphoma, 16% car-cinoma); of 40 patients with lymphoid hyperplasia, 9 later had lymphoma diagnosed.
Winterbauer RH, Belic N, Moores KD: A clinical interpretation of bilateral hilar adenopathy. Ann Intern Med 78:65–71, 1973.
An analysis of 100 patients with bilateral hilar adenopathy, in which all 30 asymptomatic patients had sarcoidosis as did 50 of 52 who had negative physical examinations.
Zornosa J, Wallace S, Goldstein HM, et al: Transperitoneal percutaneous retroperitoneal lymph node aspiration biopsy. Radiology 122:111–115, 1977.
Following lymphography, opacified lymph nodes are aspirated with a 23-gauge needle under fluoroscopic control.

Zuelzer WW, Kaplan J: The child with lymphadenopathy. Semin Hematol
12:323–334, 1975.
An excellent review of etiology in generalized and regional lymphadenopathy.

16. SKIN DISORDERS

The skin may be involved primarily by a neoplastic process (for example, squamous or basal cell carcinoma, melanoma, and mycosis fungoides) or by metastases. Certain skin lesions are associated with underlying primary malignancies, while antibiotics and anticancer drugs may produce cutaneous side-effects in patients with neoplastic diseases. Infectious complications that involve the skin may also develop in cancer patients. Finally, intense pruritus may complicate certain malignancies. These various topics will be discussed in order.

Skin Lesions Associated with Underlying Malignancies

The proximal muscle, pelvic, and shoulder girdle weakness associated with dermatomyositis usually begins insidiously and is accompanied in 40% to 50% of patients by an erythematous malar rash, with or without periorbital edema. There is no predilection for any single type of primary cancer in patients with dermatomyositis, but the association between this disorder and the development of a malignancy is greater than would be expected to occur by chance. In acanthosis nigricans, hyperpigmented symmetric lesions of the axillae, inguinal regions, and flexor surfaces are noted. This disease may be associated with an intra-abdominal malignancy, usually a gastric carcinoma, although carcinomas of the pancreas and colon have also been noted with this disorder. The erythematous, plaque-like scaly lesions of Bowen's disease, usually found in areas of sun exposure, have also been associated with underlying malignancies. The erythematous, eczematoid lesions of anogenital Paget's disease, which involve the perineum, scrotum, and labia majora, most often represent epidermal invasion by adenocarcinomas arising in either the skin adenexae, urethra, or rectum. These lesions may represent either direct extension or regional metastases from the underlying carcinoma. The localized hyperpigmented lesions characteristic of xeroderma pigmentosa or von Recklinghausen's disease may be associated with the later development of multiple skin cancers or neurofibrosarcomata, respectively.

Generalized hyperpigmentation may be caused by metastases to the adrenal glands or may be secondary to increased secretion of myelanocyte-stimulating hormone by a pituitary tumor. Although a rare event, exfoliative dermatitis has been noted both in leukemias and in the non-Hodgkin's lymphomas. In all these conditions the clinician should be alert to the possibility of an underlying malignancy. A careful history and physical examination, with appropriate radiologic and hematologic tests, may result in the correct diagnosis of the underlying neoplasm.

Drug Eruptions

Erythema nodosum, which is characterized by subcutaneous tender anterior leg nodules, may be associated in the cancer patient with bacterial, viral, or fungal infections, may herald an underlying collagen disease, or may represent a hypersensitivity reaction to sulfonamide or penicillin. Similarly erythema multiforme may be seen in patients with malignant diseases receiving penicillin therapy. This syndrome is characterized by the appearance of scattered vesicles and often a widespread cutaneous bullous eruption. Exfoliative dermatitis may result from a drug sensitivity, most commonly to penicillin, although sedatives and tranquilizers have also been implicated.

Anticancer drugs may also produce cutaneous lesions. A scarlatinaform rash from allopurinol hypersensitivity has been described. The administration of busulfan has resulted in general hyperpigmentation similar to that in Addison's disease. Bleomycin use may be associated with a widespread papillary cutaneous eruption. Severe desquamative skin reactions may occur at the irradiated site in patients receiving simultaneous radiotherapy and Adriamycin or actinomycin D, both of which apparently sensitize the skin to radiation. In all of the above dermatitides, the relationship between the cutaneous lesions and drug hypersensitivity should be recognized and appropriate dose manipulations or drug substitutions should be performed.

Cutaneous Infections
The skin may be involved by bacterial, viral, or fungal infections in cancer patients, especially those either with advanced disease or immunosuppressed by radiation therapy or chemotherapy treatments.

Herpes zoster, occurring in only 0.5% of the normal population, is noted within a year of diagnosis in 20% to 40% of patients with Hodgkin's disease. The dermatomal vesicular eruption of the evolving disease is well known, but the severe, neuritic pain preceding the eruption may confuse the diagnosis initially. Rarely, visceral herpes zoster may be its first manifestation, producing abdominal pain prior to the appearance of cutaneous vesicles. Other herpes virus infections, such as varicella and herpes simplex, may be distinguished by the widespread cutaneous involvement in the former and the localized lesion in the latter. Serologic testing of blood or vesical scrapings will allow the differentiation between the lesions in atypical cases. Herpes zoster immune globulin may prevent varicella in exposed persons.

Dissemination of herpes zoster, if it should occur, usually takes place 2 to 7 days after the appearance of the cutaneous lesions. Cytosine arabinoside has not been effective in the management of disseminated herpes zoster, while initial experience indicates that interferon is promising in preventing dissemination.

Systemic bacterial or fungal infections may also produce pyogenic cutaneous lesions. Cultures of these lesions may be necessary to make the appropriate diagnosis and select effective antibiotics.

Metastases
Cutaneous metastases may occur late in the course of disease in patients with carcinomas of the lung and breast as well as in malignant melanoma. Needle or excisional biopsy may be required to make the diagnosis.

Pruritus
Pruritus, although not found to have an adverse effect on prognosis in Hodgkin's disease, can be severe. It usually responds to successful treatment of the underlying malignancy. Pruritus is frequently seen in patients with mycosis fungoides. It may also be present in such conditions as diabetes mellitus, uremia, and other benign dermatologic disorders such as lichen planus, scabies, or pediculosis.

D.G.

Goffinet D, Glatstein E, Merigan T: Herpes zoster-varicella infections and lymphoma. Ann Intern Med 76:235–241, 1972.

In a study of 1130 patients, zoster incidence increased with extensive radiotherapy, chemotherapy, and in splenectomized patients.

Merigan T, Rand K, Pollard R, et al: Human leukocyte interferon for the treatment of herpes zoster in patients with cancer. N Engl J Med 298:981–987, 1978.

Article discusses prospective, randomized study in 90 patients. High dosage interferon limited dermatomal progression and cutaneous dissemination.

Soter N, Wilkinson D, Fitzpatrick T: Clinical dermatology (First of three parts). N Engl J Med 289:189–195, 1973.

In this first part of a three-part review of clinical dermatology, bullous lesions and skin diseases associated with underlying malignancies are discussed.

Soter N, Wilkinson D, Fitzpatrick T: Clinical dermatology (Second of three parts). N Engl J Med 289:242–248, 1973.

Skin eruptions with connective tissue diseases, drugs, and lymphomas are discussed in this second part of the series.

Soter N, Wilkinson D, Fitzpatrick T: Clinical dermatology (Third of three parts). N Engl J Med 289:296–301, 1973.

Infections and papulosquamous eruptions are discussed in the third part.

Stevens D, Jordan G, Waddell T, Merigan T: Adverse effect of cytosine arabinoside on disseminated zoster in a controlled trial. N Engl J Med 289:874–878, 1973.

In the group of 39 patients there was greater dissemination in the group that received Ara-C.

17. THYROID NODULE

Nodular goiters, about two-thirds of which are uninodular, are palpable in 4% to 8% of the adult American population. The most common causes of thyroid nodules are single or multinodular colloid cysts, followed by benign adenomas and either subacute thyroiditis or Hashimoto's disease and carcinoma. Autopsy series have revealed a 7% to 12% incidence of thyroid nodules, although many were smaller than 1.0 cm, the limit of palpability. The risk of carcinoma in unselected patients with thyroid nodules varies from less than 1% to 2–5% in various series. In selected surgical series, the cancer risk in patients with multinodular goiters is 3% to 10%, but the risk is higher (9% to 33%) in those with uninodular thyroids. However, in patients under the age of 20, the risk of a solitary nodule being malignant is very high, from 31% to 60%. The mortality from thyroid cancer is approximately 0.4% of all cancer deaths.

The incidence of thyroid nodules, both benign and malignant, is clearly increased following head and neck irradiation in childhood. A sixfold increase in the risk of thyroid cancer has been noted among children irradiated for ringworm of the scalp. The mean radiation dose to the thyroid gland in this series was only 9 rads. Similar studies, especially from the Chicago area, have also shown an increased risk of thyroid cancer among children who received therapeutic head and neck irradiation for other benign diseases.

Most thyroid nodules are asymptomatic. However, discomfort with deglutition, cervical pain, dyspnea, or an enlarged lymph node may all be associated with a mass in the thyroid. Enlarged lymph nodes are usually indicative of a malignancy but may also be present in such benign diseases as Hashimoto's thyroiditis. Diarrhea and other endocrine tumors such as pheochromocytomas or parathyroid adenomas may be associated with medullary carcinoma of the thyroid.

A detailed history and careful physical examination are important in the evaluation of a patient with a thyroid nodule. Indirect laryngoscopy should be performed to note the mobility of the vocal cords. In Hashimoto's thyroiditis, the entire gland is usually symmetrically enlarged but may be quite firm. There may also be associated lymph node enlargement. A firm, irregular thyroid mass with indistinct borders, with or without clinically enlarged cervical lymph nodes, is suggestive of carcinoma. Rapid enlargement of thyroid nodules may signify an aggressive rapidly enlarging tumor but may also be due to hemorrhage into a benign adenoma. A chest radiograph may show metastases or tracheal deviation by the mass. A soft tissue neck radiograph should also be obtained. The presence of soft tissue calcifications in the region of the thyroid may represent calcified psammoma bodies in a papillary thyroid carcinoma. A complete blood count and measurements of serum calcium and phosphorus, and serum TSH (thyroid-stimulating hormone) and thyroxin should also be obtained. An elevated serum calcitonin level may indicate a medullary thyroid carcinoma. A scintiscan is also important diagnostically. Nodules that do not take up iodine are more likely to be malignant. B-mode ultrasound and CT scans are useful in differentiating cystic thyroid masses, but their role in the evaluation of solid nodules is less clear. Needle aspiration of the thyroid for cytologic examination of cysts is a well-recognized method of diagnosis. The role of needle biopsies in the diagnostic evaluation of solid thyroid nodules is controversial, however, since there is a risk of not only seeding the needle tract by tumor (very rare) but also of missing a carcinoma with the biopsy needle.

It should be remembered that most thyroid cancers do not take up ^{123}I and that only 25% of "cold" nodules are malignant (in surgical series). Although almost all malignant thyroid nodules are "cold," a few are functional, indicating that a hyperfunctional nodule is not always benign.

"Hot" nodules are usually autonomous and do not suppress after the administration of exogenous thyroid hormone. These nodules are usually left alone if the patient is euthyroid. If the patient is older than 50 to 60, or the nodule is larger than 4 cm, or there are hyperthyroid features, surgery should be considered. In general, any nonfunctioning (or hypofunctional) nodule that is enlarging rapidly or does not decrease in size with the administration of thyroid hormone should be considered malignant and resected if possible. Patients at increased risk of developing thyroid cancers who should also be considered for surgery include those with a history of childhood head and neck irradiation, females under age 20 and over 60 with a single nonfunctioning thyroid nodule, and any male with a solitary thyroid nodule.

D.G.

Blum M, Rothschild M: Improved nonoperative diagnosis of the solitary "cold" thyroid nodule: Surgical selection based on risk factors and three months of suppression. JAMA 243:242–245, 1980.
A prospective study of 118 patients. Criteria for immediate surgery included irradiation in childhood, age less than 20 years, recent growth of hard nodule and/or adenopathy, and obstructive symptoms. Of 25 nodules removed, 15 were malignant. An additional 26 nodules were excised because they failed to shrink less than 50% with thyroid suppressive therapy; 5 of the 26 nodules were malignant.

Crile G Jr, Esselstyn CB Jr, Hawk WA: Needle biopsy in the diagnosis of thyroid nodules appearing after radiation. N Engl J Med 301:997–999, 1979.
Article discusses 576 needle biopsies performed between 1971 and 1976 at the Cleveland Clinic.

Favus M, Schneider A, Stachura M, et al: Thyroid cancer occurring as a late consequence of head and neck irradiation. N Engl J Med 294:1019–1025, 1976.
The incidence of thyroid nodules (both benign and malignant) was increased in patients who received head and neck irradiation in their childhood.

Figg D, Bratt H, VanVliet P, Deans R: Thyroid cancer: Diagnosis and management based on a review of 142 cases. Am J Surg 135:671–674, 1978.
Good discussion of evaluation and surgical results.

Modan B, Ron E, Werner A: Thyroid cancer following scalp irradiation. Radiology 123:741–744, 1977.
Thyroid cancer was increased six times when children were given radiation for tinea capitis, even though the mean thyroid radiation doses were only 9 rads.

Perlmutter M, Slater S: Which nodular goiters should be removed? N Engl J Med 255:65–71, 1956.
Literature review and discussion of incidence of cancer in uni- or multinodular goiters.

Silverberg S, Vidone R: Carcinoma of the thyroid in surgical and post-mortem material. Ann Surg 164:291–295, 1977.
In this article there was a 1% frequency of carcinomas in single nodules and 2.7% in an autopsy series.

Sokal J: The problem of malignancy in nodular goiter—recapitulation and a challenge. JAMA 170:405–412, 1959.
Review of incidence of both goiters and carcinoma in the U.S. population.

Vander J, Gaston E, Dawber T: Significance of nontoxic thyroid nodules. Ann Intern Med 69:537–540, 1968.
Article discusses 15-year follow-up of 218 patients with thyroid nodules (Framingham population of 5,127 patients).

Wessler S, Avioli L: Management of the thyroid nodule. JAMA 221:1265–1268, 1972.
Excellent discussion.

18. HOARSENESS

There are many different causes of hoarseness, but all result in difficulties of phonation due either to changes in vibratory characteristics or loss of normal approximation of the true vocal cords. Since the laryngeal mucosa is only loosely adherent, it may become edematous from allergic, traumatic, or infectious causes, with resultant hoarseness. Hoarseness may also be due to masses involving the vocal cords.

Since all the intrinsic laryngeal muscles are innervated by the recurrent laryngeal branch of the vagus nerve, with the exception of the cricothyroid (innervated by the superior laryngeal nerve), injury to the recurrent laryngeal nerve causes vocal cord paralysis, usually in the midline or paramedian position. If only the superior laryngeal nerve is paralyzed, the vocal cords cannot be tensed normally, resulting in a lower-pitched voice.

Either central nervous system or peripheral lesions may cause vocal cord paralysis and hoarseness. Approximately 90% of vocal cord paralyses are due to peripheral causes; 40% are due to neoplasms. Cancers of the lung (most common), esophagus, and thyroid may all invade and destroy the function of the recurrent nerves. Other processes, such as complications of thyroidectomy, tracheostomy, or prolonged tracheal intubation; aortic aneurysms; cervical or mediastinal tuberculosis; or such toxic causes as neuritis (alcoholic or diabetic), periarteritis, and Guillain-Barré syndrome, have all been implicated in vocal cord paralysis. In about one-fifth of cases, the cause is not found. The other 10% of vocal cord paralyses are due to central nervous system diseases such as poliomyelitis, trauma, tumors, and cerebral vascular accidents.

Even small intrinsic laryngeal lesions may produce hoarseness. Bacterial or viral laryngopharyngitis, fume inhalation, or vocal abuse (resulting in vocal nodules) may all lead to hoarseness. Laryngeal trauma, either external or internal (prolonged intubation), and miscellaneous disorders such as myxedema and rheumatoid arthritis may cause hoarseness. Tumors of the larynx produce early hoarseness and should be suspected in any adult patient with hoarseness of over 2 to 5 weeks' duration.

A careful history is important. The duration of the hoarseness, an association between laryngitis and an upper respiratory infection, or a history of voice abuse, toxic fume exposure, or inhalation reveal other benign causes of hoarseness. Recent surgery, prolonged intubation, or laryngeal trauma may also be causes. There may be a history of symptoms of hypothyroidism. A laryngeal neoplasm should be suspected in an adult smoker who becomes hoarse. In advanced cancers, dyspnea, dysphagia, hemoptysis, and head and neck pain may all be present.

The physical examination should include a complete neurologic examination to rule out central causes of hoarseness. A thorough head and neck examination is essential, including careful palpation for enlarged lymph nodes. Mirror laryngoscopy, with careful inspection of the oropharynx, hypopharynx, and larynx, should be performed. If the hoarseness has been transient and such predisposing factors as heavy smoking, vocal abuse (singers), or respiratory infection are present, voice rest may be all that is required to allow the hoarseness to resolve. If the hoarseness has not resolved or has been persistent for longer than 2 to 4 weeks, a repeat careful mirror examination should be performed. If a mass lesion of the hypopharynx or larynx is discovered, a barium swallow, laryngogram (if there are no medical contraindications), laryngotomograms, and CT scan may establish the extent of the lesion. Finally, direct laryngoscopy and biopsy should be performed. Treatment of a laryngeal or hypopharyngeal neoplasm by either radiation therapy or surgery or the two modalities in combination depends on the stage, sites of involvement, and condition and age of the patient.

D.G.

DeWeese D, Saunders W (Eds):   Textbook of Otolaryngology. St. Louis, C.V. Mosby, 1977. Pp. 102–103.
   Discusses causes of hoarseness.
Kelly D, Lee K: Differential Diagnosis in Otolaryngology, Lee, KJ (Ed). New York, Arco Publishing, 1978. Pp. 192–195.
   Book covers the differential diagnosis of hoarseness.

19. PULMONARY NODULES

Although only 5% of all primary lung cancers present as pulmonary nodules (< 4 to 6 cm in diameter), it is important to make the diagnosis early, since this small group of lung cancers are potentially the most curable. Approximately one-third of such lesions will be malignant (either primary lung cancers or metastases), while 50% will be caused by infectious or noninfectious granulomas, 7% by hamartomas, and the remainder by miscellaneous benign lesions. In patients under 30, less than 1% of solitary pulmonary nodules are malignant. The risk of cancer rises to approximately 15% for the 30- to 45-year group and is above 50% for patients over age 50.

Most pulmonary nodules are asymptomatic. If the pleura is invaded, however, localized or radicular pain may develop. Dyspnea or hemoptysis are rarely present with early, small lesions but may develop as pulmonary nodules enlarge or in the presence of multiple metastases. Occasionally a pneumothorax is the presenting sign of a pulmonary metastasis.

A detailed history may elicit symptoms suggestive of an extrapulmonary malignancy, indicating that the lung nodule is a metastasis. The patient's place of residence is important, since pulmonary fungal infections are more likely to occur in inhabitants of the Mississippi valley (histoplasmosis) and the central valley of California (coccidioidomycosis). Occupational exposure to asbestos and heavy cigarette smoking both increase the risk of lung cancer. The presence or absence of chest or bone pain, hemoptysis, weight loss, and hoarseness should be ascertained. Careful physical examination should also be carried out, including mirror laryngoscopy, head and neck and abdominal examinations, and palpation of all lymph node areas. A sputum cytologic analysis should be performed, although it may not provide the diagnosis if the nodule is peripherally located. Pulmonary tomograms may reveal lesions not noted on routine PA-lateral chest radiographs. In one series, almost 20% of patients with pulmonary metastases who had an apparent solitary lung nodule were found to have multiple or bilateral lesions on tomograms. Bronchoscopy with brush or transbronchial biopsies may yield the correct diagnosis with an accuracy of 70% to 90%. Biopsy of accessible lymph nodes and mediastinoscopy may also be performed. However, the most accurate and reasonably safe diagnostic procedure short of thoracotomy is a thin-needle aspiration biopsy of the lesion. In one study 1223 patients underwent aspiration biopsies of chest lesions, with a diagnostic yield of 86.4%. Pneumothoraces developed in almost 25% of the patients, but only a few required treatment (insertion of a pleural needle). This procedure may avoid thoracotomy, and may also provide therapeutic guidance if specific carcinoma cell types are identified. A search for a primary tumor may be carried out if metastases are identified; or if, for example, a small cell lung carcinoma is detected, thoracotomy is not necessary. However, aspiration biopsy may not provide the diagnosis in a patient who has pulmonary infiltrates rather than a nodule. It is also difficult to make the diagnosis of lymphoma (especially Hodgkin's disease) from needle aspiration cytology of a pulmonary nodule. In this situation, either a diagnostic thoracotomy or larger bore (Vim Silverman) needle biopsy is required.

It is important to diagnose primary lung carcinomas early, since early resection improves survival. In a cooperative Veteran's Hospital study, patients followed 10 years after curative resection of pulmonary nodules greater than 4.0 cm (negative mediastinal nodes) had a 20.1% survival. In a series of thoracotomies performed on 179 patients, of whom 25 had carcinomas (19 primary in the lung), only 2 deaths were noted in the latter group, and 10 patients have survived longer than 5 years.

When lung metastases are present and resection is contemplated, several considerations must be made: (1) the patient must be able to withstand a thoracotomy; (2) the primary malignancy should be controlled; (3) the lesions should not be beyond the possibility of resection; (4) there should be a lack of effective alternative forms of therapy. Metastases should be removed by wedge or segmental resection if possible, to optimally preserve functioning lung tissue.

If the free interval from diagnosis of the primary malignancy to metastases is 1 year or less, postthoracotomy survival is only 13.6%, but it increases to 41% to 44% for free intervals of 1 to 4 or 5 years, respectively.

D.G.

Chang AE, Schaner EG, Conkle DM, et al: Evaluation of computed tomography in the detection of pulmonary metastases: A prospective study. Cancer 43:913–916, 1979.
   CT scan was more sensitive than tomography; however, only 20% of the additionally detected nodules proved to be metastases.
Higgins G, Shields T, Keehn R: The solitary pulmonary nodule. Arch Surg 110:570–575, 1975.
   VA cooperative review of pulmonary nodules.
Lolli A, McCormack L, Zelch M, et al: Aspiration biopsies of chest lesions. Radiology 127:35–40, 1978.
   In 1223 patients who were biopsied, there was an 86% diagnostic yield. An incidence of 4.4% symptomatic pneumothoraces and 11 deaths were possibly related to the procedure.
Mountain C, Khalil K, Hermes K, Frazier O: The contribution of surgery to the management of carcinomatous pulmonary metastases. Cancer 41:833–840, 1978.
   The 5-year survival in patients with carcinomas who underwent surgery was 29%. Criteria for selection were: (1) ability of patient to tolerate the surgery, (2) no other disease at primary site, and (3) no metastases beyond scope of planned pulmonary resection.
Ray J, Lawton B, Magnin G, et al: The coin lesion story: Update 1976. Chest 70:332–336, 1976.
   Of 179 thoracotomies, 27 had malignancies (15%); 10 of 12 with primary lung cancer were alive at 5 years after operation.
Reynolds RD, Pajak TF, Greenberg BR, et al: Lung cancer as a second primary. Cancer 42:2887–2893, 1978.
   Of 403 patients with lung cancer, 39 had history of prior malignancy.
Willson J, Eskridge M, Scott E: Transbronchial biopsy of benign and peripheral lung lesions. Radiology 100:541–546, 1971.
   Biopsies in 189 patients showed an 80% to 90% accuracy in detecting carcinomas.

20. PLEURAL EFFUSION

Pleural fluid accumulation results from an imbalance between the filtration and resorption mechanisms present at the pleural surfaces as well as from the interaction of such factors as the magnitude of net fluid transfer, the surface area of the parietal and visceral pleura, and the competence of lymphatic drainage. A wide variety of benign conditions may cause pleural effusions, including pleural infection, cirrhosis of the liver, pancreatitis, subphrenic abscess, Meigs' syndrome, myxedema, collagen vascular disease, congestive heart failure, and pulmonary infarction. In the cancer patient, a pleural effusion may develop secondary to metastatic tumor implants on the pleural surface, obstruction of venous or lymphatic drainage, direct disruption of lymph or venous channels, postobstructive pneumonia, hypoproteinemia, lung excision (effusion ex vacuo), or irradiation (with mediastinal or pericardial fibrosis). The cause of pleural fluid accumulation should always be investigated, because a pleural effusion may represent the first clinical sign of serious and possibly fatal disease.

The most common cause of pleural effusion in patients undergoing diagnostic thoracenteses is malignancy (approximately 50%); congestive heart failure (10% to 15%) and infection (5% to 8%) account for another 20%. In most series, however, an etiology cannot be found in 15% to 30% of patients, even after extensive investigation. Since neoplasms and congestive heart failure are the most common etiologies, diagnostic studies of pleural fluid should include protein concentration and cytologic examination. Total and differential cell count, fluid concentrations of glucose, lactate dehydrogenase or carcinoembryonic antigen, and routine cultures are of lesser value except in selected cases.

Pleural fluid cytologic findings are positive in 30% to 70% of patients who have known metastatic pleural involvement. The diagnostic yield may be improved in some patients by multiple thoracenteses and of course depends upon careful histopathologic preparation of the collected fluid. Newer methods of electron microscopy and chromosomal analysis may add further diagnostic accuracy. Pleural biopsy has been used as an adjunct to fluid cytology with some success. Since this procedure has increased morbidity, it should be reserved for those patients who have suspected malignancy and negative pleural fluid cytologic findings. Direct visualization of the pleura (pleuroscopy) may increase the yield of pleural biopsy.

The malignancies most frequently associated with pleural effusions are lung cancer (25% to 40%), breast cancer (25%), and lymphoma (10% to 15%). Pleural cytology is usually positive in metastatic breast and lung cancer, whereas it is often negative in lymphoma. This is because it may be difficult to distinguish cytologically normal lymphocytes from malignant lymphoma cells; or instead of direct pleural involvement by lymphoma, there may be mediastinal disease causing lymphatic and/or venous obstruction with secondary pleural effusion formation. Carcinomatous involvement of the pleura is often the first site of documented metastatic malignancy. It carries with it an ominous prognosis: In one series the mean survial of 96 patients was only 3 months, with 95% of patients dead within the first year.

Another cause of pleural effusion is primary tumor of the pleura. Mesothelioma accounts for less than 5% of pleural neoplastic disease. It can be a benign, localized pleural tumor, or, more often, a diffusely spreading malignant disease of the pleural surface. It is associated with asbestos exposure and found most commonly in middle-aged males. Its onset is insidious, usually with dull, nonpleuritic chest pain, dyspnea, lassitude, and weight loss. The physical examination and chest x-ray reveal only the findings of a pleural effusion. Pleural cytology and biopsy are of little diagnostic value and most patients come to open biopsy procedures for diagnosis.

The therapy of pleural effusion and mesothelioma is presented in Part VII, Chapter 108.

C.P.

Black LF: The pleural space and pleural fluid. Mayo Clin Proc 47:493–506, 1972.
  An excellent review of the physiology and pathophysiology of pleural fluid formation and resorption.
Chernow B, Sahn SA: Carcinomatous involvement of the pleura: An analysis of 96 patients. Am J Med 63:695–702, 1977.
  In 46% of 96 patients a malignant pleural effusion provided the first diagnosis of cancer.

Dewald G, Dines DE, Weiland LH, Gordon H: Usefulness of chromosome examination in the diagnosis of malignant pleural effusions. N Engl J Med 295:1494–1500, 1976.
Chromosomal analysis was more frequently positive (85%) in malignant effusions from patients with leukemia or lymphoma than was cytology (31%).

Elmes PC, Simpson MJC: The clinical aspects of mesothelioma. Q J Med 69:427–449, 1976.
In this excellent analysis of 327 patients, pleural fluid cytology was positive in only 4% and percutaneous pleural biopsy in 26%, while most required open procedures for diagnosis.

Leuallen EC, Carr DT: Pleural effusion: A statistical study of 436 patients. N Engl J Med 252:79–83, 1955.
Neoplasms were the cause of pleural effusion in 52.5%, congestive heart failure in 10.1%, and infections in 8.3% of the 436 patients.

Light RW, Erozan YS, Ball WC: Cells in pleural fluid: Their value in differential diagnosis. Arch Intern Med 132:854–860, 1973.
In an analysis of 182 patients 77% of the proved malignant neoplasms had positive cytologies; differential cell counts were of no diagnostic value.

Salyer WR, Eggleston JC, Erozan YS: Efficacy of pleural needle biopsy and pleural fluid cytopathology in the diagnosis of malignant neoplasm involving the pleura. Chest 67:536–539, 1975.
Of 95 cancer patients studied, pleural fluid cytology was positive in 72% and pleural biopsy yielded an additional 18% in those with negative cytology.

Storey DD, Dines DE, Coles DT: Pleural effusion: A diagnostic dilemma. JAMA 236:2183–2186, 1976.
Of 133 unselected patients with pleural effusion, no diagnosis could be determined in 25 (19%); cytology was positive in 15% of those 136 pleural fluids studied, whereas cultures were positive in less than 3% of 143 specimens.

Theros EG, Feigin DS: Pleural tumors and pulmonary tumors: Differential diagnosis. Semin Roentgenol 12:239–247, 1977.
An excellent discussion of the radiologic features of mesothelioma.

Von Hoff DD, Li Volsi V: Diagnostic reliability of needle biopsy of the parietal pleura: A review of 272 biopsies. Am J Clin Pathol 64:200–203, 1975.
Accurate diagnoses were obtained in 48% of those patients with metastatic carcinoma and 57% of those with granulomatous disease.

21. BREAST LUMP

A mass in the breast is a common problem that may be caused by a number of processes other than carcinoma. It should be noted, however, that breast carcinoma is the most common cause of death among women between 40 and 44 years of age and has an incidence of 72/100,000 women and a mortality of 27/100,000 women. Since approximately 16% of women will develop breast cancer, and since smaller carcinomas are associated with improved survival, it is imperative to make the diagnosis of breast cancer when the lesion is in its early stages. Those having an increased risk of developing breast cancer are women with a strong family history of carcinoma of the breast, those who have already had a breast cancer, who are nulliparous, have never married, undergo early or late natural menopause, and are older than 45 to 50 years. Breast masses due to such inflammatory causes as tuberculosis and postpartum mastitis or abscess are rare at the present time. However, two other uncommon lesions, fat necrosis and sclerosing adenosis (the former primarily in obese women with large breasts), may produce firm, irregular breast masses attached to the skin. Fibrocystic disease is common in women between the ages of 25 and 45. Benign fibroadenomas are common in women between 20 and 35 years of age but are less frequently seen with advancing age. Subareolar ductal papillomas are benign but may produce bloody nipple discharge and be confused with carcinomas.

Breast masses may cause local pain or tenderness; may produce inflammation, fixation, induration, or puckering of the skin; and may cause nipple discharge or retraction. Enlarged axillary or supraclavicular lymph nodes may also be present. Skeletal pain or discomfort may suggest the presence of distant metastases.

A detailed history and careful physical examination should be performed. The length of time that the breast mass has been present is important, as well as the presence or absence of sanguineous nipple discharge; skin dimpling, retraction or fixation; and skeletal tenderness. The physical examination should consist of careful palpation of all breast quadrants (the upper-outer quadrant is the site of 50% of breast cancers, the central 20%, the lower-outer 10%, and the medial 20%) and inspection of the skin, nipple, and areola for fixation, orange peeling, or nipple retraction. Breast fixation or skin retraction may be seen with the patient upright, while the remainder of the examination may be carried out with the patient supine. Careful examination of the infraclavicular, axillary, and supraclavicular regions should also be performed. Then the nature of the breast mass should be carefully ascertained; from soft, fluid-filled cysts to moveable, firm fibroadenomas with smooth borders, and finally to the irregular, firm, poorly defined cancers. The last may be closely mimicked clinically by fat necrosis, sclerosing adenosis, and ductal papillomas.

Mammograms should be performed if cancer is suspected. They may reveal a carcinoma in the opposite breast or may aid in localizing the site for biopsy. If the patient has found a breast lump that the examiner cannot detect, the breast should be reexamined either after the next menstrual period or 1 month later. If the mass still cannot be palpated, mammography should be performed. If a mammogram is positive for carcinoma but no mass is palpable, the suspicious area should be excised using suitable localizing techniques.

If a breast mass is cystic and apparently benign, it may be aspirated. Cytologic examination should be performed if the fluid is bloody. If the mass disappears and the fluid is not bloody, the breast should be reexamined in 1 month. If a mass persists or the aspiration cytology reveals tumor cells, a biopsy should be performed. If a breast mass is clinically suspicious for carcinoma, a needle biopsy may be performed. A benign needle biopsy does not rule out a carcinoma and must be followed up by an open biopsy. Tissue samples to test for estrogen receptors should be obtained whenever possible from all patients in whom breast carcinoma is suspected.

If Paget's disease of the nipple (or nipple erosion) is present, a mammogram and biopsy should be performed. If a duct is bleeding and no mass is palpated, the duct may be cannulated and incised to locate a deeply situated mass.

A two-stage procedure, in which the biopsy (preferably an excisional biopsy) is performed first and is followed at a later date by definitive therapy based on permanent histopathologic interpretation, does not increase the risk of relapse for a patient and is highly recommended.

D.G.

Azjdela A, Ghossein N, Pilleron J, Ennuyer A: The value of aspiration cytology in the diagnosis of breast cancer: Experience at the Fondation Curie. Cancer 35:499–506, 1975.

In 1745 malignant tumors, false negative aspiration cytology rate was 3.6%. The procedure is only reliable when it gives a positive result.

Cutler S: Some epidemiologic observations on cancer of the female breast. Int J Radiat Oncol Biol Phys 2:753–754, 1977.
All aspects of epidemiology of breast cancer are covered.
Dodd G: Present status of thermography, ultrasound and mammography in breast cancer detection. Cancer 39:2796–2805, 1977.
This article analyzes risks and accuracy of all three diagnostic methods and concludes that mammography is most accurate.
Egan R: Breast biopsy priority: Cancer vs. benign pre-operative masses. Cancer 35:612–617, 1975.
17,288 breast examinations were covered. Article correlated age and clinical or radiographic presence or absence of breast masses with biopsy results.
Miller AB: Risk benefit in mass screening programs for breast cancer. Semin Oncol 5:351–359, 1978.
Article examines the roles of screening examination and mammography.
Rimsten A, Stenkvist B, Johanson H, Lindgren A: The diagnostic accuracy of palpation and fine needle biopsy and an evaluation of the combined use in the diagnosis of breast lesions. Ann Surg 182:1–8, 1975.
Correlation of clinical examination and needle aspiration cytology in 984 patients is discussed.

22. JAUNDICE

A patient with a primary malignancy may have many reasons for jaundice other than those due to the underlying neoplastic process. Jaundice may be prehepatic in origin, arising from increased red blood cell destruction (hemolysis), or may be due to such intrahepatic causes as Gilbert's disease, drug-induced impairment of hepatic bilirubin uptake, lack of bilirubin conjugation (Crigler-Najjar syndrome) or a deficiency in hepatic cell bilirubin excretion (Dubin-Johnson syndrome), cirrhosis, or hepatitis. Certain tranquilizers (Valium and Librium) or biliary cirrhosis may all produce intrahepatic cholestasis. Finally, gallstones, carcinomas of the pancreas or biliary ducts, or enlarged hepatic portal lymph nodes may all obstruct the common bile duct and produce jaundice. Primary malignant tumors of the pancreas, gallbladder, and extrahepatic bile ducts are uncommon, however, together accounting for only 5% of all malignancies. Hepatic metastases, which occur more frequently than primary, biliary obstructive tumors, are a more common cause of jaundice.

Patients with increased red blood cell destruction and low hematocrits may be dyspneic, pale, and easily fatigued. Those with a congenital lack of normal bilirubin uptake, conjugation, or excretion (Gilbert, Crigler-Najjar, or Dubin-Johnson syndromes) may appear well, whereas patients with biliary cirrhosis, hepatitis, or drug-induced cholestasis may note intense pruritus, fatigue, lethargy, weight loss, and anorexia. An impacted gallstone at the ampulla of Vater or in the common bile duct produces colicky pain and, if cholangitis is also present, fever. Pancreatic or biliary duct carcinomas may result in the insidious onset of jaundice, although 72% to 100% of patients experience anorexia, weight loss, nausea, and pain at some point in the course of their disease.

Important in the differential diagnosis of a jaundiced patient is a careful history and physical examination. For instance, a history of a preexisting malignancy may point to extrahepatic biliary obstruction. The physical examination may reveal a palpable gallbladder if a carcinoma involves the ampulla of Vater or pancreas. Occasionally masses in the epigastrium or in the region of the porta hepatis may be palpable. A complete blood count, Coombs' test, measurement of serum bilirubin (conjugated and unconjugated), and other liver function tests such as alkaline phosphatase, prothrombin time, and SGOT are all important in the differential diagnosis of jaundice. If the serum bilirubin is of the indirect-reacting type (unconjugated), prehepatic jaundice or a deficiency of hepatic biliary excretion should be suspected. Increased bilirubin production will also result in an elevated stool urobilinogen level, and the Coombs test may be positive. If the direct bilirubin level is elevated (conjugated), intrahepatic or hepatocellular jaundice may be present. Tranquilizers as a cause of intrahepatic cholestasis should be ruled out by a careful history. A liver biopsy may confirm the diagnosis of hepatocellular disease.

If the patient becomes progressively jaundiced, with the alkaline phosphatase level elevated out of proportion to that of the other hepatic enzymes, obstructive jaundice at the pancreatic, bile duct, or bile canaliculus level should be suspected. An abdominal radiograph may show calcifications indicative of a gallstone impacted in the duct. If the bilirubin values are greater than 8 mg/ 100 ml, intravenous cholangiography cannot be expected to visualize the bile ducts. In this situation gray scale ultrasound has a high degree of accuracy, almost 97%, in differentiating intrahepatic or extrahepatic jaundice. CT scans may produce a similar yield at greater cost but may aid in localizing dilated biliary radicals for transhepatic cholangiography.

Hemolysis may respond to prednisone, 60 mg/day, in divided doses. No treatment is usually required for such inborn errors of bilirubin metabolism as Gilbert's disease and the Crigler-Najjar and Dubin-Johnson syndromes. Intrahepatic cholestasis, if drug-induced, may be reversed by drug discontinuation. Chemotherapeutic agents with toxic liver side-effects, such as methotrexate and 6-mercaptopurine, should not be given (or the doses should be decreased) to patients with altered hepatic function. Since Adriamycin is excreted by the liver, its dose should also be reduced in the jaundiced patient. Obstructive jaundice resulting from enlarged nodes in the porta hepatis may be palliated by radiation therapy to the area. If a lesion of the pancreas or bile ducts is suspected, laparotomy and resection or bypass is recommended in suitable surgical candidates. It is uncertain whether postoperative irradiation leads to prolonged survival for patients after bypass procedures, but it may obtain significant palliation of pain.

D.G.

Abrams H, McNeil B: Medical implications of computed tomography. N Engl J Med 298:310–318, 1978.
CT scan effectiveness in most body sites is reviewed.
Alfidi R, Haaga J, Havrilla T, et al: Computer tomography of the liver. Am J Roentgenol 127:69–74, 1976.
CT helps to guide transhepatic needle placement for biopsy. CT is not helpful in cirrhosis when fat is not present in the liver parenchyma.
Green N, Mikkelsen W, Kernen J: Cancer of the common hepatic bile ducts—palliative radiotherapy. Radiology 109:687–689, 1973.
Four patients were discussed. All had undergone operation and bypass; one may have had tumor control. All died 7 to 17 months posttherapy, however.
Sample W, Sarti D, Goldstein L, et al: Gray scale ultrasonography of the jaundiced patient. Radiology 128:719–725, 1978.
Study covered 143 patients. The extrahepatic biliary system was demonstrated

in 38% of those with medical and 74% of those with surgical jaundice. The size of the common hepatic or bile duct (5 to 6 mm) made the differentiation. Ultrasound was the sole diagnostic procedure in 22% of patients prior to definitive surgery. If there had been prior common duct bypass surgery, ultrasound was ineffective due to gas.

Taylor K, Rosenfield A: Gray scale ultrasonography in the differential diagnosis of jaundice. Arch Surg 112:820–825, 1977.
This procedure is highly accurate in determining the intrahepatic or extrahepatic nature of jaundice.

23. HEPATOMEGALY

Hepatomegaly in a patient with a known history of a primary solid tumor may be due to liver metastases. There are many causes of hepatic enlargement, however, that are unrelated to hepatic parenchymal involvement by malignant neoplasms. It should be remembered that a palpable liver is not necessarily enlarged, since a low-lying normal liver secondary to depressed diaphragms may be felt on abdominal examination. True hepatomegaly may result from the impaired hepatic venous outflow associated with congestive heart failure or constrictive pericarditis and may also be noted when portal hypertension is present. Interruption or obstruction of biliary flow will also produce liver enlargement. Primary liver tumors, usually of hepatocellular origin, also occur but are rare, accounting for only 1% of all neoplastic diseases. Such benign liver tumors as adenomas, fibromas, hemangiomas, and cysts may cause hepatic enlargement. Fatty metamorphosis, cirrhosis, amyloid deposition, and glycogen storage disease may all result in hepatomegaly. The liver may also be involved in parasitic (*Echinococcus*), protozoal (amebic), or bacterial infections. Hepatic metastases usually develop from primary neoplasms of the colorectum, stomach, pancreas, esophagus, lung, breast, and skin (melanomas).

Most patients with hepatic metastases or primary liver carcinomas experience anorexia, malaise, fever, and weight loss. If Glisson's capsule is distended by a rapidly enlarging neoplasm or by an intrahepatic hemorrhage, the patient may have severe right upper quadrant abdominal pain. Hepatomegaly, esophageal varices, ascites, splenomegaly, and edema may all occur with severe constrictive pericarditis, heart failure, or portal vein obstruction.

A careful history and physical examination may elicit the existence of a primary malignancy or symptoms suggestive of congestive heart failure, hepatic infections, portal hypertension, biliary obstruction, or cirrhosis. It should also be ascertained whether the patient has a history of hemochromatosis, alcoholism, Thorotrast administration or vinyl chloride exposure. In the case of young women, the use of oral contraceptives (which may be related to the development of hepatic adenomas) should be documented. A venous pressure examination in the upper and lower extremities should also be carried out. Chest radiographs may provide the diagnosis by revealing cardiomegaly or congestive heart failure. Liver function tests, including those for alkaline phosphatase, SGOT, bilirubin, albumin, globulin, prothrombin time, and alpha fetoprotein (AFP), should be obtained. If all but the last are markedly abnormal, the most likely diagnoses are such intrinsic liver diseases as hepatitis, cirrhosis, glycogen storage disease, and amyloidosis. An elevation of alkaline phosphatase out of proportion to the other liver function tests (when the venous pressure is normal) suggests either a mass lesion involving the liver or biliary obstruction. Jaundice and markedly elevated alkaline phosphatase levels most commonly occur with extrahepatic biliary obstruction. A markedly elevated AFP concentration (>1000 ng/ml) is strongly suggestive of hepatocellular carcinoma.

If a hepatic mass lesion is suspected, a Tc 99m colloid liver scan should be obtained. Such scans are quite accurate in detecting hepatic defects larger than 2.5 cm. When a single focal lesion is present, however, liver scans are unreliable, unless the lesion is quite large. When hepatic CT scans, ultrasound, and radionuclide imaging are compared, similar diagnostic accuracies are noted for each of the three techniques. These various imaging modalities have an 80% to 90% accuracy rate in detecting hepatic neoplasms. The most accurate differentiation between benign and malignant hepatic tumors, however, is made by hepatic angiography. When infusion hepatic angiography and conventional angiography are combined, the diagnostic accuracy in detecting liver metastases is almost 100%. If the diagnosis remains in doubt, and acute, active hepatitis can be ruled out, a percutaneous liver biopsy and (if the latter is nondiagnostic), laparoscopically directed liver biopsies may provide the diagnosis.

Untreated patients with lymphomas and large mediastinal masses may also have elevated alkaline phosphatase values and hepatomegaly, presumably from vascular engorgement. After mediastinal irradiation and regression of the mass, this congestive hepatomegaly may resolve completely. Congestive heart failure, constrictive pericarditis, or pericardial effusion may be treated appropriately when these processes are the underlying cause of hepatomegaly. Bacterial liver infections may be managed with antibiotics, but amebic abscesses or echinococcal cysts may require surgical treatment. If a single metastatic lesion occupies only one lobe of the liver and there has been a long free interval since treatment of the primary neoplasm, partial hepatectomy may be feasible. Partial hepatectomy may also be performed for selected primary liver cancers. The treatment of hepatic metastases is discussed in Part VII, Chapter 110.

D.G.

Abrams H, McNeil B: Medical implications of computed tomography. N Engl J Med 298:310–318, 1978.
Hepatic CT scans, ultrasound studies, and radionuclide imaging are compared in this article.
Alpert E, Ferrucci J, Athanasoulis C, et al: Primary hepatic tumor. Gastroenterology 74:759–769, 1978.
A clinical conference on primary liver tumors, including work-up and etiology, is discussed.
Bleiberg H, Rozencweig M, Mathieu M, et al: The use of peritoneoscopy in the detection of liver metastases. Cancer 41:863–867, 1978.
The use of peritoneoscopy in 342 patients was analyzed.
Isselbacher KJ: Jaundice and hepatomegaly. *In* Harrison's Principles of Internal Medicine, Vol. 1. New York, McGraw-Hill, 1977. Pp. 218–223.
Differential diagnosis of hepatomegaly is provided in this chapter.
Knowles DM II, Casarella WJ, Johnson PM, Wolff M: The clinical, radiologic, and pathologic characterization of benign hepatic neoplasms: Alleged association with oral contraceptives. Medicine (Baltimore) 57:223–237, 1978.
This excellent discussion differentiates focal nodular hyperplasia from liver cell adenoma.
Marks W, Jacobs R, Goodman P, Lim R Jr: Hepatocellular carcinoma: Clinical and angiographic findings and predictability for surgical resection. Am J Roentgenol 132:7–11, 1979.

The role of angiography in both detection and assessment of operability of hepatocellular carcinoma was studied in 63 patients.

Moseley R: Primary malignant tumors of the liver. Surgery 61:674–686, 1967.
This is a good review of 47 patients with primary liver tumors.

Petasnick JP, Ram P, Turner DA, Fordham EW: The relationship of computed tomography, gray scale ultrasonography and radionuclide imaging in the evaluation of hepatic metastases. Semin Nucl Med 9:8–21, 1979.
The three studies were found to be complementary.

Rosch J, Freeny P, Antonovic R, Gutierreq O: Infusion hepatic angiography in diagnosis of liver metastases. Cancer 38:2278–2286, 1976.
In this report 68 patients were studied, with a diagnostic accuracy of 97%.

Rosenfield AT, Laufer I, Schneider PB: The significance of a palpable liver. Am J Roentgenol 122:313–317, 1974.
A scintigraphic scan-palpation correlation was found in 100 patients.

Ruiter D, Byck W, Pauwels E, et al: Correlation of scintigraphy with short interval autopsy in malignant focal liver disease. Cancer 39:172–179, 1977.
In a study of 59 patients, highest accuracy occurred with those with enlarged livers and multiple defects greater than 2.5 cm.

Viamonte M, Schiff E: Diagnostic approach to hepatic malignant neoplasms. JAMA 238:2191–2193, 1977.
This article gives a review of laboratory tests and noninvasive and invasive diagnostic methods.

24. SPLENOMEGALY

The palpable spleen presents a frequently encountered and difficult diagnostic dilemma for the clinician. As many as 5.6% of adults examined in a general outpatient clinic had palpable spleens, and an incidence of 2.86% has been reported for entering college freshmen. In these two groups the etiology of the apparent splenic enlargement could not be determined in almost 50% of the subjects. A palpable spleen is not always indicative of splenomegaly; however, the false-positive physical examination probably occurs in fewer than 2% of patients. A much more common pattern is the false-negative physical examination: splenomegaly may be detected as infrequently as one-third of the time.

The spleen normally performs a number of important functions, including hematopoesis during intrauterine life; destruction of aged and deformed erythrocytes; removal of intraerythrocytic inclusions (such as Howell-Jolly bodies); destruction of platelets and leukocytes; removal of particulates (including bacteria); production of antibody, opsonins, and lymphocytes; and release of reserved blood elements during stress. Coincident with splenic enlargement there may be excessive splenic trapping, sequestration, and destruction of the normal blood elements. Such hypersplenism is defined as circulating cytopenia of one or more of the formed blood elements, normal or increased bone marrow production, and amelioration of cytopenia following splenectomy. Although splenomegaly is usually present with hypersplenism, some consider that it is not necessary for the diagnosis. Any cause of splenomegaly may lead to hypersplenism, while splenomegaly per se is not invariably associated with the

ment of the spleen may be a primary (idiopathic) disorder or second-
tions (both acute and chronic), allergic or autoimmune disorders,

granulomatous diseases, liver disease with portal hypertension and splenic congestion, extrahepatic portal or splenic vein obstruction, lymphoreticular or hematopoetic diseases, infiltrative diseases, metastatic tumor, or splenic cyst. In many instances the associated clinical and laboratory findings lead to the underlying cause of splenic enlargement.

The clinical evaluation should include a careful history (infections, drug exposure, familial disorders, trauma, systemic symptoms) and physical examination (signs of liver disease, lymphadenopathy), and laboratory studies should begin with common diagnostic considerations (such as infectious mononucleosis in the college freshman and cirrhosis of the liver in the adult). The liver-spleen scan can demonstrate splenomegaly, liver abnormalities, increased uptake in the spleen and bone marrow in the patient with cirrhosis, uneven distribution of uptake in the infiltrated spleen, and splenic defects. Ultrasound and computed axial tomography may add information about the internal architecture of the spleen as well as other abdominal pathologic conditions. Other studies that may help to reveal the etiology of splenomegaly include skin tests, serologies, immunoprotein studies, chest x-ray, bone marrow, liver and peripheral lymph node biopsies/cultures, barium swallow to demonstrate varices, angiography of the hepatic and splenic circulation, intravenous pyelogram, and lymphography. Diagnostic fine needle splenic aspiration and/or percutaneous splenic biopsy have been used without complication in experienced hands.

Splenectomy is not commonly performed in order to establish the etiology of splenomegaly (<10% of patients undergoing splenectomy in one series). Most patients selected for diagnostic splenectomy have symptoms of chronic illness with fatigue, weakness, and fever as well as signs of hypersplenism or hepatomegaly. The diagnoses at laparotomy include lymphoma (30% to 50%), congestive splenomegaly (25%), idiopathic splenomegaly, inflammatory or infiltrative diseases, and splenic cyst. Although lymphocytic lymphoma is the most common etiology of splenomegaly at diagnostic splenectomy, fewer than 1% of patients with lymphoma require splenectomy for diagnosis. Furthermore there are few reported instances in which removal of the spleen alone led to cure of the disease. Most patients were found to have other sites of disease at laparotomy or manifested active disease shortly after splenectomy.

In patients with splenomegaly and hypersplenism, the indications for splenectomy are not only to establish an etiologic diagnosis but also to treat the circulating cytopenia. The choice of splenectomy depends on the underlying disease process as well as on the patient's general status and prognosis in addition to the degree of hypersplenism. The presence of major hemolysis with symptomatic anemia requiring transfusion, neutropenia with recurrent infection, thrombocytopenia with bleeding manifestations, and/or painful splenomegaly are all considered indications for splenectomy.

C.P.

Ahmann DL, Kiely JM, Harrison EG Jr, Payne WS: Malignant lymphoma of the spleen: A review of 49 cases in which the diagnosis was made at splenectomy. Cancer 19:461–469, 1966.
Splenectomy was performed for diagnosis in less than 1% of patients with lymphoma.
Ellis LD, Dameshek HL: The dilemma of hypersplenism. Surg Clin North Am 55:277–285, 1975.
This article discusses etiologies and indications for splenectomy.
Halpern S, Coel M, Ashburn W, et al: Correlation of liver and spleen size: Determinations by nuclear medicine studies and physical examination. Arch Intern Med 134:123–124, 1974.

Splenomegaly, as defined by scan measurements of the spleen, was correctly identified at physical examination in only 26 of 92 patients (28%) with it.

Hermann RE, DeHaven KE, Hawk WA: Splenectomy for the diagnosis of splenomegaly. Ann Surg 168:896–900, 1968.

This article presents an analysis of 52 patients in whom the causes of splenomegaly were: lymphoma (31%), congestion (25%), inflammatory disease (19%), infiltrative disease (15%), splenic cysts (6%), and miscellaneous disorders (4%).

Lipp WF, Eckstein EH, Aaron AH: The clinical significance of the palpable spleen. Gastroenterology 3:287–291, 1944.

Of 2,274 consecutive patients, 5.6% had palpable spleens; no etiology could be determined in 41.4% of those with the palpable spleen.

McIntyre OR, Ebaugh FG: Palpable spleens in college freshmen. Ann Intern Med 66:301–306, 1967.

Of 2,200 college students, 63 (2.86%) had palpable spleens; a persistently palpable spleen was documented in 18 of 39 students (30%) followed for at least 3 years.

Skarin AT, Davey FR, Moloney WC: Lymphosarcoma of the spleen: Results of diagnostic splenectomy in 11 patients. Arch Intern Med 127:259–265, 1971.

In this retrospective study 4 patients remained free of disease following splenectomy.

Soderstrom N: How to use cytodiagnostic spleen puncture. Acta Med Scand 199:1–5, 1976.

A brief description of fine needle aspiration technique and its diagnostic utility.

Spencer RP: Spleen scanning as a diagnostic tool. JAMA 237:1473–1474, 1977.

A brief review of spleen scanning is given.

Spencer RP, Pearson HA: The spleen as a hematological organ. Semin Nucl Med 5:95–102, 1975.

An excellent review.

25. GASTRIC ULCER

Benign ulcers of the stomach are caused by acid erosion of the mucosa, but the total gastric acid secretion may be either normal or decreased. Decreased tissue resistance to acid is also important in the formation of gastric ulcers. Eighty to ninety percent of benign ulcers occur on the lesser curvature of the stomach: 60% are within 6 cm of the pylorus, while 20% to 25% occur higher on the lesser curvature. Benign gastric ulcers afflict approximately 0.1% of the American population. They are difficult to cure, since 50% recur at some time after the initial healing. Even though most benign ulcers are found on the lesser curvature of the stomach, the site of involvement is not absolutely indicative of either a benign or a malignant process.

A gastric ulcer may produce typical postprandial midepigastric pain, which is usually, but not always, relieved by the ingestion of antacids, fluids, or food. Anorexia, nausea and vomiting, and marked weight loss also occur. Anemia and a positive occult stool blood test may also be noted. Ordinarily the only sign on physical examination is epigastric tenderness.

Even though declining in frequency and mortality, a gastric carcinoma must not be overlooked when a gastric ulcer is present. The risk of carcinoma is much greater in patients with pernicious anemia or those with atrophic, achlorhydric gastritis. Patients suspected of having a gastric ulcer should undergo an upper GI series. A benign gastric ulcer is usually noted as a lesser curvature out-pouching with radiating folds, with or without mucosal edema. The risk of a carcinoma even in this setting is approximately 3%, however. If the ulcer is irregular and has heaped-up margins, malignancy should be suspected. Fifty percent of gastric cancers are located in the distal stomach, while 25% involve the cardia and another 20% occur higher on the lesser curvature. The greater curvature is a site of malignant gastric ulcers 3% to 5% of the time; however, a benign ulcer is rare at this site. If an ulcer is demonstrated on a GI series, gastric secretion studies should be performed. If achlorhydria is noted, espe-cially after the administration of betazole, carcinoma must be strongly sus-pected. Fiberoptic gastroscopy is important in the evaluation of a patient with a gastric ulcer. The entire stomach can be inspected by this procedure. The edges of the ulcer should be biopsied multiple times and the edges and ulcer crater brushed through the gastroscope for cytologic evaluation. The gastroscopy may be repeated until the ulcer has healed.

If the ulcer appears benign, intensive antacid regimens should be used to ensure healing. With a rigid antacid regimen, 11% to 26% of all ulcers should be healed in 2 weeks and 60% to 85% healed 6 weeks after the institution of vigorous therapy. The upper GI series should be repeated at 3, 6, and 12 weeks or until the ulcer has healed. If the ulcer has not healed in 3 months, surgery is recommended. As already stated, 50% of benign gastric ulcers can be expected to recur. Surgery is necessary for a malignant ulcer, although the overall survival for patients with gastric carcinomas is only 10%. At the time of sur-gery, 80% of patients will have regional lymph node metastases, while 40% will have peritoneal involvement or implants and 33% will also have liver and/or lung metastases.

D.G.

Davis Z, Verheyden C, Van Heerden J, Judd E: The surgically treated gastric ulcer. Ann Surg 185:205–209, 1977.
Of 1458 patients with gastric ulcers, 595 were treated surgically. Results were good to excellent in 82%.

Englert E Jr, Freston J, Graham D, et al: Cimetidine, antacid and hospitali-zation in the treatment of benign gastric ulcer. Gastroenterology 74:416–426, 1978.
There were no significant differences between groups, but the trend was in favor of cimetidine-antacid combination; 58 to 76% of the ulcers healed by 6 weeks.

Gray G: Gastroenterology. *In* E Rubinstein and D Federman (Eds), *Scientific American Medicine.* Sci Am New York, 1978. Section 4, pp. 4II, 11–12.
Symptoms, evaluation, and treatment of gastric ulcers are reviewed.

Haenszel W, Correa P: Developments in the epidemiology of stomach cancer over the past decade. Cancer Res 35:3452–3459, 1975.
Detailed epidemiological study of decreasing incidence of gastric cancer.

26. COLON POLYP

The incidence of colon polyps of significant size (>1 cm) in the adult American population is estimated to be 5% to 15%. The incidence is higher if all polyps, including those smaller than 1 cm, are included. Most polyps are single (only

20% are multiple). Early studies of colonic sites of involvement revealed a propensity for polypoid lesions to occur in the descending colon or rectum; however, these studies were based on the results of proctoscopies and barium enemas, which demonstrate lesions in these more accessible portions of the colon. Series based on the use of colonoscopy have revealed a greater incidence of polyps in the transverse and ascending colon.

The most common colorectal polyps are neoplastic polyps, either adenomatous (pedunculated and sessile), villous, or the intermediate villoglandular type. Other types include polypoid carcinomas, juvenile polyps (hamartomas), and the pseudopolyps noted in inflammatory colonic diseases. The risk of carcinoma increases with large size, multiplicity, and certain types of polyp. Adenomatous polyps are the most common, making up 60% to 75% of all polyps, and have an associated cancer risk of 1% to 5%. Villoglandular polyps occur with a frequency of 15% to 20% and have a cancer risk of 5% to 20%. Villous adenomas, 10% to 15% of all polyps, have an associated cancer risk of 20% to 40%. Less than 1% of polyps smaller than 1 cm are malignant, but approximately 10% of polyps between 1 and 2 cm in size and almost 50% of those larger than 2 cm are malignant. Many authors believe that most, if not all, colorectal carcinomas arise from preexisting polyps. In one series, half to two-thirds of large bowel carcinomas appeared to arise from polyps, while in the remainder the association between polyps and cancer could not be determined. When routine proctoscopic examinations were performed in a large patient population, a decreased frequency in the expected number of rectal carcinomas was noted in patients who had polypectomies.

Small pedunculated polyps are usually asymptomatic. A large, stalked polyp, however, may cause intussusception, leading to colicky pain and an acute abdomen. Symptomatic polyps most commonly cause rectal bleeding, which occurs in 40% to 50% of patients. Crampy abdominal pain and change in bowel habits are less frequent. Villous adenomas, due to their large secretory surface, are associated with excessive mucous secretion, diarrhea, and electrolyte imbalance, especially hypokalemia.

Evaluation of a patient with occult or gross rectal bleeding should include proctoscopy. A yield of 1.5 cancers for 1000 examinations in patients over 40 has been estimated for this procedure. If rectal bleeding or a history of either familial polyposis, prior polyps, or a colon carcinoma is obtained, a barium enema is also indicated. The double contrast or malmö technique appears to be the most effective radiologic contrast procedure for revealing colon polyps. The CEA test is usually normal in patients with colonic polyps.

The recent use of fiberoptic colonoscopy has decreased the indications for laparotomy in patients with colon polyps. The procedure is relatively safe, has low morbidity, and rarely requires laparotomy for complications. If a polyp is removed and contains carcinoma in situ, most authors recommend no further therapy. In a patient with invasive carcinoma confined to the head of a pedunculated polyp without lymphatic invasion, colonoscopic removal may be the only procedure required. In one series 28 patients with pedunculated polyps that contained invasive carcinomas were studied. Eight patients remained well, with no evidence of cancer without undergoing laparotomy after polypectomy. The other 20 patients underwent colon resections, but only one patient developed lymph node metastases; that patient had a frankly invasive carcinoma immediately adjacent to the polyp.

Laparotomy and colon resection are recommended, however, for patients with lymphatic invasion by carcinoma, with undifferentiated invasive neoplasms, or with extension into the neck of the polyp. Laparotomy is also recommended for those with polypoid carcinomas, with involved colonoscopic resection margins, or with cancers too large to be resected endoscopically.

Periodic follow-up, with colonoscopy alternating with barium enemas at 2 or 3 year intervals, is recommended. However, if the patient is in the high-risk group (multiple polyps, prior colon cancer), yearly colonoscopies should be performed.

D.G.

Fenoglio CM, Kaye GI, Lane N: Distribution of human colonic lymphatics in normal, hyperplastic, and adenomatous tissue. Gastroenterology 64:51–66, 1973.
No lymphatics superficial to muscularis mucosae—an explanation for rare metastases from a stalked polyp.

Gilbertsen VA: Proctosigmoidoscopy and polypectomy in reducing the incidence of rectal cancer. Cancer 34:936–939, 1974.
Periodic examinations in over 18,000 patients greatly reduced the expected incidence of rectal carcinomas.

Grinnell R: The chance of cancer and lymphatic metastasis in small colon tumors discovered on x-ray examination. Ann Surg 159:132–138, 1964.
Correlation of polyp-size and risk of cancer and/or lymph node metastases was discussed.

Morson B: The polyp-cancer sequence in the large bowel. Proc Soc Med 67:451–457, 1974.
50 to 70% of colorectal cancers arise from polyps. Excellent review.

Muto T, Bussey H Jr, Morson B: The evolution of cancer of the colon and rectum. Cancer 36:2251–2270, 1975.
Article presents evidence for a slow evolution from adenomatous polyp to colorectal cancer. Malignant potential varies with size, histological type, and degree of cellular atypia.

Shatney CH, Lober PH, Gilbertsen VA, Sosin H: The treatment of pedunculated adenomatous colorectal polyps with focal cancer. Surg Gynecol Obstet 139:845–850, 1974.
Management of in situ and invasive cancers discussed.

Shinya H, Wolff WI: Morphology, anatomic distribution and cancer potential of colonic polyps: An analysis of 7,000 polyps endoscopically removed. Ann Surg 190:679–683, 1979.
An excellent analysis providing evidence for a polyp-to-cancer sequence.

Stauffer JQ: Polypoid tumors of the colon. *In* MH Sleisinger and JS Fordtran (Eds), Gastrointestinal Disease: Pathophysiology, Diagnosis, and Management. Philadelphia, W.B. Saunders, 1978. Vol. 2, Chap. 110, pp. 1771–1784.
Excellent review of the subject.

Watne AL, Lai HY, Carrier J, Coppola WT: The diagnosis and surgical treatment of patients with Gardner's syndrome. Surgery 82:327–333, 1977.
Bowel cancer occurred in 32% of 126 patients with Gardner's syndrome.

Welch CE, Hedberg SE: Polypoid Lesions of the Gastrointestinal Tract (2nd ed). Philadelphia, W.B. Saunders, 1975.
Complete review, especially good chapters on incidence and diagnosis.

Welch JP, Welch CE: Villous adenomas of the colorectum. Am J Surg 131:185–191, 1976.
In 258 patients from Massachusetts General Hospital invasive cancer occurred in 29%; 5-year survival was 52.6%.

Wheat M, Ackerman L: Villous adenomas of the large intestine. Ann Surg 147:476–487, 1958.
In this article 50 cases of villous adenomas were evaluated.

Williams CB, Hunt RH, Loose H, et al: Colonoscopy in the management of colon polyps. Br J Surg 61:673–682, 1974.
300 polypectomies were performed in 169 patients.

Winawer SJ, Leidner SD, Hajdu SI, Sherlock P: Colonoscopic biopsy and
cytology in the diagnosis of colon cancer. Cancer 42:2849–2853, 1978.
*Brush cytology in addition to biopsy increased the diagnostic yield by ap-
proximately 30% to 40% in the 40 patients studied.*

Wolff WI, Shinya H: Endoscopic polypectomy. Cancer 36:683–690, 1975.
*2000 polyps were endoscopically removed; there were no deaths and only one
complication requiring laparotomy.*

27. HEMATURIA

Hematuria, either gross or microscopic, should be considered a sign of a severe
pathologic condition of the urinary tract until proved otherwise. The bleeding
sites may be conveniently separated into (1) lesions of the upper urinary tract,
including the renal pelvis and calyces (pyelonephritis, trauma, glomerulonephritis, calculus, or tumor); (2) involvement of the lower urinary tract: bladder, prostate, and urethra (infection, calculus, tumor, trauma, benign prostatic
hypertrophy, etc.); (3) such generalized causes as hemorrhagic diatheses, sickle
cell anemia, and leukemia; (4) drug ingestion (aspirin, sulfonamides, anticoagulants, and such antineoplastic drugs as cyclophosphamide). A reddish urine,
however, may also be caused by secreted biopigments, porphyrins, cathartics,
food dyes, and hemoglobinuria.

When the cause of bleeding was assessed in 1000 patients with gross hematuria, the bladder was the source in almost 40%, the prostate in 24%, the
kidney in 15%, and the urethra in 5%. Generalized urinary tract infections or
tuberculosis were the cause of hematuria in 2%; the remainder were either of
unknown etiology (essential) or due to such systemic causes as hemophilia,
anticoagulation, or cancer therapy (chemotherapy or radiotherapy).

Microscopic hematuria is significant whether only a few or many red cells per
high-power field are present in the urinary sediment. When 200 patients with
microscopic hematuria were studied prospectively, 81% were found to have
genitourinary lesions, whereas 19% had no urologic pathology. Highly
significant urinary lesions were found in 40 of the patients (20%) and included
bladder cancers in 22, renoparenchymal disease in 7, ureteral calculi in 3,
prostatic carcinoma in 3, hydronephrosis in 3, and renal artery stenosis and
renal lymphoma in a single patient each. Overall, 13% of the patients had
neoplasms of the urinary tract and 25% had urinary infections. Since the risk of
serious genitourinary lesions is so high, especially in older adults, the presence
of painless hematuria, either gross or microscopic, should be considered to be
caused by carcinoma until a neoplasm has been ruled out.

In evaluating a patient with hematuria, a careful history is very important.
Familial renal disease, previous glomerulonephritis, a collagen vascular disorder, sickle cell anemia, the passage of stones, and drug use (including cyclophosphamide, anticoagulants, or aspirin) should all be considered. The degree
of hemorrhage, the presence or absence of pain, the passage of a stone, recent
trauma, or systemic infections are all important clues to the underlying cause
of hematuria, as are its duration and frequency. Massive bleeding usually
arises from bladder tumors, benign prostatic hypertrophy, or trauma, while
dark urine signifies old blood. Initial hematuria usually represents bleeding
from the prostatic urethra, whereas total hematuria, in which all the urine is
bloody, is most often related to bleeding from the bladder or upper urinary
tracts. Terminal hematuria often represents hemorrhage from the prostate or

bladder neck. The nature of the clot is also important. A linear, formed clot usually occurs in the urethra, whereas large, irregular, multiple clots are passed from the bladder. The physical examination should include careful palpation of the costovertebral angles, the abdomen, the suprapubic region, the genitalia, and a rectal examination. The presence or absence of systemic diseases of lymphadenopathy, petechial skin lesions, or evidence of hemorrhage elsewhere in the body should also be noted.

The laboratory examination for patients with either microscopic or gross hematuria includes a urinalysis, gram stain, and when indicated urine culture and sensitivity, excretory urogram, cystoscopy, urinary cytology, renal arteriograms, and CT scans. Examination of the urinary sediment is important. Red cell casts usually indicate parenchymal disease, while white cells and bacteria in the urine represent infectious causes for the hematuria. Hematuria with white blood cells but no bacteria may be found in such lesions as urinary calculi, bladder tumors, or interstitial cystitis. A complete blood count, platelet count, and bleeding parameters should also be obtained. Serum protein electrophoresis may be necessary to rule out sickle cell anemia. BUN, creatinine, calcium, and uric acid determinations should also be performed if urinary calculi are suspected. Urine cytology may confirm the diagnosis of genitourinary malignancy.

A careful urologic evaluation should begin with an intravenous pyelogram (IVP). Urinary calculi and renal, bladder, or prostate abnormalities may be detected by this study; and, if indicated, retrograde ureteral studies can also be performed. In a study of 200 patients with microhematuria, the IVP revealed abnormalities in 72 patients (36%). Cystoscopy, with or without retrograde examination of the ureters, is extremely important and, if the bleeding is intermittent, should be performed during an episode of hemorrhage. Hemorrhagic cystitis, bladder tumors, prostatic hypertrophy, prostatic carcinoma, or the presence of calculi may all be revealed by cystoscopy. Postirradiation or cyclophosphamide cystitis may also be diagnosed by cystoscopy. If indicated, aortograms may be performed if a renal tumor is suspected, while ultrasound or CT scans may reveal renal cysts, retroperitoneal masses invading or compressing the urinary system, or intrinsic lesions of the kidneys, ureters, bladder, or prostate.

For patients with an elevated sedimentation rate, abnormal urinary protein excretion, and progressive renal disease, renal biopsy may be indicated, especially if there is clinical suspicion of glomerular damage. In a study of 402 patients who underwent renal biopsy, 85 (21%) of the biopsies were normal. Focal proliferative glomerulonephritis was found in 54% of the patients (usually a manifestation of such systemic diseases as lupus erythematosus, subacute bacterial endocarditis, or Berger's disease); diffuse glomerulonephritis was noted in 20%; and chronic glomerulonephritis, pyelonephritis, and other renoparenchymal disorders were noted in less than 5% of the patients. The treatment in each instance depends on the underlying cause of the hematuria.

D.G.

Carlton C Jr: *In* MF Campbell and JH Harrison (Eds), Urology. Philadelphia, W.B. Saunders, 1978. Pp. 206–208.
   Differential diagnosis of hematuria is discussed.
Carson CC, Segura JW, Greene LF: Clinical significance of microhematuria. JAMA 241:149–150, 1979.
   In a study of 200 consecutive patients highly significant lesions (cancers, renal parenchymal disease, calculi, and so on) were found in 40 (20%).

Kadish HG: Determining the cause of hematuria. Postgrad Med 58:118–122, 1975.
Article describes findings in 1000 patients with hematuria.
Pollack VE, Ooi BS: Asymptomatic hematuria. Postgrad Med 62:115–120, 1977.
This excellent review includes renal biopsy results in 412 patients.
Smith D: General Urology. Los Altos, Calif., Lange Medical Publications, 1978. Pp. 32–33.
Outline of evaluation for hematuria is given.
Turner AG, Carter S, Higgins E, et al: The clinical diagnostic value of the carcinoembryonic antigen (CEA) in hematuria. Br J Urol 49:61–66, 1977.
In a prospective study in 216 patients CEA (urine or plasma) was not a useful screening test for malignancy, especially when infection was present.

28. ABNORMAL VAGINAL BLEEDING

Abnormal vaginal bleeding accompanies most organic gynecologic diseases and may be seen in patients with systemic diseases and blood dyscrasias or as the result of iatrogenic or traumatic causes. In women of childbearing age the most likely cause of abnormal vaginal bleeding is a complication of pregnancy, such as abortion, ectopic pregnancy, or trophoblastic disease. Although relatively rare in the United States (approximately 1 in 2000 pregnancies), trophoblastic disease is important to recognize because of its malignant potential and high rate of cure with chemotherapy. Typically patients present with amenorrhea and subjective symptoms of pregnancy followed by intermittent spotting and vaginal bleeding. Fetal heart tones are not heard, and pelvic ultrasound may demonstrate an enlarged uterus with "snowstorm" pattern, characteristically with multiple internal echoes reflected from numerous hydatid vesicles. Serum radioimmunoassay of β subunit chorionic gonadotropin (HCG) is elevated; after uterine evacuation, HCG can be followed for evidence of disease activity and the need for additional therapy.

Abnormal vaginal bleeding in the premenarchal or adolescent menstruating female may result from vaginal adenosis or adenocarcinoma. In utero exposure to diethylstilbestrol has been associated with these diseases, and exposed patients should have a complete gynecologic evaluation. In addition to Papanicolaou smears of the cervix and vagina, any areas not staining with iodine should be examined by biopsy. The risk of adenocarcinoma is low (less than 4 in 1000 persons exposed); however, vaginal adenosis occurs in at least 35%. To date, there is no evidence that adenosis is a premalignant condition, although it is recommended that affected patients be followed closely.

During menopause, vaginal bleeding may be secondary to malignancy in as many as 10% to 25% of patients. Endometrial and cervical cancer account for most cases, in a ratio of 1:1. Benign etiologies of vaginal bleeding include estrogen administration and adenomatous hyperplasia, atrophic endometrium, uterine adenomyosis, endometrial and cervical polyps, leiomyomas, and cervicitis. The diagnosis of cervical cancer can usually be made by Papanicolaou smear, biopsy of areas failing to stain with iodine, and culposcopy. On the other hand, endometrial cancer presents a more difficult diagnostic problem. Papanicolaou smear is positive in only half of cases of known carcinoma, and in many cases the uterus is not enlarged. Consequently it is necessary to identify patients at high risk and not to be satisfied with the results of Papanicolaou smears alone. Obesity, hypertension, diabetes mellitus, late menarche and infertility, prolonged menopausal exposure to diethylstilbestrol, and endometrial adenomatous hyperplasia have all been associated with increased risk. Outpatient diagnostic procedures that can be performed following a negative Papanicolaou smear include endometrial aspiration and/or biopsy, Gravlee jet washing, and vacuum curettage. Fewer than 10% of patients with endometrial cancer will be left undiagnosed after one of these studies and will require a formal diagnostic dilatation and curettage under anesthesia.

C.P.

Creasman WT, Weed JC Jr: Screening techniques in endometrial cancer. Cancer 38:436–440, 1976.
A good review of the diagnostic accuracy of Papanicolaou smear, endometrial biopsy, Gravlee jet washer, and vacuum curettage.
Goldfarb JM, Little AB: Abnormal vaginal bleeding. N Engl J Med 302:666–669, 1980.
An excellent review of benign causes in premenopausal women.
Gusberg SB: The individual at high risk for endometrial carcinoma. Am J Obstet Gynecol 126:535–542, 1976.
A general discussion with extensive references.
Herbst AL, Norusis MJ, Rosenow PJ, et al: An analysis of 346 cases of clear cell adenocarcinoma of the vagina and cervix with emphasis on recurrence and survival. Gyn Oncol 7:111–122, 1979.
Emphasizes the need for early detection and aggressive surgery. Actuarial survival of greater than 87% at 5 years with Stage I disease. Local excision only was associated with recurrence in 33% of 17 patients as compared to 8% of 117 patients with radical surgery.
Keirse MJNC: Aetiology of postmenopausal bleeding. Postgrad Med J 49:344–348, 1973.
In this good analysis of 160 patients evaluated at a general hospital malignancy accounted for 24% of the cases of bleeding.
Kobayashi M: Use of diagnostic ultrasound in trophoblastic neoplasms and ovarian tumors. Cancer 38:441–452, 1976.
A good review.
Poskanzer DC, Herbst AL: Epidemiology of vaginal adenosis and adenocarcinoma associated with exposure to stilbestrol *in utero*. Cancer 39:1892–1895, 1977.
A brief review of the subject is given.
Procopé, B-J: Aetiology of postmenopausal bleeding. Acta Obstet Gynecol Scand 50:311–313, 1971.
In an analysis of 1,085 women malignancy was found in 28%.
Stafl A: Colposcopy. Clin Obstet Gynecol 18:195–213, 1975.
A good description of this technique and its diagnostic utility.
Wright VC: Vaginal metastases of hypernephroma. Case report and summary of world literature. Can Med Assoc J 100:816, 1969.
Metastatic cancer is an unusual cause of abnormal vaginal bleeding.
Ziel HK, Finkle WD: Increased risk of endometrial carcinoma among users of conjugated estrogens. N Engl J Med 293:1167–1170, 1975.
An analysis of 94 patients found that the risk of endometrial cancer increased with duration of exposure.

Although the chance of detecting an ovarian malignancy is only 1 in 10,000 asymptomatic patients examined, the routine pelvic examination remains the only sure method of detecting an adnexal mass. In order to be palpated abdominally in an adult, an ovarian tumor must be at least 15 cm in diameter.

During the menstruating years, ovarian enlargements are usually due to physiologic cysts measuring less than 10 cm. They are most often unilateral and resolve spontaneously within 2 to 3 months or after administration of birth control pills. A malignant tumor should be suspected if the mass is larger than 10 cm, solid rather than cystic, bilateral, does not resolve after 2 to 3 months, or develops while the patient is taking birth control pills. Benign causes of an adnexal mass include endometriosis, pelvic inflammatory disease, diverticulitis, pelvic kidney, and pedunculated uterine leiomyoma. Unlike the premenopausal patient with a physiologic ovarian cyst, malignancy is the most common cause of ovarian enlargement in the prepubertal or postmenopausal age group. Germ cell neoplasms make up the majority of childhood tumors, whereas epithelial malignancies and metastatic cancer to the ovary predominate after menopause.

The normal ovary (measuring $3.5 \times 2 \times 1.5$ cm) shrinks with age, so that within 5 years after clinical menopause it is no longer palpable on pelvic examination ($2 \times 1.5 \times 0.5$ cm). Therefore, in the postmenopausal patient, a palpable ovary is pathologically enlarged, even if it is only the size of a "normal" premenopausal ovary.

Other pathologic findings on pelvic examination may be tumors or irregularity in the cul-de-sac, bilateral masses, or the presence of ascites. In spite of clinically advanced disease many patients have few symptoms, complaining only of abdominal discomfort, dyspepsia, or increasing abdominal girth. High-risk patients are those between the ages of 40 and 65 years and women with prior ovarian dysfunction, infertility, early menopause, or a family history of ovarian cancer.

If a malignant ovarian mass is suspected, Papanicolaou smear and/or culdocentesis may yield positive cytologic findings. Prior to exploratory laparotomy, all patients should have a thorough physical examination, with sigmoidoscopy, blood counts, chemistries, and urinalysis as well as chest x-ray and IVP. Other radiographic studies, such as an upper GI series, barium enema, lymphogram, ultrasound, and computed axial tomography, may be useful in identifying the extent of disease. Serum levels of alpha fetoprotein, carcinoembryonic antigen, or Regan isoenzyme may be elevated. Peritoneal and/or pleural fluid should be tapped for cytologic analysis.

Although preoperative studies may suggest malignancy, laparotomy is frequently necessary to establish a diagnosis and to evaluate the extent of disease. In addition to tumor biopsy, removal of the bulk of the disease, and usually a total abdominal hysterectomy and bilateral salpingo-oophorectomy, there must be a careful evaluation of the peritoneal surface (with aspiration of ascitic fluid for cytologic examination, peritoneal washings, blind biopsies, and visualization of both diaphragmatic surfaces and abdominal gutters), the gastrointestinal tract, and the retroperitoneum. Oophorectomy alone can be considered only in selected prepubertal and premenopausal patients in whom disease appears confined to one ovary.

In summary the indications for exploratory laparotomy include any adnexal mass detected before puberty, after menopause, or while taking birth control pills; a solid tumor at any age; a cystic mass larger than 10 cm; a cystic mass (4 to 10 cm) present for more than 3 months during menstruation; and an ovary of normal premenopausal dimensions in a postmenopausal woman.

C.P.

Barber HRK, Graber EA: The PMPO syndrome (postmenopausal palpable ovary syndrome). Obstet Gynecol 38:921–923, 1971.
This report emphasizes that a "normal"-sized premenopausal ovary is pathological when found in a postmenopausal woman.

Day TG, Smith JP: Diagnosis and staging of ovarian carcinoma. Semin Oncol 2:217–222, 1975.
An excellent review.

Fraumeni JF, Grundy GW, Creagan ET, Everson RB: Six families prone to ovarian cancer. Cancer 36:364–369, 1975.
Article emphasizes need for close medical surveillance of susceptible family members.

Greenwald EF: Ovarian tumors. Clin Obstet Gynecol 18:61–86, 1975.
A comprehensive review outlining etiology, histopathology, clinical evaluation, staging, and therapy.

McGowan L, Bunnag B, Arias LB: Peritoneal fluid cytology associated with benign neoplastic ovarian tumors in women. Am J Obstet Gynecol 113:961–966, 1972.
Culdocentesis yielded peritoneal fluid for cytology and cytogenetic analysis in 40 patients with benign ovarian tumors.

Norris HJ, Jensen RD: Relative frequency of ovarian neoplasms in children and adolescents. Cancer 30:713–719, 1972.
Malignancies accounted for 55% of ovarian tumors in 353 patients; germ cell neoplasms were most frequent (58%), while epithelial neoplasms were uncommon (19%).

Prem KA: The ovarian mass: An approach to diagnosis and treatment. *In* JS Najarian and JP Delaney (Eds), Advances in Cancer Surgery. New York, Stratton, 1976. Pp. 597–602.
Article discusses the surgical indications for laparotomy and appropriate operative staging procedures.

Samaan NA, Smith JP, Rutledge FN, Schultz PN: The significance of measurement of human placental lactogen, human chorionic gonadotropin, and carcinoembryonic antigen in patients with ovarian carcinoma. Am J Obstet Gynecol 126:186–189, 1976.
Elevated serum levels were frequently found (45% to 72%); however, they did not correlate with the extent of clinical disease activity.

Spanos WJ: Preoperative hormonal therapy of cystic adnexal masses. Am J Obstet Gynecol 116:551–556, 1973.
Of 286 menstruating patients with adnexal masses who were treated with combination estrogen-progestogen therapy for 6 weeks, in only 81 did the mass persist, requiring surgical exploration.

Walsh JW, Rosenfield AT, Jaffe CC, et al: Prospective comparison of ultrasound and computed tomography in the evaluation of gynecologic pelvic masses. Am J Roentgenol 131:955–960, 1978.
Ultrasound and computed tomography were not *found to be complementary studies in the 24 patients studied.*

Webb MJ, Decker DG, and Mussey E: Cancer metastatic to the ovary: Factors influencing survival. Obstet Gynecol 45:391–396, 1975.
In this analysis of 357 patients metastatic adenocarcinoma of the breast (31%) and gastrointestinal tract (47%) were most common.

30. TESTICULAR MASS

A testicular mass in a young adult should initially be considered malignant. In a recent retrospective review, 37 of 100 patients with testicular carcinomas were initially misdiagnosed as having epididymitis or epididymo-orchitis (23 patients), or, less commonly, torsion of the testicle, hydrocele, strangulated hernia, or hematocele. Although rare in general (less than 1% of all malignancies), testicular germ cell neoplasms are one of the most common tumors in the 18 to 35 age group.

It is commonly believed that testicular carcinomas are painless, but various authors estimate that 25% to 40% of patients with these malignancies will at some time have mild to moderate testicular pain. Therefore testicular pain should not lead to a delay in diagnosis. Patients may also note the rapid onset of gynecomastia (HCG-secreting tumors), feminization (Leydig cell tumors), or precocious puberty (Sertoli's cell tumors). Cough (pulmonary metastases), abdominal pain (lymph node or retroperitoneal soft tissue metastases, hydronephrosis), or weight loss may all occur with testicular neoplasms.

A detailed history may suggest the correct diagnosis in a patient with a testicular mass. In particular a history of gynecomastia, precocious puberty, feminization, prior tuberculosis, syphilis, or treated leukemia (the testicle is a sanctuary site) is important. Simultaneous parotitis may suggest mumps orchitis. Physical examination may reveal an abdominal, inguinal, or supraclavicular mass. The scrotum and both testicles should be carefully evaluated; the contour, degree of fixation of the mass, its consistency, and the consistency of the epididymis and vas deferens should all be noted. The anatomic relationship of the epididymis and testicle are important—in spermatic cord torsion, the epididymis is located anteriorly instead of in its usual position posterior to the testicle. A "beaded" vas deferens may be characteristic of tuberculosis, while the presence of a spermatocele, hematocele, varicocele or hernia should all be apparent from the physical examination. In a testicular carcinoma, testicular sensation is usually impaired and the testis is "heavy," while the spermatic cord is normal to palpation. However, in epididymitis, the testicle and spermatic cord are tender and the testis is not positioned low in the scrotum. A patient with acute epididymitis and/or orchitis usually has a prior history of urinary tract infection, while pyuria and pus in prostatic secretions should make the diagnosis more certain. A painful testicular mass may also represent mumps orchitis or torsion of the spermatic cord. The testicle should also be transilluminated. Hydroceles transilluminate, but since teratocarcinomas occasionally have multiple fluid-filled transilluminating cystic areas also, they can be confused with a simple fluid collection. The hydrocele should be aspirated and the testicle re-examined if it cannot be palpated through the cyst.

A complete blood count and urinalysis are indicated, along with liver functions and such tumor marker studies as chorionic gonadotropin (HCG) and alpha fetoprotein (AFP). A prospective pretherapy study, in groups of patients with either testicular neoplasms or benign testicular lesions, revealed that no HCG or AFP elevations occurred in 24 patients with benign testicular diseases. However, elevated markers in patients with testicular masses are highly suggestive of a malignant germ cell neoplasm. Overall approximately 10% of testicular carcinomas are associated with elevated markers.

Pre-orchiectomy diagnostic studies should include chest radiographs, an excretory urogram and, if indicated, an inferior vena cavagram. Ureteral and/or renal displacement secondary to retroperitoneal masses may be demonstrated by the latter two studies. CT scans may demonstrate enlarged celiac lymph nodes or laterally situated retroperitoneal tumor masses at the level of the renal pelvis. If the diagnosis of testicular carcinoma is made, a lymphangiogram should be performed.

If acute epididymitis is suspected (marked epididymal tenderness, fever, pyuria), a two-week course of antibiotic therapy is indicated. If the patient has improved on this regimen, the diagnosis of malignancy is unlikely. However, in all instances of suspicion of a testicular malignancy, an inguinal orchiectomy should be performed. Histopathologic tumor type, stage, and sites of involvement are all important in determining whether surgery, radiotherapy, or chemotherapy will be used singly or in combination in treating the neoplasm.

D.G.

Fraley EE: The testicular mass: An approach to diagnosis and treatment. *In* JS Najarian and JP Delaney (Eds), Advances in Cancer Surgery. New York, Stratton, 1976. Pp. 589–596.
A short review of testicular masses is given.
Hill JT: Misdiagnosis of testicular tumours. J R Soc Med 71:737–740, 1978.
In the 100 patients with testicular neoplasms who were reviewed, 37% of the neoplasms were initially misdiagnosed, usually as epididymo-orchitis.
Moore MR, Garrett PR Jr, Walton KN, et al: Evaluation of human chorionic gonadotropin and alpha fetoprotein in benign and malignant testicular disorders. Surg Gynecol Obstet 147:167–174, 1978.
There were no elevated markers in 24 patients with benign testicular lesions (determinations performed pre-therapy). Elevated markers and a testicular mass indicates presence of a malignant germ cell tumor.
Smith D: General Urology. Los Altos, Calif., Lange Medical Publications, 1978. Pp. 298–303.
Concise description of the evaluation of testicular masses.
Whitmore WF Jr: Tumors of the testis. *In* MF Campbell and JH Harrison (Eds), Urology. Philadelphia, W.B. Saunders, 1978. Vol 2, pp. 1210–1218.
Differential diagnosis of testicular mass is described.

31. PARANEOPLASTIC SYNDROMES: ECTOPIC HORMONE PRODUCTION

The clinical manifestations of ectopic hormone production can precede, lead to, or follow a diagnosis of malignancy. In any case the incidence of clinically apparent ectopic humoral syndromes is low and is usually associated with lung cancer (Cushing's syndrome 3%, inappropriate ADH 8%, hypercalcemia 15%, gynecomastia 0.5%). On the other hand inappropriately elevated plasma hormone levels may be present without concomitant clinical signs or symptoms; and although the true incidence is unknown, it has been reported in approximately 50% of patients with small cell carcinoma.

An ectopic hormone is a polypeptide that is synthesized and usually secreted by tumor tissue, and that tissue from which the tumor is derived does not normally produce that hormone. Pearse and others have postulated that such ectopic hormones are produced by those neoplastic cells that are embryologically related to precursors of normal endocrine tissues but not directly derived from them. Cells of neuroectodermal origin share the ability to take up and decarboxylate amine precursors, and the APUD (amine precursor uptake and decarboxylation) cells of Pearse are those that are thought to produce ectopic hormones in malignancy. Another proposed mechanism is random genetic "derepression" with neoplastic change and the subsequent production of ectopic hormones. This hypothesis, however, does not account for the relatively tumor-specific nature of these humoral syndromes.

The diagnostic criteria of ectopic hormone production include association with a clinical endocrine syndrome, association with elevated plasma hormone levels, failure of homeostatic suppression of hormone concentrations, fall in hormone levels and/or regression of clinical manifestations of hormone excess following effective tumor therapy, no fall in hormone levels nor regression of syndrome following removal of normal gland of origin, arteriovenous gradient across the tumor bed, and production of hormone in vitro by tumor explants or dispersed cells. Ectopic hormone production is frequently not documented because the clinical manifestations of the humoral syndrome may be subtle or entirely absent. The malignancy may be rapidly progressive so that the hormone's clinical effects do not become apparent; the ectopic hormone may be an inactive form of the native hormone; the ectopic hormone may suppress the normal gland, resulting in normal hormone levels; or there may be intermittent ectopic hormone secretion.

The ectopic humoral syndromes that have been discussed so far are hypercalcemia (Part I, Chapter 10), inappropriate ADH secretion (Part I, Chapter 12), and hypoglycemia (Part I, Chapter 13). The production of ectopic placental lactogen, growth hormone, prolactin, thyrotropic substances, erythropoietin, and calcitonin has been reported rarely.

Ectopic ACTH production is most frequently documented in small cell carcinoma of the lung. In addition it has been reported in endocrine carcinomas of foregut origin (islet cell carcinoma, carcinoid, thymoma, medullary carcinoma of the thyroid), pheochromocytoma, neuroblastoma, and ovarian tumors (arrhenoblastoma, adenocarcinoma). Patients with rapidly progressive lung cancer and ectopic ACTH usually do not present the classic clinical features of Cushing's syndrome, whereas those with slow-growing tumors of foregut origin and ectopic ACTH frequently do. There may be moon facies, hirsutism, ecchymoses, truncal obesity, plethora, straiae, severe muscle weakness and wasting particularly in the lower extremities, peripheral edema, hyperpigmentation, hypertension, and symptoms of diabetes. Hypokalemic alkalosis is common, and the plasma cortisol and urinary 17-hydroxycorticoids are elevated. The normal diurnal variation in plasma cortisol is absent, and exogenous glucocorticoids fail to suppress ACTH production. Treatment of ectopic ACTH production requires effective tumor eradication. Palliative therapies may include metyrapone, amino-glutethimide, and mitotane (o,p'-DDD) to suppress abnormal glucocorticoid production.

Ectopic chorionic gonadotropin (HCG) has been reported most frequently in lung cancer and hepatoma. HCG production in tumors of trophoblastic origin (choriocarcinoma, hydatidiform mole, embryonal carcinoma of the testis) is not ectopic but "eutopic," since the tumor cell of origin normally produces HCG. Clinical manifestations include precocious puberty, gynecomastia, and testicular atrophy. Occasionally there may be symptoms of hyperthyroidism secondary to massive concentrations of HCG in trophoblastic disease.

Changes in ectopic hormone levels may be used for tumor localization, as an indicator of tumor responsiveness, or for detection of recurrent disease. As an aid to early cancer detection, ectopic hormone levels may prove to be of value, as exemplified by the presence of "big" ACTH in lung cancer patients.

C.P.

Azzopardi JG, Williams ED: Pathology of "nonendocrine" tumors associated with Cushing's syndrome. Cancer 22:274–286, 1968.
   In this literature review small cell carcinoma of the lung and endocrine tumors of foregut origin were associated with the syndrome most frequently.

Blackman MR, Rosen SW, Weintraub BD: Ectopic hormones. Adv Intern Med 23:85–113, 1978.

An excellent review with extensive references.

Braunstein GD, Vaitukaitis JL, Carbone PP, Ross GT: Ectopic production of human chorionic gonadotrophin by neoplasms. Ann Intern Med 78:39–45, 1973.

In an analysis of 60 patients with nontesticular neoplasms and detectable hCG carcinomas of the stomach, liver, and pancreas were most frequent.

Gailani S, Chu TM, Nussbaum A, et al: Human chorionic gonadotrophins (hCG) in non-trophoblastic neoplasms: Assessment of abnormalities of hCG and CEA in bronchogenic and digestive neoplasms. Cancer 38:1684–1686, 1976.

An elevated plasma hCG was found in 54 of 320 cancer patients (17%) and in only 1 of 70 control subjects.

Gewirtz G, Yalow RS: Ectopic ACTH production in carcinoma of the lung. J Clin Invest 53:1022–1032, 1974.

"Big" ACTH was detected in all but 1 of 28 tumor specimens.

Levine RJ, Metz SA: A classification of ectopic hormone-producing tumors. Ann NY Acad Sci 230:533–546, 1975.

A good discussion.

Pearse AGE: The cytochemistry and ultrastructure of polypeptide hormone-producing cells of the APUD series and the embryologic, physiologic and pathologic implications of the concept. J Histochem Cytochem 17:303–313, 1969.

An elaboration of the APUD hypothesis is given.

Rees LH, Ratcliffe JG: Ectopic hormone production by non-endocrine tumours. Clin Endocrinol 3:263–299, 1974.

An excellent clinical review.

Wolfsen AR, Odell WD: ProACTH: Use for early detection of lung cancer. Am J Med 66:765–772, 1979.

Of 74 patients with newly diagnosed lung cancer, 53 had proACTH elevations.

32. PARANEOPLASTIC SYNDROMES: CUTANEOUS, CONNECTIVE TISSUE, OSSEOUS, AND NEUROMUSCULAR DISORDERS

The remote effects of cancer include a broad spectrum of cutaneous and connective tissue and osseous and neuromuscular disorders. The most common skin changes are acanthosis nigricans, tylosis, poikiloderma, erythema gyratum repens, chronic generalized pruritus, and exfoliative erythroderma. In most instances the cutaneous disorder precedes the diagnosis of malignancy, and an associated malignancy is documented in 10% to 50% of cases. By definition "malignant" acanthosis nigricans is always associated with neoplasia. The disease presents with papillary hypertrophy, hyperkeratosis, and hyperpigmentation distributed symmetrically over the nape of the neck, perineum, medial aspects of the thighs, and dorsa of the hands and feet. These verrucous lesions may be intensely pruritic. Other etiologies of acanthosis nigricans include family predisposition (often with juvenile onset), obesity, and drug ingestion (estrogens, nicotinic acid). The incidence of associated malignancy in all cases of acanthosis nigricans is approximately 20%, and those cancers most frequently identified are stomach, lung, and breast.

The connective tissue disorders, dermatomyositis, scleroderma, and disseminated lupus erythematosus, have all been reported to have an increased risk of associated malignancy. It is best documented for dermatomyositis, in which the incidence of cancer is approximately 15%. Like the cutaneous disorders, the onset of dermatomyositis usually precedes the diagnosis of malignancy, sometimes for up to a year or more. Cancers of the stomach, lung, breast, and ovary, as well as lymphomas, are most commonly found. Dermatomyositis presents with both skin and muscle manifestations. There is an erythematous, violaceous rash on the sun-exposed surfaces of the body, particularly the face, neck, arms, and dorsa of the hands, which may desquamate and become pruritic. The eyelids are characteristically heliotrope in color, and the skin over the knuckles becomes red and atrophic. There is also proximal muscle weakness of the extremities, with pain and muscle wasting. The diagnosis is made on clinical examination. Laboratory studies may document elevated serum muscle enzymes (creatine phosphokinase) and increased urinary creatine, while electromyography will demonstrate signs of primary muscle degeneration and atrophy, and a muscle biopsy typically shows fibrosis, muscle fiber degeneration, some muscle regeneration with basophilia and varying fiber size, and an interstitial and perivascular round cell infiltrate. The clinical course of dermatomyositis may improve dramatically with effective tumor therapy and may not recur in spite of recurrent malignancy. On the other hand dermatomyositis may become manifest only after treatment of a malignancy or may resolve spontaneously in spite of continued malignant disease. Corticosteroids may improve dermatomyositis, as may adrenalectomy or hypophysectomy, but this connective tissue disorder may be progressive and prove fatal. The etiology of dermatomyositis is unknown; however, its association with malignancy has raised many hypotheses, including the presence of a tumor-derived substance that is toxic to skin and muscle; a hypersensitivity reaction resulting from a "misdirected" immune response to tumor antigens or a cross-reactivity of tumor, muscle, and skin antigens; and one agent (toxin, virus) that causes both dermatomyositis and its associated malignancy.

The osseous disorder, hypertrophic pulmonary osteoarthropathy (HPO), is associated with malignancy in almost all cases. Approximately 80% of patients have lung cancer, 10% have pleural tumors (mesothelioma), and 5% have other intrathoracic malignancies. Patients with chronic suppurative lung diseases and congenital cyanotic heart disease account for the other 5%. Interestingly, HPO is rarely caused by pulmonary metastases from extrathoracic neoplasms. The disorder is manifested by clubbing of the fingers and toes; nonpitting swelling over the ends of the long bones with associated bone tenderness; symmetric arthritis of the wrists, ankles, and knees; and frequent autonomic changes of sweating, flushing, and blanching. Patients often have gynecomastia; and if HPO is extensive, there may be involvement of the ribs, clavicles, scapulae, pelvis, and malar bones, with a superficial resemblance to acromegaly. X-rays reveal subperiosteal proliferation of new bone at the distal ends of the long bones, metacarpals, and metatarsals. Clubbing of the fingers alone, without evidence of periosteal new bone formation, does not connote cancer and may be seen in many cardiorespiratory disorders; furthermore, only 10% of patients with lung cancer will have HPO. The serum alkaline phosphatase is normal, while the bone scan may be positive in areas of new bone formation and arthritis. As with dermatomyositis, the symptoms of HPO may resolve with effective tumor therapy. In addition there are reports of dramatic improvement of arthritis and periostitis with vagotomy. As with dermatomyositis, the etiology of HPO is unknown, and similar hypotheses have been put forward for it. Ectopic growth hormone production by tumor tissue, resulting in new bone growth, is an idea favored by many; however, no firm data support this hypothesis, and there are some negative studies.

Nonmetastatic neuromuscular disorders are reported to affect up to 7% of all cancer patients and are most common in patients with carcinomas of the lung, ovary, and stomach. Symptoms generally precede the diagnosis of cancer and may be present for as long as 2 years. These disorders may affect virtually every level of the nervous system as well as muscles and the neuromuscular junction. They include parenchymatous cerebellar degeneration, encephalomyelopathy, progressive multifocal leukoencephalopathy, polyneuropathy (motor, sensory or mixed), carcinomatous myopathy, and the Eaton-Lambert syndrome.

The Eaton-Lambert or "myasthenic" syndrome is a disorder of the neuromuscular junction. It is identified in approximately 1% of all lung cancer patients and may be seen in at least 6% of those with small cell carcinoma. Patients are typically male, 40 to 70 years of age, with a history of weakness and easy muscle fatigue. There may also be complaints of dysphagia, hoarseness, slurred speech, and ptosis, although oculobulbar involvement is much less common than in myasthenia gravis; as well as dry mouth, impotence, and peripheral paresthesias. On physical examination there is proximal muscle weakness out of proportion to muscle bulk, delay in developing motor force, and reduced or absent muscle stretch reflexes. Electromyography demonstrates postactivation facilitation, while direct muscle fiber stimulation and nerve conduction velocity are normal. Muscle biopsy also gives normal results. In contrast to myasthenia gravis there is a poor response to edrophonium chloride and an unusual sensitivity to curare and other muscle-relaxant drugs. The cause of the Eaton-Lambert syndrome is impaired release of acetylcholine quanta from the nerve terminal (as seen in botulism), and it has been hypothesized that this is mediated by a tumor toxin. Guanidine hydrochloride has been reported to be of benefit in improving the symptoms and signs of the syndrome.

C.P.

Barnes BE: Dermatomyositis and malignancy. Ann Intern Med 84:68–76, 1976.
A literature review of 258 cases of dermatomyositis associated with malignancy.
Engel WK: Remote effects of focal cancer on the neuromuscular system. Adv Neurol 15:119–147, 1976.
A comprehensive review.
Ennis GC, Cameron DP, Burger HG: On the aetiology of hypertrophic pulmonary osteoarthropathy in bronchogenic carcinoma: Lack of relationship to elevated growth hormone levels. Aust NZ J Med 3:157–161, 1973.
Abnormalities of growth hormone metabolism did not correlate with the presence of osteoarthropathy.
Hammarsten JF, O'Leary J: The features and significance of hypertrophic osteoarthropathy. Arch Intern Med 99:431–441, 1957.
A clinical analysis of 22 patients with this syndrome.
Ishikawa K, Engelhardt JK, Fujisawa T, et al: A neuromuscular transmission block produced by a cancer tissue extract derived from a patient with the myasthenic syndrome. Neurology 27:140–143, 1977.
An in vitro study demonstrating inhibition of acetylcholine release by a cancer tissue extract.
Newbold PCH: Skin markers of malignancy. Arch Dermatol 102:680–692, 1970.
An overview of the subject.
Oh SJ, Kim KW: Guanidine hydrochloride in the Eaton-Lambert syndrome: Electrophysiologic improvement. Neurology 23:1084–1090, 1973.
A report of three patients with Eaton-Lambert syndrome.

Penn AS: Myasthenia gravis, dermatomyositis, and polymyositis: Immuno-pathological diseases. Adv Neurol 17:41–61, 1977.
This article discusses etiologies of these diseases.
Rosenthall L, Kirsh J: Observations on radionuclide imaging in hypertrophic pulmonary osteoarthropathy. Radiology 120:359–362, 1976.
Bone scans revealed subperiosteal new bone formation in 4 patients studied.
Rowland LP, Clark C, Olarte M: Therapy for dermatomyositis and polymyositis. Adv Neurol 17:63–97, 1977.
An excellent clinical review.
Tierny LM Jr: Dermatomyositis. West J Med 124:316–322, 1976.
A clinical review.

PART III. THE PRIMARY OR REGIONAL MALIGNANCY

To make a correct diagnosis of cancer, an adequate tissue sample must be obtained. The diagnosis may be made by exfoliative cytologic analysis (of sputum, urine, or cervix Papanicolaou smear), by either punch, incisional, or excisional biopsies, or through needle biopsy techniques. A thin needle may allow aspiration cytologic specimens to be obtained from such inaccessible sites as lung nodules and para-aortic lymph nodes. Expert histopathologic interpretation of biopsy material is also very important. If pathologists are alerted before the biopsy is performed, the best use may be made of the material: examples are (1) performing estrogen-receptor assays from breast biopsies; (2) making touch preparations in certain non-Hodgkin's lymphomas; and (3) obtaining fresh tissue for electron microscopy to clarify whether undifferentiated lymphoma or metastatic nasopharyngeal cancer is present in a cervical lymph node specimen. Since tumor grading and cell type are often important prognostic indicators, skilled interpretation of the biopsy material is very important.

After the diagnosis of cancer has been made, careful but prompt staging of the extent of involvement is carried out. A detailed history and physical examination are essential, and signs or symptoms indicative of metastatic spread of the cancer must be sought. Any coexisting primary neoplasms, commonly found in patients with head and neck carcinomas, should be detected. The performance status should also be evaluated, since the patient's functional level is a major determinant of the outcome of treatment. Careful laboratory, clinical, and radiographic evaluations are made to determine the functional status of the patient and the presence or absence of regional or distant metastases. Such special procedures as lymphangiograms, CT scans, or special nuclear scintiscans may all be indicated. For certain neoplasms, additional diagnostic surgery may be required; for example, the staging laparotomy performed on patients with Hodgkin's disease, which includes splenectomy, bone marrow, liver, and select lymph node biopsies. Biopsy sites or areas of residual neoplasms should be *marked* at the time of surgery with metallic clips to facilitate later radiation therapy. When the staging evaluation has been completed, the disease can be staged according to the TNM system (see Part VIII) or other staging systems. The primary tumor can be staged either by size in centimeters (oral cavity, for example), by number of lymph node regions involved (lymphomas) or by number of anatomic sites involved by the neoplasm (carcinoma of the larynx or nasopharynx). In general, when primary neoplasms are localized and small, the prognosis is usually better than for larger primary neoplasms or those with regional lymphatic involvement. For most cancers, regional lymph node involvement worsens the prognosis by 50%.

An advantage obtained from careful staging is the availability of prognostic information: it is easier to estimate the patient's chances for cure. Careful staging also assists in planning adequate treatment that will encompass all known local and regional cancer. Furthermore, staging allows the results of treatment to be evaluated, facilitates interinstitutional data comparison, and helps clinicians set up and carry out clinical investigations of cancer management.

After the initial evaluation and staging are completed, the therapeutic goals should be assessed in each particular instance. Is the treatment goal palliation of bone pain, impending fracture, or other local problems? Is the treatment to be with curative intent? Is local control of the primary cancer the major therapeutic endeavor? Since the first treatment course for many cancers determines the outcome, and as salvage of an initial treatment failure is not always possible, an optimum therapeutic plan needs to be arrived at for the initial treatment course. Therefore a combined approach by surgical, radiation, and medical oncologists in conjunction with other physicians skilled in the treatment of a particular neoplasm is very important. The optimum therapeutic goal is to cure the cancer but also to maintain optimal tissue and organ function and avoid severe injury to normal tissues, both acutely and long after the treatment has been completed.

The type of therapy to be carried out depends in general on how aggressive the cancer is likely to be, what its potential is for spread both regionally and distantly, the morbidity and mortality expected from the therapeutic plan, and the cure rate expected on the basis of prior experience with tumors of similar grade, size, and stage.

The potentially curative therapeutic modalities at present are surgery, radiotherapy, and chemotherapy. Some others, which are either experimental or have a poorly defined role at present in cancer management, are immunotherapy, hyperthermia, laser treatment, and cryosurgery. Of the available curative modalities, the oncologic team must decide whether they can be more effectively used individually or combined for a particular carcinoma, on the basis of its expected behavior and stage. In general terms, surgery is an excellent means of debulking cancers, and radiation therapy is able to sterilize residual foci of carcinoma in the resection bed. Radiotherapy can also sterilize subclinical neoplastic foci in lymph nodes. The sequence of radiotherapy and surgery must also be determined, whether initial surgery and postoperative irradiation will be used, or vice versa. Finally, it must be determined whether the use of adjuvant chemotherapy is indicated for a particular cancer.

After the treatment course has been completed, regular, careful follow-up examinations are important, not only to detect failures early, when salvage treatment may be possible, but also to discover normal tissue reactions or sequelae early, so that corrective treatment may be instituted. A standard follow-up interval for determining cure in most malignancies is 5 years from the time of treatment. However, in many epithelial malignancies of the head and neck and in some lymphomas (Hodgkin's disease and diffuse histiocytic lymphoma), most relapses occur within the first 3 years after treatment. Longer follow-up to determine cure may be necessary for other cancers, such as those of the breast and salivary glands and malignant melanoma.

D.G.

34. SKIN CANCER—PRIMARY OR REGIONAL

Skin cancers are the most common of all malignancies, causing 25% of all cancers in males and 11% in females. Over a lifetime, 40% to 50% of the population will be afflicted with skin cancers. Almost 95% of these neoplasms are either squamous or basal cell carcinomas. Even though the lesions are readily curable when small, approximately 3000 deaths per year occur from these malignancies, usually in neglected cases. Several other cutaneous malignancies, such as adenocarcinomas of sweat glands, mycosis fungoides, and Kaposi's sarcoma, will be discussed below.

The association between skin cancers and environmental carcinogens was first established when chimney sweeps were noted to have a high incidence of scrotal cancers. Other carcinogens such as arsenic (20- to 40-year latent period), methylcholanthrene, benzpyrene, coal tars, and pitch all promote cutaneous carcinogenesis. Sun exposure also plays a major role, exemplified by a greatly increased frequency of skin cancers in people living in Australia and Texas. Patients with a genetic inability to repair DNA strand breaks (xeroderma pigmentosa) also may develop multiple skin cancers. There are also ethnic variations and susceptibility to skin cancers. Those of Scotch and Irish descent are at an increased risk, whereas blacks have a reduced incidence of skin cancers. It is probable that increased melanin pigment somehow protects DNA from the effects of ultraviolet radiation.

Several lesions are *precancerous*. Actinic keratoses are scaly, hyperkeratotic lesions that involve the sun-exposed face, neck, and dorsum of the hands; if they become thicker and erythematous over many years, carcinoma may be present. In persons chronically exposed to arsenic, characteristic keratoses develop, consisting of hard, yellowish callouses on the palms and soles. The solar keratotic changes are absent in arsenical keratosis, but hyperkeratosis is present. Bowen's disease, a form of carcinoma in situ of the skin, may ultimately produce ulcerating lesions or may be confused with eczema. The risk of a systemic primary malignancy in association with Bowen's disease may be as high as 25%. Radiation dermatitis from excessive doses of iodizing radiation is characterized by cutaneous atrophy, telangiectasia, and ultimately ulceration. There is a possibility of malignant change after a long latent period of 20 or more years. Erythroplasia of Querat, a plaque-like dermatosis of the glans penis, is also a premalignant lesion.

Squamous cell carcinomas occur in areas of solar exposure such as the face (orbital, lip, forehead, and nasal regions) and the dorsum of the arms and hands. These tumors arise from the superficial, keratinizing layers of the skin. They are elevated, scaly, keratotic annular lesions that may scab, ulcerate, bleed, and then scab again. Squamous carcinomas may metastasize to lymph nodes, but the risk is low except under special circumstances. The following are all associated with an increased risk of lymph node metastases: tumors arising in irradiated skin or involving mucocutaneous junctions; Bowen's disease or erythroplasia of Querat; cutaneous leg ulcers or other preexisting lesions; and anaplastic or large tumors or those invasive below the level of the sweat glands.

Basal cell carcinomas occur primarily in the skin of the head and neck (91%). They most commonly involve the central face, including the nose, forehead, cheeks, canthi, and eyelids. At least four kinds of basal cell carcinoma exist: nodular ulcerative, which begin as a papule, ultimately ulcerate with a depressed center, appear pearly or yellow with a central crusting over the area of ulceration, extend and invade horizontally into surrounding tissues; pigmented basal cell, which are similar to the nodular ulcerative type except that they contain increased pigment; sclerosing (morphea), which infiltrate extensively horizontally, have poorly defined margins, and are associated with dense scarring that makes the extent of the lesion difficult to estimate; and superficial, which primarily involve the trunk and appear as a red, scaly, patchy, pigmented, slowly advancing superficial lesion. Basal cell carcinomas may be confused with seborrheic keratoses or hyperplasia, warts, cutaneous ulcers, and scars (morphea type).

A careful history may determine prior arsenical use, radiation therapy for benign disease, or chemical or extensive sun exposures. The regional lymph nodes should be examined in patients with suspected squamous carcinomas. If the lesion is large and fixed to underlying structures, radiographs should be obtained to rule out involvement of bone or cartilage.

Actinic keratoses may heal and disappear with frequent use of petroleum jelly and ordinarily do not need to be biopsied. However, a suspected skin cancer should be biopsied, either by a full-thickness punch, the simplest technique, or by the excisional method if the lesion is smaller than 2.0 cm. For a larger lesion, an incisional or punch biopsy will establish the diagnosis and allow a therapeutic decision to be made.

Basal and squamous carcinomas may be treated successfully by a wide variety of techniques, including excision, cautery, radiotherapy, combined surgery and irradiation, chemosurgery, and immunotherapy. Very small cutaneous cancers may be treated by cautery alone. However, other techniques, such as surgery, radiation therapy, and chemosurgery, are recommended for lesions of the nasal tip or alae, canthi, or those extending into bone or cartilage. Lesions may also be excised with 1- to 2-mm margins, the procedure of choice for cancers located near cartilage or bone or at mucocutaneous junctions. Excision should also be considered for young patients, who may risk potentially serious long-term sequelae from radiation therapy. The advantages of excision are that a cancer may be resected with a margin of normal tissue, the procedure is performed quickly, and there is no long-term potential for tissue injury. Excision is also the procedure of choice for the rare adenocarcinomas of sweat glands.

Radiotherapy produces cure rates similar to those for surgery, but the treatment course is longer if good cosmesis is to be obtained. Superficial x-rays of 100 kV to 200 kV are generally used, but other techniques available to the radiation therapist such as radioactive contact applicators and removable interstitial implants (iridium 192) allow more sharply localized treatment without the deeper penetration characteristic of external beam irradiation. Radiotherapy can effectively treat skin cancers in sites where surgery may be deforming, such as the nose, eyelids, and canthi. A cure rate of 95% for carcinomas of the eyelids by radiation has been reported. When tumor has invaded bone or cartilage, radiotherapy is relatively ineffective and may result in osteoradionecrosis or chondritis. If the cartilage is not invaded, however, carefully directed radiation therapy may produce an excellent result without severe tissue loss and deformity (e.g., ear pinna). Surgery and radiotherapy may be combined for patients with neglected, large, basal or squamous cancers, those which are deeply invasive into bone, or those with lymph node metastases.

Chemosurgery by the Mohs technique involves initially using a keratolytic agent, then applying zinc chloride paste and an occlusive dressing. The tissues are then excised and fixed and a frozen section is performed; the procedure is repeated many times until the cut margins are free of tumor. This procedure is time-consuming and costly but is very effective in producing 5-year cure rates of 95% to 97% for both squamous and basal cell carcinomas. A modification of the technique involves excising small areas without zinc chloride fixation and obtaining multiple frozen sections until clear margins are obtained. Topical 5-fluorouracil (5-FU) may clear actinic keratoses but is not indicated for actual cutaneous carcinomas. Other techniques, such as immunotherapy with dinitrochlorobenzene (DNCB), depend on a local hypersensitivity reaction to eradicate the neoplasm. These are not as useful in most cutaneous cancers as surgical or radiotherapeutic approaches. With careful evaluation and treatment, 80% to 90% cure rates can be expected for squamous carcinomas and over 90% in basal cell cancers.

Kaposi's sarcoma is a rare cutaneous malignancy, which affects persons of Jewish or Mediterranean extraction, presenting as multiple skin and subcutaneous purplish nodules involving the lower extremities. The neoplasm affects the skin alone in most instances but may ultimately metastasize to lymph nodes. In younger patients the lymph nodes occasionally are involved without skin lesions, indicating a poor prognosis. Radiation therapy is the treatment of choice, as the lesions are radiosensitive. Fractionated doses of 2000 rads over 1 to 2 weeks or single doses of 800 rads emitted from 250 kV or megavoltage units have been effective in clearing the lesions. Since Kaposi's sarcoma is a disease of the subcutaneous tissue, however, most 2-to-5 mV electron beams do not penetrate deeply enough to control the malignancy, and photon beams are required. In a series of 34 patients with Kaposi's sarcoma in which 12 patients were treated with extended field megavoltage irradiation (covering most of the involved extremity), 10 patients responded completely, providing long-term local control of the neoplasm.

Mycosis fungoides (MF) is a T-cell lymphoma, originating in multiple foci in the skin. It may involve only the skin for many years but can ultimately spread to lymph nodes and visceral sites. When visceral involvement is widespread, MF is invariably fatal, either through repeated infection or through extensive lymphomatous infiltration of many sites. There are four cutaneous presentations of mycosis fungoides: limited plaque, which has the best prognosis for complete remission and long survival; the stage with intermediate prognosis, or generalized plaque; erythematous, with generalized infiltration of the skin and intense pruritus and ichthyosis, which may be associated with circulating peripheral MF cells (Sezary's syndrome); and the tumor stage, with extensive skin involvement by thick, ulcerating infected lesions, which has the worst prognosis. A skin biopsy must be performed to make the diagnosis. The morphologic hallmark of mycosis fungoides is Pautrier's abscesses, characterized by atypical histiocytes that infiltrate the dermis and focally invade the epidermis.

Mycosis fungoides may be treated palliatively by superficial, 100 kV x-rays. However, the completeness of the initial remission is directly related to the extent of skin irradiated and to the radiation dose. Complete remissions have been obtained in over 90% of patients who received 3000–3600 rads to the entire integument over a 9-week course with a 2.5 mV electron beam, while only 18% of patients receiving doses of 800 to 1000 rads had complete remissions. Patients with dermatopathic changes in palpable lymph nodes have a worse prognosis than those with clinically normal lymph nodes. The skin may also be treated with topical nitrogen mustard, in which a 20 mg/100 ml solution is prepared by diluting 10 mg of Mustargen in 50 ml of water before applying it to the entire skin except for the scalp, eyelids, and perineum. The latter three areas are painted with a more dilute solution. The skin is then dried. Daily cutaneous treatments with topical nitrogen mustard produce slightly longer relapse-free intervals than the electron beam alone. Currently a randomized study in which half of patients with MF who are receiving electron beam irradiation will also receive adjuvant topical nitrogen mustard is in progress at the Stanford Medical Center.

Primary cutaneous involvement by lymphoma is rare, occurring in fewer than 5% of patients with diffuse non-Hodgkin's lymphomas. After a biopsy has established the diagnosis, an evaluation for systemic involvement should be performed, with chest radiographs, lymphangiogram if there are no medical contraindications, bone marrow biopsy, and such laboratory tests as CBC, 12-panel screening battery, and erythrocyte sedimentation rate. If no visceral involvement is found, the affected region may be irradiated, but if widespread cutaneous lymphoma is present, combined chemotherapy and/or palliative irradiation are indicated depending on the histopathologic diagnosis.

D.G.

Edelstein L, Whelan C, Levene M: Cancer of the skin. *In* Cancer. American Cancer Society, Boston, 1978. Pp. 91–98.
  Good review of skin cancer diagnosis and treatment.
Fitzpatrick P, Jamieson D, Thompson G, Allt W: Tumors of the eyelids and their treatment by radiotherapy. Radiology 104:661–665, 1972.

In 477 tumors that were irradiated there was a 95% control rate with excellent cosmetic results.

Freeman R, Knox J, Heaton C: The therapy of skin cancer. Cancer 17:535–538, 1964.

A comparison of surgery, radiation therapy, and curettage in therapy of skin cancers is made in this article.

Holeck M, Harwood A: Radiotherapy of Kaposi's sarcoma. Cancer 41:1733–1738, 1978.

34 patients were treated with radiotherapy. Extended field radiotherapy apparently gave improved long-term control.

Hoppe RT, Cox RS, Fuks Z, et al: Electron-beam therapy for mycosis fungoides: The Stanford University experience. Cancer Treat Rep 63:691–700, 1979.

Remission induction and survival inversely correlated with the extent of skin involvement (plaque limited best, tumorous worst).

Klein E, Burgess G, Helm F: Neoplasms of the skin. *In* Cancer Medicine, JF Holland and E Frei III (Eds). Philadelphia, Lea & Febiger, 1974. Pp. 1789–1822.

Good description of etiology and differential diagnosis of skin cancers.

Mohs F: Chemosurgery for skin cancer. Arch Dermatol 112:211–215, 1976.

Over 9000 lesions were removed by either zinc chloride or fresh tissue chemosurgical techniques. The 5-year cure rates were 97% to 99%.

Price N, Hoppe R, Constantine V, Fuks Z, Bagshaw M: The treatment of mycosis fungoides. Cancer 40:2851–2853, 1977.

There was a slightly prolonged disease-free survival when topical nitrogen mustard and electron beam therapy were used compared to electron beam alone. Basis for randomized protocol studying topical nitrogen mustard as a postelectron beam adjuvant is presented.

VonEssen C: Roentgen therapy of skin and lip carcinoma. Am J Roentgenol 83:556–570, 1960.

Excellent discussion of dose-time-volume relationships in radiotherapy treatment of the skin.

35. MELANOMA—PRIMARY OR REGIONAL

Approximately one-third of melanomas arise from a preexisting nevus, while the remainder originate in melanocytes in the skin. The head and neck is the most common site of involvement, followed in order by the trunk, lower extremities, and upper extremities. Sun exposure is probably important in the etiology of melanomas, as the lesions are particularly common in Australia and rare in blacks. The slightly increased familial risk of developing melanomas suggests that there may be a partial genetic basis for the disease.

There are three main types of melanoma. Lentigo maligna make up 10% of melanomas and occur primarily in the elderly. These neoplasms have irregular edges, are plaque-like, and grow slowly and horizontally. Superficial spreading melanomas, 60% of melanomas, also grow horizontally in the skin but may also be plaque-like or have an irregular advancing border and an uneven surface. When a melanoma is growing vertically, it becomes nodular (30% of melanomas). The latter two lesions occur at a median age of 50 (range, 15 to 80). Few melanomas are noted in prepubertal patients. Melanomas may be pruritic and may bleed easily, ulcerate, change color, or enlarge. The best clinical indication of malignancy is variegation of color, with red, white, and blue shades in the tumor with gradations of brown to black. The redness is due to inflammation, the blue to light diffraction by deep-lying pigmentation, and the whiteness to areas of spontaneous tumor regression. Complete regressions are rare. Satellite nodules may also develop. If metastases are present, enlarged lymph nodes, cough, bone pain, or central nervous system symptoms may be noted.

In the evaluation of a suspicious lesion, the regional lymph nodes should be carefully palpated. The characteristics of the lesion, especially pigment changes, color gradations, and the presence of satellite lesions, should be noted. A chest radiograph, multipanel chemical screening battery, and complete blood count are essential.

Melanomas may be confused with junctional nevi, black seborrheic keratoses, lentigos, pigmented basal cell carcinomas, and vascular malformations. Amelanotic melanomas are very difficult to diagnose. In the case of a large lesion, a punch biopsy may make the diagnosis, but a smaller nodule may be excised. The most important classification system correlates prognosis with *levels of invasion*: (I) confined to the epidermis; (II) extended into papillary dermis (survival greater than 90%); (III) at the interface between the papillary and reticular dermis (70% survival); (IV) extended into the reticular dermis (55%); (V) invading the dermal fat (10% survival). Also, when a melanoma is thicker than 15 mm, there is a much lower chance of survival.

Therapy for melanomas is primarily surgical. In general the primary lesion is removed with 3- to 5-cm margins. If the regional lymph nodes are clinically involved and there are no distant metastases, node dissection is performed. With lymph node involvement, however, there is only a 20% to 30% chance of long-term survival. A European randomized study in 553 patients with clinically negative lymph nodes showed that prophylactic lymph node dissection (at the time of the original diagnosis of melanoma) yielded no better survival than therapeutic dissections performed when the lymph nodes became palpable for levels III, IV, and V melanomas. Most authors agree that lymph node dissection is also not necessary for patients with levels I and II melanomas and clinically normal lymph nodes. Prophylactic neck dissections may be indicated, however, for level III, IV, or V melanomas originating in head and neck sites.

Radiation therapy has only a palliative role in the treatment of melanoma. In a recent randomized study in which 56 patients either received lymphadenectomy alone or postoperative irradiation to the resection bed, there were no differences in local control rates or survival between the groups. Age, sex, and number of involved nodes seemed to be more important factors than the addition of radiation therapy. Conventional radiation at 200 rads per fraction may not reproducibly control melanomas, but radiation may have an increased effect when large fractions (600 rads) are used in treating cutaneous metastases.

The most effective single chemotherapeutic agent for melanoma is DTIC, which may produce a 20% response rate, usually lasting less than 6 months. Thirteen percent response rates have been reported for the nitrosureas alone. When bleomycin, velban, and DTIC are combined, 25% to 30% objective, short-term responses have been reported.

Other modalities, such as hyperthermic perfusion of extremity melanomas, have produced inconsistent results. When tissue hyperthermia to 42°–43° C was combined with fractionated irradiation of subcutaneous metastases, the combination of these two modalities had a greater effect than radiation alone. This combination of hyperthermia and radiation may be important in future treatment of melanomas. Scarification and intralesional BCG applications have produced regression of cutaneous but not visceral melanomas. Since partial and occasionally complete spontaneous remissions occur in melanoma, the immune system appears to be important in the control of the disease, but unfortunately immunotherapy has yet to produce either cures or long-term palliation in disseminated disease. In a recent study of 71 patients with levels III, IV, and V melanomas who were randomly allocated postoperatively to receive either DTIC, BCG, or BCG-DTIC in combination, the group receiving the combination had significantly fewer relapses and better short-term survival (at 2 years). Perhaps combined modality approaches will ultimately produce improved survival in melanoma.

Since late recurrences do happen (>13% after 5 years), subjects must be followed closely for many years. Complete resection of late-appearing metastases may result in the salvage of 20% to 30% of such patients and should be considered for patients with localized relapses after a long free interval.

D.G.

Breslow A: Thickness, cross-sectional areas and depth of invasion in the prognosis of cutaneous melanoma. Ann Surg 172:902–908, 1970.
Article shows correlation of thickness of melanoma (in mm) with survival.

Clark W Jr, Ainsworth A, Bernardino E, et al: Primary human melanomas. Semin Oncol 2:83–103, 1975.
Article describes levels of invasion and gives excellent description of three types of melanomas.

Creagan E, Cupps E, Ivins J, et al: Adjuvant radiation therapy for regional nodal metastases from malignant melanomas. Cancer 42:2206–2210, 1978.
Fifty-six patients with biopsy-proved lymph node metastases randomly received lymphadenectomy alone or postlymphadenectomy radiotherapy to the area. Age, sex, and number of positive nodes were the important variables; radiotherapy probably did not add to the cure rate.

Habermalz H, Fischer J: Radiation therapy of malignant melanoma. Cancer 38:2258–2262, 1976.
Article shows possible advantage for high dose per fraction radiotherapy (600 rads) compared to conventional 200 to 300 rad fractions in cutaneous lesions.

Harris M, Roses D, Culliford A, Gumport S: Melanoma of the head and neck. Ann Surg 182:86–91, 1975.
Article discusses management of melanomas of head and neck in 94 patients.

Kim J, Hahn E, Tokita N: Combination hyperthermia and radiation therapy for cutaneous malignant melanoma. Cancer 41:2143–2148, 1978.
Hyperthermia to 42.5° and fractionated irradiation produced more complete regressions than radiotherapy alone.

Lure J: Chemotherapy of melanoma. Semin Oncol 2:179–185, 1975.
Review of melanoma chemotherapy, including drug combinations.

Mihm M, Fitzpatrick T, Lane-Brown M, et al: Early detection of primary cutaneous malignant melanoma. N Engl J Med 289:989–996, 1973.
Color atlas of melanomas.

Rosenberg SA: Surgical treatment of malignant melanoma. Cancer Treat Rep 60:159–163, 1976.
A surgeon's overview of primary therapy for melanoma.

Sim FH, Taylor WF, Ivins JC, et al: A prospective randomized study of the efficacy of routine elective lymphadenectomy in management of malignant melanoma: Preliminary results. Cancer 41:948–956, 1978.
Interval to metastases and survival not significantly improved by lymphadenectomy.

Veronesi U, Adamus J, Bandiera D, et al: Inefficacy of immediate node dissection in stage I melanomas of the limbs. N Engl J Med 297:627–630, 1977.
In a randomized European study in 553 patients there was no survival ad-

vantage for patients undergoing prophylactic inguinal lymph node dissection over therapeutic dissection when nodes became clinically involved.

Wood W, Cosimi A, Carey R, Kaufman S: Randomized trial of adjuvant therapy for "high risk" primary malignant melanoma. Surgery 83:677–681, 1978.

Seventy patients with level III, IV and V melanomas were randomly allocated postresection to receive either DTIC, BCG, or BCG-DTIC combined. The group receiving the drug combination had significantly fewer relapses and better survival (2-year results).

36. CENTRAL NERVOUS SYSTEM—PRIMARY OR REGIONAL

Brain tumors make up 2% to 5% of all malignancies, have a peak age incidence of 40 to 60 years, and cause approximately 8000 deaths per year. In childhood the peak age incidence of brain tumors is 6 years, with 60% to 70% of the tumors arising in the posterior fossa. Twenty-one percent of all childhood tumors occur in the central nervous system.

Eighty percent of all central nervous system tumors involve the brain. Fifty percent of these are gliomas, ranging from benign astrocytomas (grade I cystic astrocytomas and optic nerve gliomas) to the more malignant astrocytomas, grades II, III, and IV. The most malignant tumor, glioblastoma multiforme, accounts for 25% of all brain neoplasms. Oligodendrogliomas make up 2% of brain tumors. Ependymomas, also 2% of all brain tumors, usually arise from cells lining the ventricles of the brain. Medulloblastomas, 2% of adult brain tumors, are more common in children (20% of pediatric brain tumors). Other childhood neoplasms that arise in the brain are astrocytomas (30%), ependymomas of the fourth ventricle (12%), optic gliomas (5%), and craniopharyngiomas (from Rathke's pouch). Meningiomas most frequently involve the anterior base of the skull or the parasagittal region and compose 15% of all brain tumors. Pituitary tumors (also 15%) are of three cell types: chromophobe adenomas, 60% of which secrete prolactin; basophilic adenomas (Cushing's syndrome); and eosinophilic adenomas (associated with acromegaly). Twenty percent of brain tumors are metastatic lesions from neoplasms of the breast, lung, kidney, melanomas, and the gastrointestinal tract. Sixty percent are multiple. Other brain tumors, including chordomas (from notochordal remnants) and pineal tumors (pinealomas and dysgerminomas), are rare.

Spinal cord tumors make up the remaining 20% of central nervous system neoplasms. Twenty-five percent of these are intradural, intramedullary tumors, usually gliomas (66% ependymomas, 33% astrocytomas). Fifty percent of spinal cord tumors are intradural and extramedullary neoplasms: meningiomas and schwannomas. Extradural extramedullary spinal cord tumors are usually metastatic lesions. Rarely, cysts or chordomas are found.

Brain tumors cause differing symptoms, depending on the anatomic location of the neoplasm and its rate of growth. All result in impaired neurologic function and commonly produce relentlessly progressive symptoms. Changes in affect, lethargy, or visual or hallucinatory changes may be noted. Intracerebral masses typically cause morning headaches. At least one-half of cerebral gliomas are associated with pathologic reflexes (Babinski, hyperreflexia) or seizures. Approximately one-third of adult onset seizure disorders are due to malignant tumors. If a tumor blocks a ventricle or the aqueduct, or enlarges rapidly, increased intracranial pressure may result in progressive headache, vomiting, and papilledema. Galactorrhea may be produced by chromophobe adenomas of the pituitary. An acoustic neuroma may result in unilateral deafness. A careful neurologic examination should be performed to evaluate station and gait, coordination, reflexes, sensorium, presence of cranial nerve abnormalities, visual fields, hearing, and the presence of pathologic reflexes or papilledema.

Treatment Evaluation

The evaluation should include skull radiographs, which may show suprasellar calcification (craniopharyngioma), a pineal shift (intracerebral mass), or pressure erosion of the calvarium (meningioma), for example. Chest radiographs should be obtained to rule out a primary lung neoplasm. A CT brain scan is the best and least invasive screening test to detect a primary brain tumor. The CT scan is approximately equal in sensitivity to a radionuclide brain scan for detecting equal-sized masses but provides more data on the etiology of a mass, since it may be used to distinguish between edema, cystic areas, solid masses, and hemorrhagic zones. The CT scan also determines the anterior and anterolateral extent of pituitary tumors better than pneumoencephalography and cerebral angiography. The CT scan, however, may not reveal very small lesions of the brain and may be difficult to perform on uncooperative patients. Arteriograms have been used less frequently since the introduction of CT scans but are still important preoperatively in determining the vascular supply of a tumor. Pneumoencephalograms are also used less frequently but are still important in demonstrating the extent of suprasellar extension in pituitary tumors. Ventricular air injections may delineate posterior fossa masses. A lumbar puncture is contraindicated when there is increased intracranial pressure, unless a catheter has been placed superiorly to equalize pressure and prevent herniation of the cerebellar tonsils. An endocrine evaluation may be necessary if a pituitary tumor is suspected, with determination of serum prolactin or growth hormone levels or dexamethasone suppression, serum cortisol, or urinary 17-keto- and hydroxysteroid tests as indicated.

If a spinal cord tumor is suspected, a careful neurologic examination should be performed to localize the possible site of involvement. A lumbar myelogram is then necessary to determine the site of the block and is usually supplemented by a cisternal injection to delineate the superior extent of the block.

A tissue diagnosis should be obtained, if possible. In a few sites, radiotherapy may be given without a histopathologic diagnosis—in the pineal, thalamic, and brain stem regions, where a biopsy is hazardous, for example. Expert interpretation of histopathologic specimens is necessary.

Surgery is the most important modality in the management of resectable brain tumors. The resection, if possible, should be performed without causing severe neurologic impairment. If a total resection of the tumor cannot be carried out safely, then either a biopsy or a partial resection should be performed.

Treatment Results

Astrocytomas

The survival of patients with completely resected grades I and II astrocytomas approaches 100%. If the astrocytomas are incompletely resected, postoperative irradiation has resulted in 5-year survivals of 58% and 25% for those with grade I and grade II astrocytomas, respectively. The tumor bed (with margins) receives approximately 5500 rads in 5½ to 7 weeks.

Patients with grade III malignant astrocytomas have a better prognosis than those with glioblastoma multiforme (grade IV). A 5-year survival of 10% to 22% is possible with postoperative whole brain radiation doses of 4000–4500 rads, followed by a 1500–2000 rad booster dose to the resection bed, over 6 to 8 weeks. Radiation therapy in glioblastoma multiforme appears to prolong functional survival for up to 3 years, but most patients are dead by 5 years. Chemotherapy with such single agents as the nitrosureas and procarbazine or a combination of procarbazine, CCNU, and Velban (PCV) may produce short responses and slightly prolonged survivals. However, when the results of postoperative radiotherapy alone, CCNU alone, or the two combined were randomly compared in patients with glioblastoma multiforme, no significant differences were noted between the groups. Survival *has* been significantly prolonged when the hypoxic cell sensitizer metronidazole and radiotherapy were given, rather than postoperative irradiation alone. Fast neutron irradiation has also been studied in 15 patients with grade III and IV astrocytomas postoperatively. Survival in the group that received neutron irradiation was probably *shortened* in comparison to survival with conventional radiotherapy treatments, presumably due to coagulation necrosis in the tumor area with resultant early deaths.

Oligodendrogliomas
Patients with oligodendrogliomas, slow-growing neoplasms, have an approximate 30% to 40% 5-year survival when treated by surgery alone. If radiotherapy is added following incomplete resection, 50% to 80% survival may be expected. Approximately 5500 rads are delivered to the tumor bed with margins in 5.5 to 7 weeks.

Ependymomas
Most ependymomas cannot be completely resected, and postoperative irradiation is required. The spinal axis should be irradiated if the patient has a high grade tumor (ependymoblastoma) since there is a 20% risk of CSF tumor cell seeding. Other patients who should receive spinal axis irradiation are those with known metastatic seeding or with positive CSF cytologic findings. Four thousand rads are delivered to the whole brain and spinal axis in 4 to 5 weeks, followed by a 1500 rad boost in 2 weeks to the area of the primary neoplasm. The match line between adjacent radiotherapy fields is moved each week to avoid areas of over- or underdosage. Surgery alone results in 20% to 27% 5-year survivals, but the addition of postoperative irradiation has improved these results to 50% to 75% at 5 years.

Medulloblastomas
Few long-term survivors were reported prior to postoperative irradiation of medulloblastomas. The median survival without radiotherapy was only 13 months. Since there is a 33% risk of CSF seeding by tumor cells in medulloblastomas, whole-brain and spinal axis irradiation to 4000 rads with a 1500-rad tumor boost are recommended. Five-year survival rates of 40% to 60% have been reported with combined resection and irradiation. Since medulloblastoma is primarily a childhood neoplasm, pituitary deficiency (especially decreased growth hormone) may be produced 2 to 10 years after irradiation. If recognized early, hormone replacement may allow normal growth and development. Combination chemotherapy as a surgical-radiation adjuvant is currently being studied in patients with medulloblastomas.

Pineal Tumors
Because of their deep midline location, pineal tumors are rarely biopsied. Pineal neoplasms are most commonly dysgerminomas. Approximately 5000 rads are delivered to the pineal area in 5 to 6 weeks. Since CSF seeding can

occur, a cytologic examination should be performed. Craniospinal axis irradiation is indicated if malignant cells are present in the spinal fluid. Seventy to eighty percent 5-year survivals have been obtained with radiotherapy alone.

Meningiomas

When meningiomas can be completely resected, failures are rare. There were no recurrences in 84 patients at the University of California, San Francisco, Medical Center who were treated by complete surgical resection alone. Patients with incompletely resected meningiomas, however, should be considered for postoperative irradiation. Of 92 patients with incompletely resected meningiomas, 58 underwent surgery alone and, of these, 74% ultimately developed a recurrence. The recurrence rate among the 34 patients who received postoperative irradiation was reduced to only 30%.

Brain Stem Tumors

Biopsies are usually not performed for brain stem lesions. Radiation therapy is recommended, encompassing the tumor with margins and delivering 5500 rads in 5 to 7 weeks. Most tumors are gliomas, and a high percentage are glioblastoma multiforme (in autopsy series). Approximately 70% of patients will have postirradiation neurologic improvement, and 40% survivals at 5 years have been obtained.

Pituitary Tumors

Small pituitary tumors may be irradiated if there are no visual field defects, no rapid decreases in visual acuity, and no suprasellar extension greater than 1.0 cm. Radiotherapy alone can control 60% to 80% of chromophobe adenomas. After irradiation, approximately 40% of patients with eosinophilic adenomas will have a noticeable decrease in acromegalic facies, while stabilization of the acromegaly should occur in the remainder. Radiotherapy also controls almost 100% of patients with Cushing's syndrome secondary to a basophilic adenoma of the pituitary. Elevated prolactin and growth hormone levels decrease more rapidly after transsphenoidal hypophysectomy, however. Growth hormone titers may return to normal in as many as 92% of patients with eosinophilic adenomas. Excellent results were obtained when transsphenoidal hypophysectomy was used to treat patients with small prolactin-secreting chromophobe adenomas (3 to 9 mm): 16 of 17 women began menstruating or became pregnant postoperatively. Only 2 of 7 patients with larger tumors resumed menstruation. Transient postoperative complications such as inappropriate ADH hormone release, CSF leak, and diplopia may occur after transsphenoidal hypophysectomy. Postoperative irradiation is recommended after incomplete resection of a pituitary tumor, in large nonsecretory neoplasms, and for craniopharyngiomas.

The treatment of metastatic spinal cord tumors has been detailed in Part I, Chapter 5. Resection by microsurgical techniques has given the best results in extramedullary tumors such as meningiomas and schwannomas. The results after surgery alone are poor for intramedullary tumors such as astrocytomas and ependymomas. Postoperative irradiation to 4000–5000 rads in 5 to 6 weeks is recommended, and 5-year survivals of 60% for spinal cord gliomas have been obtained with these combined techniques.

D.G.

Bloom H, Wallace E, Henk J: The treatment and prognosis of medulloblastoma in children. Am J Roentgenol 105:43–62, 1969.
In 82 patients there were 32% 5-year and 26% 10-year survival rates.

Bradfield J, Perez C: Pineal tumors and ectopic pinealomas. Radiology 103:399–406, 1972.
In this article 18 cases are discussed in detail.

Jelsma R, Bucy P: The treatment of glioblastoma multiforme of the brain. J Neurosurg 27:388–400, 1967.
This classic neurosurgical article correlates length and quality of survival with extent of resection, use of steroids, and/or radiotherapy.

Laramore G, Griffin T, Gerdes A, Parker R: Fast neutron and mixed (neutron/photon) beam teletherapy for grades III and IV astrocytomas. Cancer 42:96–103, 1978.
Neutron treatments led to shortened survival.

Levin V, Wilson C: Chemotherapy: The agents in current use. Semin Oncol 2:63–67, 1975.
Article gives description of single agents and combination chemotherapy of brain tumors.

Marks J, Gado M: Serial computed tomography of primary brain tumors following surgery, irradiation and chemotherapy. Radiology 125:119–125, 1977.
Article gives CT findings during clinical courses of 55 patients.

Marsa G, Goffinet D, Rubenstein L, Bagshaw J: Megavoltage irradiation in the treatment of gliomas of the brain and spinal cord. Cancer 36:1681–1689, 1975.
With this treatment there was a 47% 5-year survival for patients with medulloblastomas.

Pistenma D, Goffinet D, Bagshaw M, et al: Treatment of chromophobe adenomas with megavoltage irradiation. Cancer 35:1574–1582, 1975.
Sixty-two patients were irradiated, alone or postoperatively. Indications for initial surgery were: (1) visual field defects, (2) deteriorating visual acuity, and (3) greater than 1 cm suprasellar extension.

Sheline G: Radiation therapy of brain tumors. Cancer 39:873–881, 1977.
Extensive review of results of radiotherapy for all brain tumors.

Sheline G: Radiation therapy of tumors of the central nervous system in childhood. Cancer 35:957–964, 1975.
Extensive review.

Urtasun R, Band P, Chapman J, et al: Radiation and high dose metronidazole in supratentorial glioblastomas. N Engl J Med 294:1364–1367, 1976.
Survival was significantly prolonged with radiation therapy and hypoxic cell sensitizer combined compared to radiation therapy alone.

Wara W, Sheline G, Newman H, et al: Radiation therapy of meningiomas. Am J Roentgenol 123:453–458, 1975.
If resection was incomplete, postoperative radiotherapy delayed or prevented recurrence regardless of histological type of meningioma.

Weir B, Band P, Urtasun R, Blain G: Radiotherapy and CCNU in the treatment of high grade supratentorial astrocytomas. J Neurosurg 45:129–134, 1976.
Postoperative treatment was randomly allocated to: (1) radiation therapy alone, (2) CCNU alone, (3) radiation therapy and CCNU. No significant differences between the groups.

Wilson CB: Current concepts in cancer: Brain tumors. N Engl J Med 300:1469–1471, 1979.
Review of all modalities of treatment.

Approximately 5% to 10% of all malignancies involve head and neck sites. In 1977 there were an estimated 9200 new cases of laryngeal cancer, 4500 tongue cancers, 6600 pharyngeal neoplasms, and 8700 salivary gland or floor of mouth malignancies. These cancers predominantly affect males and usually occur in the 50- to 60-year age group. Tobacco and alcohol abuse are common among subjects with squamous carcinomas. Partially due to these factors there is also a high risk (15% to 20%) that second primary neoplasms will develop. Survival is further decreased by intercurrent deaths common to this age group. The use of snuff or betel nut, and, rarely, syphilis or the Plummer-Vinson syndrome have been associated with oral cancers. Racial factors are also important, since the incidence of nasopharyngeal malignancies is greatly increased in those of Chinese descent.

The use of excessive tobacco or alcohol should be noted. Hemoptysis or epistaxis, pain anywhere in the head and neck, dysphagia, trismus, loose teeth, visual or related problems, and stridor or hoarseness are all important symptoms of head and neck cancers. A physical examination should include careful palpation of all lymph node areas and the thyroid gland. Cranial nerve function should be checked. A laryngeal click is a normal finding and when absent suggests a postcricoid mass. Systematic inspection of the oral cavity and oropharynx and a mirror inspection of the hypopharynx, nasopharynx, and larynx should be carried out. Tongue and vocal cord mobility and palatal symmetry should all be determined. Palpation of the oral cavity and the oropharynx is very important, especially in detecting infiltrative lesions that frequently invade the base of the tongue.

A blood count, serologic test for syphilis, and liver and renal function tests should be obtained. A chest radiograph is mandatory. Special radiographic studies include mandible views for patients with oral cavity and oropharyngeal lesions, sinus series, and possibly skull radiographs for those with suspected sinus tumors. Tomograms may also be important in demonstrating the presence or absence of bone destruction. In suspected nasopharyngeal malignancies, a base skull radiograph should be performed with tomograms, if necessary, along with consideration of a nasopharyngogram. In lesions of the hypopharynx and oropharynx, a lateral soft tissue x-ray of the neck may show a mass at the base of the tongue or extension into the pre-epiglottic space. For laryngeal malignancies, laryngotomograms or preferably laryngograms should be performed prior to direct laryngoscopy and biopsy. A laryngogram is more accurate in assessing the extent of disease than laryngotomograms, but the former should not be performed in patients with large, bulky lesions or a compromised airway, since any edema induced by the study may result in airway obstruction. CT scans may be important in assessing the extent of involvement of sinus or nasopharyngeal malignancies and are also being evaluated for patients with laryngopharyngeal cancers. Liver and bone scans should be performed if indicated. Patients with suspected laryngopharyngeal cancers should have a direct laryngoscopy. Finally, a biopsy should be performed either with a punch under local anesthesia or by incision or excision, depending on the size and anatomic location of the lesion. When the evaluation has been completed, the biopsy obtained, and the histopathologic findings reviewed, the patient may finally be staged by the TNM system (see Part VIII).

The initial treatment decision and therapeutic course are critically important in cases of head and neck cancer. In many instances recurrent cancers cannot be eradicated and the resultant cosmetic and functional distortions are agonizing to both patient and family. Therefore a combined modality, multidisciplinary approach to treatment planning should be carried out. An early decision must be made as to whether a lesion may be cured or if a palliative approach is indicated and which treatment modality or combination of modalities will give the best results with maximum preservation of function.

In general, radiation therapy and surgery are equally effective for small primary cancers in most head and neck sites. It is generally agreed that heavy smokers and drinkers are more effectively managed by surgery. For more extensive carcinomas (T_3 and T_4) combined surgery and radiotherapy are recommended. With these cancers, the tumor is debulked surgically either before or after it is irradiated. The cervical lymph nodes are also resected and/or irradiated. An advantage of radiation therapy to the neck is that contralateral lymph nodes may also be treated. An important concept is that even though the neck examination is normal, cervical lymph nodes may harbor subclinical metastases which, if untreated, would produce clinical lymphadenopathy. Elective lymph node irradiation with doses of 4500–5000 rads has been found to be very effective and may reduce the risk of development of lymph node metastases from 20–75% to less than 5%. In patients with clinically palpable, single cervical lymph nodes less than 3 cm in greatest dimension, 75% or more can be controlled by radiation alone. When the lymph nodes are larger or multiple lymph nodes are involved ($N_{2,3}$), however, combined surgery and radiotherapy are needed. The recurrence rates for patients with N_1, N_2, and N_3 cervical lymph node involvement have been reduced from 14%, 26%, and 34% with surgery to 2%, 11%, and 25% with combined surgery and radiotherapy.

The chemotherapy of head and neck cancers has been disappointing, in that the few prospective studies performed to date have shown no survival advantage for the groups receiving chemotherapy. The most commonly used agents have been methotrexate, hydroxyurea, and more recently *cis*-diammine dichloroplatinum (CDDP) and bleomycin either alone or in combination. The most active agent is apparently CDDP which can produce objective responses in 33% to 60% of patients. The responses may be long-lasting; complete remissions of 6 months or more have been reported. This agent is now being used as a surgical-radiotherapy adjuvant in a randomized trial for patients with advanced, operable cancers. CDDP may be associated with ototoxicity or nephrotoxicity as well as severe nausea during its administration, which somewhat limits its potential as an adjuvant.

Oral Cavity
Tongue
Tongue lesions, usually found along the lateral free margin, frequently ulcerate, produce local pain, and, if enlarged, result in speech defects. Smaller lesions ($T_{1,2}$) may be managed either by surgery or by radiation therapy alone. They may be irradiated with external beam or by interstitial implantation. Both modalities produce 70% to 85% cure rates. Larger lesions usually require combined surgical and radiation treatment, with an expected control rate of 30% to 40%. Lymph node involvement decreases the expected cure rates by approximately 50%. The cervical lymph nodes should be electively irradiated in all patients with initially normal neck examinations except in those with very small (T_1) primary cancers.

Floor of Mouth, Buccal Mucosa
Floor of mouth and buccal mucosa lesions also produce speech changes and local pain. They are managed similarly to lesions of the tongue, except that floor of mouth lesions encroaching upon the mandible are usually treated surgically because of both the risk of mandibular osteoradionecrosis from irradiation and a lesser chance for cure with this modality. Often a radical or modified neck

dissection is performed in continuity with resection of the primary site, but again, if N_2 or N_3 lymphadenopathy is noted, postoperative irradiation should be used. Five-year survivals of 70% for small lesions and less than 33% for patients with bulky cervical lymph nodes or $T_{3,4}$ primaries are reported. Small buccal lesions may be treated by interstitial implants or local resection with or without a skin graft. Larger lesions require combined surgery and radiotherapy treatment, with chances for cure similar to those for other oral cancers.

Oropharynx
Tonsil
Small tonsillar cancers may produce localized pain or pain referred to the ear. When advanced, hemoptysis, dysphagia, or trismus may all be noted. Smaller primary lesions $(T_{1,2})$ may be managed by irradiation, but larger cancers usually require combined surgery and radiotherapy. A neck dissection may be performed in continuity with resection of the primary, but elective or therapeutic neck irradiation may also be carried out. Five-year cure rates of 60% to 75% for small lesions and 20% to 35% for large cancers are reported.

Base of Tongue
Speech problems, referred ear pain, dysphagia, hemoptysis, and unexplained neck mass may all be due to base of tongue cancers. Cancers involving this site present difficult therapeutic problems, in that surgical margins may not be free, there is a high risk of bilateral lymph node metastases and postoperative aspiration, and swallowing and speech difficulties commonly occur. Radiation therapy has been the preferred method of treatment, although reports of successful massive base tongue resections have also appeared. Five-year survival for even the smallest lesions is usually 50% to 60% and decreases to 20% to 30% for those with massive primary sites or involved lymph nodes.

Palate
Palate cancers may produce local pain, dysphagia, or trismus if the lesions are extensive and invade the pterygopalatine fossa. Smaller lesions may be treated by radiotherapy or surgery, but large lesions require combined treatment with an expectation of a 60% to 70% cure rate for small lesions and 30% for larger ones.

Nasopharynx
Nasopharyngeal cancers usually present with lymph node metastases or nasal obstruction but may also produce cranial nerve deficits resulting in visual changes, epistaxis, or localized pain. The jugular foramen syndrome, with paralysis of cranial nerves IX through XII, may also develop. These lesions are managed by high-dose, large-volume irradiation, to 6600–7000 rads in 6 to 8 weeks. Bilateral cervical lymph nodes are also completely irradiated, even when findings in the neck are clinically negative, since there is a very high incidence of occult metastases. Five-year survivals of 80% for small lesions and 0% to 10% for those with bony destruction (T_4) are reported.

Glottic Larynx
Small glottic cancers produce hoarseness early, but as they enlarge may also induce dysphagia, hemoptysis, stridor, or ear pain. For $T_{1,2}$ glottic cancers with normal vocal cord mobility, radiotherapy is the treatment of choice and will cure 90% and 70% of cancers, respectively. Surgical salvage after relapse is also very effective in cases of $T_{1,2}$ glottic cancers. With larger glottic cancers $(T_{3,4})$ combined surgery and radiotherapy are used, with an expected cure rate of at least 50%. Lymph node metastases are very rare in glottic malignancies.

Supraglottis

Small lesions, especially on the suprahyoid epiglottis, may be managed by radiotherapy alone. Larger tumors may be treated by supraglottic or total laryngectomy and postoperative radiation to the tumor bed and bilateral necks.

Hypopharynx

Hypopharyngeal lesions may produce an asymptomatic neck mass, hoarseness, stridor, dysphagia, hemoptysis, and referred ear pain. Except for very small, exophytic lesions, carcinomas of the pyriform sinus are managed by combined preoperative or postoperative irradiation and laryngopharyngectomy. Five-year survivals, even with the most favorable lesions, are usually 50% or less but decrease to 30% or less for larger lesions or when cervical adenopathy is present.

Sinus

Sinus carcinomas may result in obstructive symptoms, epistaxis, visual changes, trismus, loose teeth, or malar masses if they enlarge or invade soft tissues. Sinus tumors are best managed by resection and postoperative irradiation. A 50% cure rate can be obtained for the most favorable lesions, but lower results are noted in cases of extensive tumors and bone involvement.

Salivary Gland

Salivary gland malignancies are treated surgically. Benign mixed tumors and adenomas may be encountered. Malignant tumors, such as mucoepidermoid, adenoidcystic (invade the nerves), acinic cell (metastasize), and malignant mixed adeno- and squamous cell carcinomas, may all be encountered. Superficial parotidectomy is performed on patients without facial nerve involvement and with a superficial parotid mass, but a total parotidectomy is necessary, with nerve grafting, if the facial nerve is involved. Postoperative irradiation should be considered for patients with malignant tumors, invasion of surrounding structures, including nerves and/or bone, and for those with positive surgical margins or recurrent tumors. The local failure rate for highly malignant tumors may be reduced from 36% to about 10% with postoperative irradiation.

For most head and neck cancers cure is measured in terms of 5-year survival. Most squamous carcinomas relapse in the first 3 years after therapy, however, and it is rare for recurrences to take place later. Follow-up intervals of 1 to 2 months for the first year, with progressively longer intervals between visits up to 5 years, are recommended. After 5 years, annual examinations should be sufficient.

D.G.

Fletcher G, Jesse R: The place of irradiation in the management of the primary lesion in head and neck cancers. Cancer 39:862–872, 1977.
Recommends radiation therapy alone for small lesions and combination of radiation therapy and surgery for T_{3-4} cancers and malignant salivary gland tumors.
Fletcher G, Jing B: The Head and Neck. Chicago: Year Book Medical Publishing, 1968.
Anatomy, workup, and treatment techniques and results for radiation therapy and surgery are all presented.
Hoppe R, Goffinet D, Bagshaw M: Carcinoma of the nasopharynx: 18 years experience with megavoltage radiation therapy. Cancer 37:2605–2612, 1976.
Excellent results obtained in early stages. High radiation doses and large treatment volumes used.

Jesse R, Fletcher G: Treatment of the neck in patients with squamous cell carcinoma of the head and neck. Cancer 39:868–872, 1977.
Radiation therapy after radical neck dissection reduces neck recurrence rate for patients with $N_{2,3}$ nodal status.

Lindberg R: Distribution of cervical lymph node metastases from squamous cell carcinoma of the upper respiratory and digestive tracts. Cancer 29:1446–1449, 1972.
Classic mapping of lymph node involvement at presentation.

Randolph V, Vallejo A, Spiro R, et al: Combination therapy of advanced head and neck cancer. Cancer 41:460–467, 1978.
Bleomycin plus cis-diamminedichloroplatinum combination produced 71% objective responses in 21 patients.

Rubin P: Cancer of the head and neck. Hypopharynx and larynx. JAMA 221:1252–1260, 1972.
Five authors cover management by radiation therapy and surgery.

Vandenbrouck C, Sancho H, LeFur R, et al: Results of a randomized clinical trial of preoperative irradiation versus postoperative in treatment of tumors of the hypopharynx. Cancer 39:1445–1449, 1977.
In 49 patients randomized, there were fewer complications, better survival, and shorter hospital stays in patients who received postoperative irradiation.

Wang C: Radiation therapy for head and neck cancers. Cancer 36:748–751, 1975.
Review of management at Massachusetts General Hospital.

38. THYROID CANCER—PRIMARY OR REGIONAL

The evaluation of a patient with a thyroid nodule is covered in Part II, Chapter 17.

Thyroid cancer makes up about 1.3% of all cancers and causes 0.4% of all deaths due to malignant disease. Irradiation of the head and neck in childhood is important in the etiology of thyroid cancer; 25% of patients thus irradiated will develop thyroid nodules, and 25% of the nodules will be malignant, with a latency period of 5 to 25 years. Prolonged stimulation of pituitary TSH (thyroid stimulating hormone) production may also play a role in the ultimate development of thyroid cancer. There is an increased familial incidence of medullary carcinoma but not of the other histopathologic types of thyroid cancer.

Thyroid cancer spreads locally either by direct intraglandular extension or through lymphatic channels in the gland. In addition there may be direct invasion of adjacent tissues. Regional or distant spread occurs through extraglandular lymphatics or hematogenously.

Thyroid cancer may present as a neck mass or may be associated with hoarseness (present in 10% of patients with papillary and 55% with anaplastic carcinomas, respectively). Dyspnea is rare in papillary carcinomas (3%) but is frequently noted in patients with anaplastic cancers (43%). Stridor and dysphagia may also be present in advanced cases.

The presence or absence of the above symptoms should be noted, as well as any childhood head and neck irradiation. Mirror laryngoscopy should be carried out to ascertain vocal cord mobility. The neck should be carefully examined for the presence of enlarged lymph nodes. Examination of the thyroid may reveal a firm intraglandular mass, fixation to surrounding structures, or failure of the thyroid to move normally with swallowing.

There are several forms of thyroid cancer, each with a different prognosis. Differentiated thyroid cancers are the most common. Papillary carcinomas (50% to 60% of adult thyroid cancer, 70% of cancer in children) usually have a long noninvasive period and are found in younger patients. Perhaps 5% of these lesions will eventually become invasive, anaplastic tumors. Psammoma bodies are usually present. Papillary carcinomas may present in lymph nodes. Follicular carcinomas, with a peak incidence at age 40, make up 20% to 30% of adult thyroid cancers. Although follicular cancers may involve lymph nodes, they usually metastasize hematogenously. Poorly differentiated follicular carcinomas with vascular invasion have a worse prognosis. Mixed papillary and follicular cancers may be less frequently noted. Undifferentiated giant cell, small cell, and spindle cell cancers make up 10% to 15% of thyroid malignancies. All are invasive, may metastasize, and are highly lethal. Medullary carcinomas, accounting for 5% of thyroid cancers, arise from parafollicular C cells, have an increased familial incidence, and commonly present with lymph node metastases. A unique biologic marker (calcitonin) accompanies these carcinomas. Medullary cancers may be associated with other endocrine abnormalities, such as pheochromocytomas and parathyroid adenomas. Hurthle cell cancers are usually encapsulated, can be invasive, and occur in 5% to 10% of patients. Rarer neoplasms, such as lymphomas (fewer than 1% of non-Hodgkin's lymphoma presentations), squamous carcinomas, and metastases, may also involve the thyroid. Inferior cervical lymph nodes involved by Hodgkin's disease and the non-Hodgkin's lymphomas may encroach upon the thyroid and simulate a thyroid mass without directly invading the gland.

The minimum recommended surgical procedure for a thyroid nodule is lobectomy and frozen section examination. If a papillary or noninvasive follicular carcinoma is present, most surgeons also resect the isthmus with or without a portion of the opposite lobe. This procedure is sufficient for low-risk patients (those younger than 40 years of age with small papillary or mixed lesions). The risk of multifocal involvement of the opposite thyroid lobe is 10% to 25%, but few cancers in the contralateral lobe ever become clinically apparent (5.7% in one series). This low risk is probably due to the widespread postoperative use of thyroid hormone to suppress the gland. If invasive follicular carcinoma is present, either a total thyroidectomy or a subtotal contralateral thyroid lobectomy is recommended, as these ablative procedures also allow future ^{131}I therapy to be given if necessary. Total thyroid lobectomy is also recommended for patients with a palpable nodule in the contralateral lobe, for those with a past history of childhood head and neck irradiation (increases the risk of multicentricity), and for those with familial medullary carcinomas (also increased risk of multicentricity). If possible, anaplastic carcinomas should be resected in toto. It should be remembered that postoperative hypoparathyroidism is increased from 0.6% with a lobectomy to at least 4% following total thyroidectomy.

Most surgeons sample adjacent cervical lymph nodes at the time of the initial thyroid lobectomy. Patients whose neck examination is negative have an overall risk of approximately 7% to 15% of ultimately developing clinically apparent lymph node involvement. Modified neck dissections are recommended for large medullary carcinomas or poorly differentiated follicular cancers, as well as for patients with palpable lymph nodes. The sternocleidomastoid muscle can usually be preserved in these instances. Patients with extensive cervical disease should have a classic radical neck dissection.

External beam radiotherapy may slow the growth rate of anaplastic thyroid carcinomas and may also be useful in palliation of painful metastases. The use of radiation therapy may also be considered for patients with residual carcinomas who have no iodine uptake on subsequent scans.

Postoperatively, especially for patients over 40, those with involved cervical lymph nodes, or those with follicular carcinomas, ^{131}I tracer studies with whole body scans at 48 to 72 hours and ablation should be considered. Under the age of 40 routine postoperative ablation appears to produce no better survival rates than surgery alone. A tracer ^{131}I dose of approximately 1 mCi is given, and if foci of uptake are noted, these are ablated with 30 to 50 mCi of [131]I. Following this ablation, thyroid hormone is given for 2 to 3 months, then discontinued for 1 month, after which a total body thyroid scan is done after the ingestion of 1 to 5 mCi of [131]I. If uptake is noted, 75 to 200 mCi are given at 3- to 4-month intervals until ablation or until a total of approximately 500 mCi ^{131}I is given. Following ablation, the thyroid is suppressed by the administration of either T_3 or T_4 and reevaluated periodically by withdrawing exogenous thyroid hormone and rescanning at 6- to 12-month intervals for a total of three negative scans.

D.G.

Aldinger K, Samaan N, Ibanez M, Hill C Jr: Anaplastic carcinomas of the thyroid. Cancer 41:2267–2275, 1978.
   Article covers 84 patients with 7.1% 5-year survival and median 6.2 month survival.
Black M: Management of carcinoma of the thyroid. Ann Surg 185:133–144, 1977.
   Excellent review of recommended surgical procedures and results.
Blahd WH: Treatment of malignant thyroid disease. Semin Nucl Med 9:95–99, 1979.
   Reviews the role of radioactive iodine.
Cady B, Sedgwick C, Meissner W: Changing clinical, pathologic, therapeutic and survival patterns in differentiated thyroid carcinoma. Ann Surg 184:541–553, 1976.
   Article presents 15-year follow-up of 631 patients with thyroid cancer at Lahey Clinic.
Hill C Jr: Medullary carcinoma of the thyroid. Am Fam Physician 7:99–105, 1973.
   Review article.
Varma V, Beierwaltes W, Nofal M, et al: Treatment of thyroid cancer: Death rates after surgery and after surgery followed by 131-I. JAMA 214:1437–1442, 1970.
   263 patients with thyroid cancers received postoperative [131]I. A decreased mortality was noted in patients older than 40 compared to when surgery was used alone.

---

39. BREAST CANCER—PRIMARY OR REGIONAL

Carcinoma of the breast is the most common neoplasm in white women over age 40. Seventy-five percent of such carcinomas occur in women over 50. The incidence of breast cancer is 72 in 100,000 women, while 25 in 100,000 die each year. The female–male ratio is 100 : 1. The risk that bilateral breast cancers will develop is 4% to 10%. The risk is increased in nulliparous patients, in those with a family history of breast carcinoma, and in women whose first child was born late in life.

The sequential evaluation of a breast mass is described in Part II, Chapter 21. A small breast mass is usually asymptomatic, but as it enlarges it may produce breast fixation, skin retraction, ulceration, erythema, local pain, nipple discharge or retraction, or enlargement of axillary lymph nodes. If metastases have occurred, bone pain (osseous metastases), cough (pulmonary metastases and/or a malignant pleural effusion), and fatigue and weight loss (liver metastases) may all occur.

A careful history, including symptoms referable to the breast mass, a possible family history of breast carcinoma, and any symptoms suggesting distant metastases should be obtained. The physical examination should include lung auscultation and liver and bone palpation, in addition to a careful breast examination. Cystic-appearing structures should be transilluminated, while the nature of the mass and any associated skin or muscle fixation or the presence or absence of nipple discharge and crusting should all be noted. Mammograms should be obtained to rule out the possibility of a contralateral breast cancer and to localize the mass better prior to biopsy. A complete blood count and liver chemistry panel should also be obtained, as well as a bone scan if the mass is suggestive of malignancy. A histopathologic diagnosis may be obtained by aspiration cytology or through cutting needle, excisional, or incisional biopsies. Tissues should be assayed for estrogen receptors. In the case of premenopausal women for whom breast irradiation rather than a mastectomy is planned, the axillary lymph nodes should be biopsied; if they contain metastatic carcinoma, the use of adjuvant chemotherapy should be considered.

Seventy-five percent of breast cancers are ductal adenocarcinomas. The remainder include lobular (8%), medullary (4%), colloid (3%), papillary (1%), mucinous (2%), and intraductal carcinomas (comedo, 4%) or Paget's disease (2%). Breast cancers are further classified histopathologically according to one of four types. Type I is nonmetastasizing (not invasive). Examples are Paget's disease, papillary carcinoma, and lobular carcinoma in situ. Type II is rarely metastasizing (always invasive). Examples are colloid carcinoma, medullary carcinoma, and well-differentiated adenocarcinomas. Type III is moderately metastasizing (always invasive). Examples are adenocarcinomas, and intraductal carcinomas with stromal invasion. Type IV, highly metastasizing (always invasive), include undifferentiated carcinoma or any in types I, II, and III with blood vessel invasion.

A histopathologic diagnosis should be obtained prior to definitive treatment. Since breast cancers have been shown to be multicentric in at least 25% of cases, this fact should be kept in mind when planning treatment. Absolute contraindications to radical mastectomy [Haagensen, 1975] are (1) satellite nodules, (2) arm edema, (3) parasternal nodules, (4) extensive breast edema, (5) biopsy-proved supraclavicular lymph node involvement, (6) inflammatory carcinoma, or (7) distant metastases. Mastectomy is also contraindicated if two or more of the following grave signs are present: (1) skin ulceration, (2) limited edema (one-third of breast), (3) axillary lymph nodes larger than 2.5 cm, (4) fixed axillary lymph nodes, and (5) chest wall fixation.

Early Cancers—Stage I (T_1N_0) and Stage II ($T_{0,1}N_1$ and T_2N_1)

Either a radical or a modified radical mastectomy is the standard treatment for stages I and II breast cancer. Not only have the largest number of patients been treated by mastectomy, but also longer follow-up information is available than for any other procedure. After triple biopsy of (1) the breast, (2) high axillary lymph nodes, and (3) the upper intercostal lymph nodes, Haagensen found a 10-year survival of 70.6% in patients with stage I breast cancers. With radical mastectomy, 10-year survivals of 66% with negative axillary nodes and 35% with lymph node involvement are reported. With modified radical mastectomy, survival at 10 years for those with involved lymph nodes may be slightly below 35%. Postoperative irradiation to the internal mammary and supraclavicular regions and to the chest wall has been recommended for patients with involved axillary lymph nodes, medially located carcinomas, large primary cancers, and skin or pectoral involvement by carcinoma. Administration of 5000 rads in 5 weeks to these regions greatly reduces the risk of local recurrence. A recent prospective, randomized trial showed that regional irradiation after mastectomy resulted in both significantly fewer relapses and increased survival in patients treated with cobalt 60 irradiation.

Adjuvant chemotherapy is now widely used postoperatively in patients with involved axillary lymph nodes. Three regimens have been shown to be effective: L-PAM (phenylalanine mustard) for 5 consecutive days every 6 weeks for 2 years or until relapse, CMF (cyclophosphamide-methotrexate-5 FU monthly for 12 months), and cyclophosphamide for 6 days postoperatively have all resulted in significantly improved survival compared to control groups that received no chemotherapy. The first two studies, however, showed sustained improvement in relapse-free survival only in the premenopausal age group: at 4 years, 75% vs. 40% for CMF vs. no adjuvant therapy, and 65% vs. 43% for L-PAM vs. placebo.

A possible alternative to radical mastectomy in patients with early stage breast cancers is wedge or excisional biopsy of the primary cancer and irradiation of the breast and regional lymph nodes (internal mammary, supraclavicular, and axillary). In this treatment 4500–5000 rads are given at 900–1000 rads per week with external megavoltage radiation techniques. The entire breast is initially irradiated to treat possible multicentric foci of carcinoma as well as the primary neoplasm. The tumor bed then receives either additional external beam irradiation or a temporary, removable iridium 192 interstitial implant. An additional 2000–3000 rads is administered to a localized breast volume by either of these techniques. Fewer patients have been treated by excision and irradiation and there is shorter follow-up than in the mastectomy series; however, 5-year relapse-free survivals of 91% and 60% for stages I and II breast cancers, respectively, in 150 patients have been reported. In another series of 82 patients, local control was obtained in 95% following wedge resection and external beam irradiation. Therefore this alternative form of therapy may be a substitute for mastectomy, but longer follow-up will be needed to assess its value accurately. A recent report from the National Surgical Adjuvant Breast Project (NSABP), in which operable breast cancers were treated randomly by either radical mastectomy, total mastectomy and regional irradiation, or total mastectomy alone followed by axillary dissection if the lymph nodes ultimately became involved, has shown no statistical advantage for any of the methods.

Advanced Cancers—Stage III ($T_3N_{1\,2}$) and Stage IV

For patients with stage III carcinomas, either preoperative irradiation or simple mastectomy and postoperative irradiation (with adjuvant chemotherapy) are recommended, depending on the local extent of the breast cancer. In these initially inoperable cancers, without demonstrable metastases, cure is unlikely but local control may be obtained by combinations of surgery and irradiation.

In patients with stage IV breast cancers (with distant metastases), irradiation of the primary carcinoma is recommended, while hormonal manipulations or chemotherapy are necessary for systemic management (covered in greater detail in Part IV, Chapter 62). Palliative irradiation of painful sites, pathologic fractures, or long bone or vertebral metastases should also be performed. Inflammatory breast cancers are managed locally by irradiation of the breast, chest wall, and regional lymph nodes. Surgery is contraindicated. Chemotherapy and hormone ablation are also used. Again, local control or palliation may be obtained, but cure is unlikely.

D.G.

Bonadonna G, Valagussa P, Rossi A, et al: Are surgical adjuvant trials altering the course of breast cancer? Semin Oncol 5:450–464, 1978.
This excellent discussion presents an update on the CMF trial.

Fisher B, Montague E, Redmond C, et al: Comparison of radical mastectomy
with alternative treatments for primary breast cancer. Cancer 39:2827–
2839, 1977.
*There were no significant differences (average, 36 months follow-up) in pa-
tients with operable breast cancers randomized between radical mastectomy,
total mastectomy and radiotherapy, or total mastectomy and axillary dissection if necessary when enlarged nodes become evident.*

Fisher B, Sherman B, Rockette H, et al: L-Phenylalanine mustard (L-PAM) in
the management of premenopausal patients with primary breast cancer:
Lack of association of disease-free survival with depression of ovarian function. Cancer 44:847–857, 1979.
An update of the L-PAM vs placebo trial.

Fletcher G, Montague E, Nelson E: Combination of conservative surgery and
irradiation for cancer of the breast. Am J Roentgenol 126:216–222, 1976.
*There was 95% local and regional freedom from relapses with local excision
and careful postoperative irradiation (5000 rads).*

Haagensen C: Treatment of curable carcinoma of the breast. Int J Radiat
Oncol Biol Phys 2:975–980, 1975.
Article covers ten-year survival results of radical mastectomy.

Harris JR, Levene MB, Hellman S: The role of radiation therapy in the primary treatment of carcinoma of the breast. Semin Oncol 5:403–416, 1978.
An excellent summary.

Host H, Brennhovd I: The effect of post-operative radiotherapy in breast
cancer. Int J Radiat Oncol Biol Phys 2:1061–1067, 1977.
*Stage II patients irradiated with cobalt-60 had significantly fewer relapses and
better survival than patients not irradiated postoperatively.*

Nissen-Meyer R, Kjellgren K, Malmio K, et al: Surgical adjuvant chemotherapy. Cancer 41:2088–2098, 1978.
*There were significantly fewer recurrences in the group randomly receiving a
consecutive 6-day postmastectomy course of cyclophosphamide (30 mg/kg of
body weight).*

Peters M: Wedge resection with or without radiation in early breast cancer.
Int J Radiat Oncol Biol Phys 2:1151–1156, 1977.
*There was no difference in 30-year survivals between those undergoing mas-
tectomy vs excision and radiation therapy (matched pairs).*

Weichselbaum R, Marck A, Hellman S: The role of postoperative irradiation
in carcinoma of the breast. Cancer 37:2682–2690, 1976.
Article discusses postmastectomy irradiation in 352 patients.

40. SMALL CELL CARCINOMA OF THE LUNG—PRIMARY OR REGIONAL

Small cell carcinoma of the lung represents 20% to 25% of all lung cancers. If
left untreated, it is the most rapidly fatal of all histologic types, with a median
survival of 6 to 20 weeks. The disease is associated with a male predominance,
rapid onset of symptomatology, paraneoplastic syndromes, central thoracic location, early metastases, low resectability, and 5-year survival of less than 1%.

The World Health Organization's classification recognizes four histologic
subtypes of small cell carcinoma: fusiform, polygonal, lymphocyte-like, and

mixed cell. The most common subtype is the lymphocyte-like, which includes 40% to 50% of all patients. To date there are no conclusive data indicating differences in presentation or survival according to histologic subtypes. Ectopic hormone production is frequently documented in small cell carcinoma, and electron microscopy reveals the presence of cytoplasmic neurosecretory granules, unlike other lung cancers. Because these microscopic characteristics are similar to those of other cell types of neuroectodermal origin, it has been proposed that small cell carcinoma is related to other amine-secreting tumors (APUDomas). Ectopic hormones found in association with small cell carcinoma include antidiuretic hormone, adrenocorticotrophic hormone, melanocyte-stimulating hormone, and calcitonin.

At presentation extrathoracic disease is documented in as many as 70% to 80% of patients with careful staging. Sites of metastatic involvement may include peripheral lymph nodes, bone marrow, bone, liver, soft tissue, brain, and contralateral lung. Unlike other lung cancers, small cell carcinoma is associated with bone marrow involvement in up to 40% to 50% of patients. Likewise, brain metastases may be identified in up to 10% of patients at diagnosis and are frequently asymptomatic. In addition to the physical examination, staging procedures that may be useful in defining disease extent include chest x-ray, full lung tomography, bronchoscopy, mediastinoscopy, bone scan, bone x-rays to define areas of concern on scan, liver function tests, liver scan, liver biopsy, bone marrow aspirate and biopsy, and brain scan or computerized tomography.

Rarely, patients with small cell carcinoma are found to have solitary peripheral pulmonary lesions. In one series 11 such patients underwent curative resection, and 4 survived 5 years. This setting appears to be the only one in which surgery may offer curative potential in small cell carcinoma. In contrast to these results were the findings of a prospective comparison of surgery and irradiation in the treatment of "resectable" small cell carcinoma. Here the 5-year survival was 1% with surgery and 4% with irradiation, and the average survival for those patients receiving radiation therapy was significantly longer (284 days) than for surgery alone (199 days).

Whether chemotherapy can improve the poor results of surgery or radiation therapy in "resectable" small cell carcinoma has not been extensively tested in prospective trials. However, chemotherapy has been shown to be highly effective for unresectable limited disease and for extensive small cell carcinoma (see Part VI, Chapter 90), and the approaches used for unresectable disease would also apply to "resectable" small cell carcinoma. Because the results of radical surgery are so poor in patients with "resectable" disease, surgery should only be used as a diagnostic and staging tool except perhaps in the rare patient with a solitary peripheral pulmonary lesion.

C.P.

Higgins GA, Shields TW, Keehn RJ: The solitary pulmonary nodule: Ten-year follow-up of Veterans Administration–Armed Forces cooperative study. Arch Surg 110:570–575, 1975.
Of 11 patients with peripheral small cell carcinomas, 36.4% survived 5 years following resection.
Hirsch F, Hansen HH, Dombernowsky P, Hainau B: Bone-marrow examination in the staging of small-cell anaplastic carcinoma of the lung with special reference to subtyping: An evaluation of 203 consecutive patients. Cancer 39:2563–2567, 1977.
Bone marrow involvement was found in 17.2% of patients; marrow aspiration was more sensitive than biopsy but neither procedure was adequate alone.

Jacobs L, Kinkel WR, Vincent RG: "Silent" brain metastasis from lung carcinoma determined by computerized tomography. Arch Neurol 34:690–693, 1977.

Three patients (6% of 50 studied) had metastases demonstrated by CT scan although brain scans and skull films were normal.

Margolis R, Hansen HH, Muggia FM, Kanhouwa S: Diagnosis of liver metastases in bronchogenic carcinoma: A comparative study of liver scans, function tests, and peritoneoscopy with liver biopsy in 111 patients. Cancer 34:1825–1829, 1974.

Liver metastases were documented in 8 of 19 patients with small cell carcinoma but in only 2 of 79 patients with other histologies.

Matthews MJ, Kanhouwa S, Pickren J, Robinette D: Frequency of residual and metastatic tumor in patients undergoing curative surgical resection for lung cancer. Cancer Chemother Rep 4:63–67, 1973.

Within 30 days of "curative" surgery, 12 of 19 patients were found to have distant metastatic disease.

Miller AB, Fox W, Tall R: Five-year follow-up of the Medical Research Council comparative trial of surgery and radiotherapy for the primary treatment of small-celled or oat-celled carcinoma of the bronchus. Lancet 2:501–505, 1969.

Five-year survival was 1% for those undergoing surgery and 4% for those having irradiation; average survival was significantly longer in those with radiation therapy (284 days) than with surgery (199 days).

41. NON-SMALL CELL CARCINOMAS OF THE LUNG—PRIMARY OR REGIONAL

There are at least 80,000 new cases of lung cancer each year in the United States, representing 22% of all cancer in males (33% of the deaths) and 6% of female malignancies (11% of total deaths due to cancer). The male-female ratio is 4 : 1. Lung carcinoma has a peak incidence at 50 to 60 years. Less than 1% of these neoplasms occur in patients under 30, while 10% are found in those over 70. Lung cancer is related to cigarette smoking, asbestosis, and exposure to nickel, arsenic, and other metals as well as radioactive ores. The four histopathologic lung cancer types are (1) squamous carcinoma (30% of all lung cancers), which remains localized longer than the other subtypes but involves the pleura in 30% of patients and the lymph nodes in 65%; (2) adenocarcinoma (30% of lung cancers), which metastasizes earlier and at presentation has metastasized to the lymph nodes in 80%, the pleura in 60%, and the central nervous system in 37% of patients; (3) giant cell carcinoma (15% of all lung cancers), which is similar to adenocarcinoma in frequency of metastases; and (4) small cell carcinoma (25% of all lung cancers), in which lymph node metastases are present in 95% of patients at presentation, while pleural, central nervous system, and bone marrow examinations are positive for small cell carcinoma in 35%, 30%, and 50% of patients, respectively.

Such pulmonary symptoms as hemoptysis, cough, increased sputum production, dyspnea, hoarseness, or obstructive pneumonia may all be associated with lung cancer. The signs and symptoms of paraneoplastic syndromes (described in Part II, Chapters 31 and 32) may also be present. Diplopia, headache, bone pain, or unexplained weight loss may indicate metastases.

The history and physical examination are important in the evaluation of a patient with suspected lung cancer. A history of heavy smoking combined with any of the above symptoms suggests the diagnosis. A careful chest examination should be carried out, and the regional lymph nodes, including the supraclaviculars, should be palpated. Vocal cord mobility should be ascertained, and hepatic palpation, neurologic examination, and spine percussion done. Digital clubbing and cigarette stains indicate heavy tobacco use. Laboratory studies include a complete blood count and chemical screening panel, including liver and renal function tests. If indicated, liver, brain, and bone scans are also performed. With full lung tomograms, the pulmonary hilae can be evaluated, and pulmonary nodules, not visible on ordinary radiographs, may be noted. Fluoroscopy may be needed to evaluate decreased diaphragmatic motion secondary to phrenic nerve involvement. Sputum cytologic analyses (multiple) provide the diagnosis of cancer in approximately 60% of patients.

A scalene lymph node biopsy is diagnostic in 20% of patients, and when positive indicates inoperability. Lymphatics from the left lower lobe and all right pulmonary lobes drain to the right scalene region. Combined sputum cytology and scalene lymph node biopsy provide the correct diagnosis in approximately 73% of patients. Bronchoscopy, biopsy of visible lesions (46% yield), bronchial washings (44% cytologic yield), and brush biopsies (81% accuracy with central carcinomas) may also be necessary. Since 75% of patients with lung cancer have mediastinal lymph node involvement, mediastinoscopy may either provide the diagnosis or prove inoperability if high paratracheal or contralateral lymph nodes are found to be involved. Bilateral mediastinal lymph nodes contain metastases in 16% of patients with squamous carcinomas, 50% to 68% of those with large cell cancers, 70% of those with small cell carcinomas and 50% to 60% of patients with adenocarcinomas. If the pulmonary lesion is accessible and (preferably) peripheral, needle aspiration biopsy may provide the diagnosis in 80% to 85% of the cases. If a pleural effusion is present, a positive cytologic examination of the fluid indicates inoperability. A prethoracotomy biopsy of accessible sites (bone marrow biopsy in small cell carcinoma, for example) should also be carried out. The diagnosis of lung carcinoma may therefore be made without thoracotomy in approximately 50% of patients. A thoracotomy may ultimately be necessary for diagnosis, however.

Lung cancer is a devastating malignancy, with few 5-year survivors in advanced stages. Fifty percent of lung cancer patients are initially inoperable, while another 25% are found to have unresectable carcinoma at surgery. Only 20% survive 1 year. The 5-year survival is just 5%. The mean survival is only 6 to 9 months. For every stage, poor prognostic features are weight loss greater than 10% to 12%, low Karnofsky status, and age greater than 70 years. Sixty percent of patients with small, peripheral (coin) lesions may be expected to survive 5 years. For those with larger lesions, but on which segmental resection may still be performed, 5-year survivals of 40% have been obtained, with an operative mortality of 3%. For still larger lesions that require lobectomy, 30% 5-year survivals are obtained (operative mortality 5%), while only 20% of patients with larger, central lesions that require pneumonectomy survive 5 years. There is a 14% operative mortality in this group.

Surgery is the preferred method of treatment for localized non-small cell lung carcinomas. The prognosis is best for patients with peripheral lesions who can be treated by lobectomy or a segmental resection and have no involvement of the mediastinal lymph nodes. The prognosis is worse for patients with metastases to the pulmonary hilar nodes who require a pneumonectomy. Five-year survivals are 44% to 53% for stage I cancers (negative nodes), 28% to 31% for stage II carcinomas, and only 0% to 8% for patients with stage III cancers. The prognosis for those with squamous carcinomas may be better than for large cell or adenocarcinomas, since 46% of patients with the former cell type in autopsy series have only residual carcinoma in the thorax and no apparent metastases. Potential surgical complications include arrythmia, empyema, pulmonary embolus, bronchopleural fistula, and postoperative respiratory failure.

Radiotherapy is useful in non-small cell lung carcinomas for (1) palliative treatment of unresectable cancers (5% to 8% 5-year survival) (2) patients medically unfit for resection (22% 5-year survival at best), (3) those with involved supraclavicular lymph nodes, (4) preoperative treatment for Pancoast's tumors (34% survival), and (6) local palliation (e.g., SVC syndrome). Relative contraindications to radiation therapy include the presence of tracheoesophageal fistulae, multiple distant metastases, or severe respiratory insufficiency. Local recurrences after high-dose irradiation range from 9% to 30%. For unresectable carcinomas, doses of 5000–6000 rads in 5 to 7 weeks are used, with limitation of the spinal cord dose to 4000 rads or less. Several studies have shown that split course irradiation, in which 2000–3000 rads are delivered in 2 weeks, followed by a break in treatment and an additional 2000–3000 rads 3 weeks later if metastases have not developed in the interval, may be equal to or better than consecutive radiation treatments.

Preoperative irradiation, except for Pancoast's tumor, has not produced increased survival in several prospective, randomized studies, even though greater resectability was noted in the group that received preoperative radiotherapy. When 568 patients randomly received either surgery alone or preoperative irradiation and surgery, no differences in any variables were noted between groups. When pleural, mediastinal, or lymph node involvement is present, postoperative irradiation may prolong survival. In one series a 5-year survival of only 16% was noted with surgery alone (15 of 94 patients), but 39 of 125 patients (31%) treated by combined surgery and radiation survived 5 years. Resection and/or debulking of the primary cancer, and removal of involved lymph nodes followed by radiotherapy, is the preferred treatment approach for patients with locally advanced carcinomas. Complications of radiation therapy may include tracheitis, esophagitis, radiation pneumonitis, and more rarely radiation pericarditis or myelitis.

Since metastases are noted at presentation in 50% of patients with lung cancers and ultimately develop in 90%, chemotherapy either with single agents or with combinations of drugs has been attempted many times in non-small cell lung carcinomas. In metastatic disease, responses range from 0% to 35%, are short, and have rarely been found to prolong survival significantly. Active agents alone or in combination are cyclophosphamide, the nitrosoureas, procarbazine, and Adriamycin (see Part IV, Chapter 64). Adjuvant chemotherapy, following surgical resection and/or irradiation, has not been shown to improve relapse-free survival or survival.

A significantly reduced rate of local failure and prolonged survival in patients with stage I lung carcinomas was noted when bacillus Calmette-Guérin (BCG) was instilled intrapleurally at thoracotomy in a randomized study of 60 operable patients (9 in 22 recurrences without BCG vs. 0 in 17 in the BCG group). No differences were noted when patients with more advanced carcinomas than stage I received BCG.

D.G.

Gildberg E, Shapiro C, Glickman A: Mediastinoscopy for assessing mediastinal spread in clinical staging of lung carcinoma. Semin Oncol 1:205–215, 1974.
Good review article.
Green N, Kurohara S, George F, Crews Q Jr: Postresection irradiation for primary lung cancer. Radiology 116:405–407, 1975.

This is one of several studies showing benefit of postoperative radiation therapy if lymph nodes are involved (219 patients).

Lee R, Carr D, Childs D Jr: Comparison of split-course radiation therapy and continuous for unresectable bronchogenic carcinoma: 5 year results. Am J Roentgenol 126:116–122, 1976.

The split course and continuous radiation therapy are equally effective.

Legha S, Muggia F, Carter S: Adjuvant chemotherapy in lung cancer. Cancer 39:1415–1424, 1977.

In this critical analysis of adjuvant chemotherapy trials there is little therapeutic gain to date.

Livingston R: Combined modality approaches in lung cancer. *In* Adjuvant Therapy of Cancer. Amsterdam, North Holland Publishing, 1977. Pp. 191–205.

Excellent review article.

McNeally M, Mauer C, Kausel H: Regional immunotherapy of lung cancer with intrapleural BCG. Lancet 1:377–379, 1976.

Article covers 60 patients. In stage I there were 0 in 17 relapses with BCG and 9 in 22 relapses in control patients. No benefit gained from BCG in the more advanced stages.

Paulson D: Selection of patients for surgery of bronchogenic carcinoma. Ann Surg 39:1–5, 1973.

Article provides a basis for improved clinical selection of thoracotomy candidates.

Perez C: Radiation therapy in the management of carcinoma of the lung. Cancer 39:901–916, 1977.

Excellent review article.

Roswit B: The survival of patients with inoperable lung cancer: A large scale randomized study of radiation therapy vs. placebo. Radiology 90:688–697, 1968.

There was no difference in survival although there was better local control in irradiated group.

Warram J: Preoperative irradiation of cancer of the lung: Final report of a therapeutic trial. Cancer 36:914–925, 1975.

568 operable patients were randomized to surgery alone or preoperative radiation therapy (minimum 4000 rads in 4 weeks) and surgery. There were no significant differences in survival or local relapses or metastases among the groups. In another study, the cancers of 152 of 425 "inoperable" patients became resectable and were randomized to surgery or additional irradiation; no significant differences in survival were noted.

42. ESOPHAGEAL CANCER—PRIMARY OR REGIONAL

Carcinoma of the esophagus, with an incidence in the United States of 2.5 cases per 100,000 population, causes 2% of all cancer deaths. There is a 3 : 1 male preponderance. The disease usually occurs in men over 60. Fifty percent of the cancers involve the lower third of the esophagus, 35% the middle, and 15% the upper or cervical esophagus. The neoplasms are usually squamous carcinomas except for gastroesophageal junction involvement by adenocarcinomas. There are marked geographic differences in incidence of carcinoma of the esophagus. In Japan there are 46 such cancers per 100,000 population (twenty times the American figure). The incidence is also markedly increased in China and South

Africa. Preexisting lye strictures, the Plummer-Vinson syndrome, and tobacco and alcohol abuse are all important etiologic factors in esophageal cancer.

The most common symptom, present in over 90% of patients with esophageal carcinomas, is dysphagia. There is usually marked weight loss. Pain from extraesophageal extension or metastases may also occur. There may also be cough and hemoptysis with a tracheoesophageal fistula, aspiration secondary to esophageal obstruction, or hoarseness secondary to mediastinal invasion and recurrent laryngeal nerve injury. An enlarged supraclavicular lymph node may also be the first manifestation of esophageal cancer.

As part of the physical examination, vocal cord mobility should be noted, and the regional lymph node areas should be palpated. Spine percussion may elicit pain from osseous metastases. The presence or absence of hepatomegaly should also be determined. A chest radiograph may reveal a mediastinal mass, pulmonary metastases, or thoracic vertebral compression fracture. A barium esophagogram should be obtained if esophageal carcinoma is suspected. Esophagoscopy and either punch or brush cytologic biopsies should be performed to make the diagnosis of esophageal cancer. Bronchoscopy and mediastinoscopy should both be considered. In a series of staging laparotomies, the celiac lymph nodes were not involved in any patients with cervical esophageal carcinomas, but 45% of those with midesophageal cancers and 55% of those with lower third lesions had positive nodes. When preoperative irradiation is to be used, a staging laparotomy is probably not indicated, as the liver and lymph nodes may be palpated and biopsied at the time of planned postirradiation resection.

Since esophageal carcinomas commonly extend to the mediastinal and celiac lymph nodes, only 25% to 40% of patients have resectable cancers. Ominous prognostic signs include complete esophageal obstruction, marked weight loss and cachexia, hemoptysis, esophageal perforation, deep wall invasion (which predisposes to wide submucosal lymphatic spread), and certain sites of involvement: patients with upper esophageal carcinomas have the worst prognosis.

Surgery is the treatment of choice for resectable lesions of the distal third of the esophagus. Esophagogastrectomy and single stage esophagogastrostomy are the most commonly performed procedures. Five-year survivals of 0% to 15% are obtained. Resection relieves dysphagia in approximately 90% of cases but has an operative mortality of 5% to 15%. The surgical results are poor for carcinomas of the upper half of the esophagus. Cervical esophageal cancers may invade the trachea or larynx. These tumors may be resected with staged reconstruction, or the esophagus may be resected and the stomach rerouted superiorly through a substernal tunnel to reduce the operative morbidity, and then anastomosed. In advanced cancers, palliation may be obtained by passing a Celestin esophageal tube. Seventy-five percent of patients treated in this way have noted improved swallowing and better palliation than could be obtained from a gastrostomy.

Radiation therapy may have either a curative or a palliative role in the treatment of carcinoma of the esophagus. If the primary lesion is larger than 10 cm, or if there are distant metastases, a tracheoesophageal fistula, suspected perforation, or lung extension, radiotherapy has only a palliative role in management. Radiation alone sterilizes approximately 30% to 50% of esophageal cancers but may make 40% to 67% of the lesions resectable. Radiotherapy does not palliate dysphagia as well as surgery, however (20% to 50% and 90% palliation, respectively). The best results with radiation therapy alone were achieved by Pearson [1969], who delivered 5000 rads in 4 weeks to the esophagus and found a 20% 5-year survival. Preoperative irradiation doses of 5000–6000 rads in 5 to 7 weeks, followed by esophagogastrectomy 3 to 8 weeks later if there are no celiac lymph node or liver metastases, has resulted in a 23% 5-year survival (6 of 26 patients). In a larger series of patients who received preoperative irradiation, a 14% 5-year survival was noted. Nakayama has also reported improved survival with a short preoperative radiation course (2000 rads in 5 fractions) followed by immediate esophagectomy and staged reconstruction. Possible complications of high-dose irradiation are pericarditis, pneumonitis, tracheitis, myelitis, delayed esophageal strictures, hemorrhage, and esophagobronchial fistulae. For resectable, smaller lesions, most authors recommend a combined radiation therapy–surgical approach. For advanced or locally advanced lesions, palliative irradiation or Celestin tube placement should be considered. To date there has been little gain from the use of chemotherapy in cancer of the esophagus.

D.G.

Doggett R, Guernsey J, Bagshaw M: Combined radiation and surgical treatment of carcinoma of the thoracic esophagus. Front Radiat Ther Oncol 5:147–154, 1970.
When celiac lymph nodes were biopsied the following was found: 0 in 9 positive, upper esophageal lesions; 9 in 20 (45%), middle third; 6 in 11 (55%), lower third.

Fraser R, Wara W, Thomas A, et al: Combined treatment methods for carcinoma of the esophagus. Radiology 128:461–465, 1978.
Preoperative radiation doses were 5000-6000 rads, and the resectability rate was 67%. Article recommends preoperative radiation and resection 3 to 8 weeks later only if celiac lymph nodes and liver are uninvolved at laparotomy.

Goodner J: Surgical and radiation treatment of cancer of the thoracic esophagus. Am J Roentgenol 105:523–528, 1969.
In 260 patients at Memorial-Sloan Kettering there was a 6.1% 5-year survival.

Marks R Jr, Scruggs H, Wallace K: Preoperative radiation therapy for carcinoma of the esophagus. Cancer 38:84–89, 1976.
Preoperative radiation was planned in 332 patients; 101 had resections, with a 5-year survival of 13.6%. There was 5% survival in patients whose carcinomas were not resectable.

Pearson J: Value of radiotherapy in management of esophageal cancer. Am J Roentgenol 105:500–513, 1969.
20% of patients treated by 5000 rads to esophagus over 4 weeks without surgery were 5-year survivors.

Rubin P: Cancer of the gastrointestinal tract: II. Esophagus. JAMA 227:175–185, 1974.
Five authors describe surgery alone, radiation alone, the two modalities combined, and results of pretreatment laparotomies.

---

43. STOMACH CANCER—PRIMARY OR REGIONAL

For unknown reasons the incidence of stomach cancer has decreased in the United States over the last four decades from a peak of 35 cases per 100,000 males and 19 per 100,000 females in the 1930s to 8 and 4 per 100,000 respectively at the present time. There is still a high incidence of stomach cancer in Japan. In the United States the disease peaks at ages 50 to 59. The risk of gastric cancer is increased in males, in those living in colder climates, in lower socioeconomic classes, possibly in those with A blood group, and in patients with pernicious anemia and achlorhydria. At least 95% of gastric cancers are adenocarcinomas. There are four general types: superficial spreading, linitis plastica, ulcerating, and polypoid. The remaining malignant primary gastric tumors are lymphomas and leiomyosarcomas.

The location of gastric carcinomas in the stomach, the symptoms caused by these neoplasms, and their diagnostic evaluation are discussed in Part II, Chapter 25.

Unfortunately lymph nodes are involved in 80% of patients with gastric cancers, while 40% have peritoneal involvement and 33% have hepatic metastases at the time of diagnosis. The surgical procedure of choice is radical subtotal gastrectomy, in which the stomach, regional lymph nodes, omenta, and spleen, as well as the tail of the pancreas, if necessary, are resected. Gastrointestinal continuity is restored by a Billroth I or II anastomosis. A total gastrectomy may be necessary for more advanced lesions, but this procedure is associated with decreased survival and increased mortality as well as postoperative pernicious anemia and iron deficiency anemia. If an obstructive gastric lesion is present or there is recurrent hemorrhage, a palliative gastric resection may be indicated. The survival for all patients undergoing gastric resections is only 10% but ranges from 60% for the small number of patients with uninvolved regional lymph nodes to few or no survivors with patients with lymph node involvement.

Radiation therapy has only a palliative role alone in the treatment of gastric cancer. Doses of 5000–5500 rads may be delivered but rarely control unresected gastric carcinomas. When lower radiation doses (3500–4000 rads in 3½ to 4 weeks) were used to treat locally unresectable gastric cancers, with and without intravenous 5-fluorouracil, 15 mg/kg, on the first three radiation days, significantly prolonged survival was noted for the group that received combined radiation and 5-FU.

Gastric lymphomas are rare (5% of gastric malignancies) but may mimic primary adenocarcinomas of the stomach. These lesions should be resected by a subtotal gastrectomy. In 50 consecutive cases of gastric lymphoma, survivals of 90% to 80% were obtained for patients with only mucosal or submucosal involvement, respectively. For patients with penetration of the gastric wall by lymphoma or regional lymph node involvement, survival decreased to 24% and 32%, respectively. Local recurrences were also apparently decreased by postoperative irradiation. A standard lymphoma evaluation consisting of chest radiographs, lymphangiogram, bone marrow biopsy, and excretory urography is recommended for those with gastric lymphomas. Radiotherapy portals should cover at least the entire upper abdomen, delivering 4000–4400 rads to the resection bed and regional lymph nodes in 5 to 6 weeks, while at the same time giving 2000–2200 rads to the remainder of the liver and 3500–4000 rads to the bowel.

Leiomyosarcomas are rare, accounting for only 1% to 3% of gastric malignancies. They are best managed by gastrectomy, but radiation therapy and chemotherapy (Adriamycin-DTIC) may palliate symptomatic local or metastatic neoplasm.

D.G.

Buchholtz TW, Welch CE, Malt RA: Clinical correlates of resectability and survival in gastric carcinoma. Ann Surg 188:711–715, 1978.
   In a 10-year follow-up study of 201 patients actual survival was 11% and 7% at 5 and 10 years, respectively.
del Regato JA, Spjut HJ: Cancer of the digestive tract/stomach. *In* L Ackerman and JA del Regato (Eds), Cancer: Diagnosis, Treatment and Prognosis. St. Louis, Mo., C.V. Mosby, 1977. Pp. 463–493.
   Thorough review of the subject.

Lim F, Hartman A, Tan E, et al: Factors in the prognosis of gastric lymphomas. Cancer 39:1715–1720, 1977.
50 cases of gastric lymphoma were analyzed. Prognosis was worse when there was penetration through serosa or regional lymph node involvement.

Mayo H Jr, Owens J, Weinberg M: A critical evaluation of radical subtotal gastric resection as a definitive procedure for antral gastric carcinoma. Am J Surg 141:830–839, 1955.
In this large series there were no survivors if regional nodes were involved by carcinoma.

Moertel C, Reitemeier R, Childs D Jr, et al: Combined 5-FU and supervoltage radiation therapy of locally unresectable gastrointestinal cancer. Cancer 2:865–867, 1969.
Article discusses a randomized study of 3500–4000 rads vs similar radiation doses plus 5-FU, 15 mg/kg, given intravenously, on the first 3 days of irradiation. Significantly prolonged survival was noted in the 5-FU–XRT group.

44. COLORECTAL CANCER—PRIMARY OR REGIONAL

Carcinoma of the colon and rectum is a common malignancy, second only to lung cancer in the number of deaths due to cancer (51,000 yearly). It is most commonly diagnosed in patients over 60 years of age. The male-female ratio is approximately equal. Most colon cancers are adenocarcinomas, but squamous carcinomas and, rarely, cloacogenic carcinomas are found in the rectum. Fifty percent of these cancers occur in the rectum, 20% in the sigmoid colon, and 16% in the cecum.

There is evidence that colorectal carcinomas can arise from neoplastic colonic polyps. In addition, patients with hereditary familial polyposis have a greatly increased risk of developing colon cancers. There is also an increased cancer risk in ulcerative colitis, which varies with the age of the patient and with the duration and extent of colonic involvement by the colitis. Dietary factors may also be important in the etiology of colorectal carcinoma, as there is a markedly decreased frequency of these neoplasms in Africans and others whose diets are high in fiber. Symptoms from colorectal cancers depend on the anatomic site of involvement. Cecal lesions may be asymptomatic for long periods of time, but may ultimately cause anemia and occult rectal bleeding, progressive weight loss, and right lower quadrant abdominal pain or a palpable mass. Rarely, ileocecal obstruction may be produced. Left colonic carcinomas usually produce obstructive symptoms, with weight loss, decreased stool caliber, abdominal pain, fatigue, and often gross blood from the rectum. Rectal carcinomas cause not only decreased stool caliber but also gross rectal bleeding and tenesmus.

The diagnostic evaluation of colon polyps is described in Part II, Chapter 26. When a colon carcinoma is suspected, a history of the above symptoms may be elicited, or the patient may have familial polyposis or ulcerative colitis. The examination should include careful assessment of hepatic size and a search for abdominal masses. The inguinal, iliac, and supraclavicular lymph node regions should all be palpated. A rectal examination, with a test for fecal occult blood, is mandatory. A barium enema should be performed, with air contrast enhancement if necessary. Proctoscopic examination may allow visualization and biopsy of the lesion. A chest radiograph may reveal metastases. Patients with bulky colorectal masses should be considered for excretory urography and cystoscopy. Colonoscopy may also be necessary. A complete blood count and chemical screening battery, including liver function tests, should be performed. Liver and bone scans are obtained if indicated. Carcinoembryonic antigen (CEA) is not specific for colorectal cancer but may be elevated in 40% of patients with localized carcinomas, in 50% with lymph node involvement, and in 80% to 90% with metastases. An elevated CEA titer in the immediate postoperative period suggests the presence of metastases or residual carcinoma. If the CEA titer rises during follow-up, it may signify recurrent carcinoma.

Colorectal carcinomas are managed primarily by surgery. Polyps and villous adenomas should be resected, and total colectomy should be considered for patients with familial polyposis and perhaps for those with ulcerative colitis. Carcinoma of the colon does not extend longitudinally along the bowel wall to the extent that esophageal carcinoma does, averaging only 1 to 2 cm from the primary mass, but does invade regional tissues and extend through the bowel wall (50% to 70% of patients). It also frequently metastasizes to lymph nodes (50% to 60%). Residual masses or areas at risk for recurrence should be marked at surgery with metallic clips for later radiotherapeutic localization. A left colectomy is ordinarily performed for carcinomas of the cecum or ascending colon. A left colectomy and partial transverse colectomy are carried out for hepatic flexure cancers, while a transverse colectomy is necessary for lesions of that segment of colon. For splenic flexure or sigmoid lesions, a left colectomy is performed; and for more distal lesions an anterior resection is carried out if a 4 cm distal margin can be obtained. The adjacent mesentery and associated lymph nodes are also resected with the specimen. Low rectal carcinomas are usually managed by an abdominoperineal resection. An en bloc resection of involved organs is performed at the time of the initial colectomy, which should be carried out by the "no-touch" technique. In massive or obstructive lesions a colostomy may be necessary for fecal diversion.

Only 60% to 70% of patients with colorectal carcinomas are operable, and the overall 5-year survival after surgery is 27% to 30%. The prognosis is excellent for patients with uninvolved lymph nodes whose tumor is confined to the bowel wall, with survival approaching 100% in this small group. Of patients with negative lymph nodes but extension through the bowel wall (Duke's B_2), approximately 70% will relapse without further treatment. When the tumor has both extended through the wall and involved the lymph nodes, 85% of patients will relapse. Additional therapy should be considered for patients with advanced carcinomas that have extended through the bowel wall and/or metastasized to regional lymph nodes. For patients undergoing "second-look" operations after colectomy, Gunderson [1974] determined that, when patients relapsed, 92% of failures occurred locally, with or without distant metastases. Distant metastases only were noted in just 8% of the patients.

Radiation therapy of the primary cancer may be used palliatively when a patient has refused surgery, in inoperable or poor-risk patients, or when a painful, obstructive mass is present. In one series, 9 of 16 inoperable cancers were made resectable by radiation doses of approximately 5000 rads in 5 to 6 weeks, and a 23% 5-year survival rate was obtained. In another series of 65 selected patients with inoperable colorectal carcinomas, radiotherapy alone produced 29% 5-year survivals. Therefore, radiotherapy of the primary neoplasm may be used palliatively but is not a substitute for resection of operable lesions. In a Veterans Administration study, low-dose preoperative radiotherapy (2000–2500 rads) significantly increased survival (41%) of patients who received abdominoperineal (AP) resections as compared to those who received AP resections alone (28%). Higher preoperative radiation doses of 4000 to 4500 rads have caused no increased morbidity and may also have prolonged survival (in nonrandomized studies). A lower than expected incidence of lymph node involvement was noted in the surgical specimens from the irradiated patients.

Postoperative irradiation should be considered for patients with locally advanced colorectal cancers, based on the data of Gunderson, where the risk of local recurrence is high: in stage B_2 (negative nodes, extension through bowel wall), C_1 (positive nodes, wall intact), and C_2 (positive nodes, extension through wall). Local recurrences were markedly reduced in 62 patients given 5000 rads to the tumor bed in 5 to 6 weeks postoperatively, as compared to those patients who did not receive postoperative irradiation. The radiation fields for both preoperative and postoperative irradiation include the pelvis and in most cases the para-aortic lymph nodes.

Inferior rectal carcinomas may also be managed by cautery, interstitial radioactive source implants, or contact teletherapy. In France, Papillon [1975] has devised a 50 kV superficial treatment source with a special rectoscope that delivers 10,000–15,000 rads in four equal weekly 2500–4000-rad doses. Selection criteria for this treatment include (1) well-differentiated carcinomas only, (2) accessible lesions no further than 12 cm from the anal verge, (3) lesions smaller than 3×5 cm in greatest dimension, and (4) cancers clinically confined to the bowel wall. Poorly differentiated, large, or deeply invasive lesions have a high risk of lymph node metastases and are not suitable for this therapy. In Papillon's series 101 of 133 patients are without evidence of diseases 5 years after irradiation, and 3 of the 11 with local failures were salvaged by resection.

Adjuvant trials using postoperative chemotherapy have failed to show consistent advantage for either single or multiple drugs in preventing local relapses or improving survival. 5-FU, either intravenously or orally, produced only transient responses in a small proportion of patients. However, when 5-FU, 15 mg/kg, was given intravenously on the first three days of a 4000-rad radiation course, a significantly prolonged survival for patients with advanced colorectal cancers was noted.

Immunotherapy with BCG has been tried in both controlled and nonrandomized studies. Again, it has been difficult to prove a definite advantage for BCG in controlled postoperative trials. A single study with limited follow-up revealed improved relapse-free survival for postoperative BCG or BCG–5-FU compared to *historical controls*. However, other prospective trials have failed to show that immunotherapy improves either the results of surgery or adjuvant postoperative chemotherapy.

Follow-up examinations should involve a search for either local, regional, or distant relapses. Periodic chest radiographs, liver function studies, and stool occult blood tests at each rectal examination are all important. Serial CEA examinations may be performed, with sudden titer elevations in the postoperative period suggesting recurrent carcinoma. Barium enema and proctoscopy may be alternated with colonoscopy on a yearly basis.

D.G.

Gunderson L, Sosin H: Areas of failure found at reoperation (second or symptomatic look) following "curative surgery" for adenocarcinoma of the rectum. Cancer 34:1278–1291, 1974.
In 92% of failures local relapse was part of the recurrence. Only 8% had distant metastases without a local recurrence. Patients with B_2, C_1, and C_2 cancers have a 70 to 85% risk of local recurrence.
Higgins G Jr: Surgical considerations in colorectal cancer. Cancer 39:891–895, 1977.
Review article.
Higgins G, Humphrey E, Jules G, et al: Adjuvant chemotherapy in the surgical treatment of large bowel cancer. Cancer 38:1461–1467, 1976.
Adjuvant 5-FU did not significantly improve postoperative survival.

Kligerman M: Pre-operative radiation therapy in rectal cancer. Cancer 36:691–695, 1975.
Administration of 5500 rads probably improved survival and also reduced the expected number of lymph node metastases and deeply invasive cancers.

Kligerman M: Irradiation of the primary lesion of the rectum and rectosigmoid. JAMA 231:1381–1384, 1975.
Good review article.

Mavligit G, Burgess J, Seibert G, et al: Prolongation of post-operative disease-free interval and survival in human colorectal cancer by BCG or BCG plus 5-FU. Lancet I:871–876, 1975.
Use of BCG or BCG plus 5-FU, when compared to historical controls, apparently improved both short-term (less than 30 months) relapse-free survival and actuarial survival.

Papillon J: Resectable rectal cancers. Treatment by curative endocavitary irradiation. JAMA 231:1385–1387, 1975.
Of 133 patients 101 were alive without evidence of disease at 5 years. 3 of 11 local failures were salvaged by subsequent resection. Author followed strict criteria for selection of contact radiotherapy.

Romsdahl M, Withers H: Radiotherapy combined with curative surgery. Arch Surg 113:446–453, 1978.
62 patients who received 5000 rads in 6 weeks postoperatively had fewer local recurrences than resected patients not given radiation.

Roswit B, Higgins G, Keehn R: Pre-operative irradiation for carcinoma of the rectum and sigmoid. Cancer 35:1597–1602, 1975.
Improved results were noted in a controlled trial but only in patients who underwent A-P resections.

Turnbull R: Cancer of the colon. The influence of the "no-touch" technique on survival rates. Ann Surg 166:420–427, 1967.
The "no-touch" technique of colon resection may improve survival and decrease distant metastases.

Urdaneta-Lafee N, Kligerman M, Knowlton A: Evaluation of palliative irradiation in rectal carcinoma. Radiology 104:673–677, 1972.
9 of 16 inoperable patients underwent resection after irradiation. There was a 23% 5-year survival.

Wanebo HJ, Rao B, Pinsky CM, et al: Preoperative carcinoembryonic antigen level as a prognostic indicator in colorectal cancer. N Engl J Med 299:448–451, 1978.
Recurrence rate was higher and disease-free interval shorter with CEA > 5 ng/ml.

45. PANCREATIC CANCER—PRIMARY OR REGIONAL

Pancreatic carcinoma is a common malignancy (23,000 new cases in 1979) with a very poor prognosis. It ranks fifth in the number of cancer deaths (20,200 yearly), behind lung, colorectal, breast, and prostate carcinomas, respectively. Carcinoma of the pancreas has a peak age of 60 years and there is a 3 : 1 male preponderance. 90% of the neoplasms are adenocarcinomas, 66% arising in the head and 33% in the body and tail of the pancreas. Islet cell tumors are less common pancreatic neoplasms. Most islet cell tumors are functional (10% malignant, 10% multiple), although a few are nonsecreting (50% of these are malignant). Non-islet cell tumors and cystadenocarcinomas also occur but are quite rare. Pancreatic carcinoma may have an etiologic association with excessive tobacco use, calcific pancreatitis, and exposure to certain chemicals such as benzidene, but a proved cause-effect relationship has yet to be shown.

The symptoms of pancreatic carcinoma depend on the anatomic site of involvement. Those neoplasms that involve the pancreatic head and/or the ampulla of Vater result in progressive jaundice usually, a palpable gallbladder in 50% of cases, and epigastric pain in 33% of the patients. The stool test for occult blood may be positive. Patients with carcinomas in the body of the pancreas may experience back pain, while those with lesions in the tail may have no symptoms until the mass is quite large. All pancreatic carcinomas may be associated with weight loss, nausea and vomiting, anorexia, phlebitis, mild diabetes, and perhaps steatorrhea.

Islet cell tumors may produce morning fatigue, malaise, and restlessness, but severe hypoglycemic symptoms resulting in coma may also occur. The fasting blood sugar is usually less than 50 mg/ml during an attack, but consciousness is promptly restored by administration of glucose. Non-beta cell tumors may cause the Zollinger-Ellison syndrome, consisting of multiple peptic ulcers that often occur in such unusual locations as the small bowel, with or without diarrhea. There are also large volumes of fasting gastric juice and a marked increase in gastric acid output.

A careful history should elicit the above symptoms. Physical examination may ascertain the presence of an abdominal mass, hepatomegaly, enlarged lymph nodes, or occult stool blood as well as evidence of phlebitis. The WBC, PCV, amylase, and lipase examinations are usually normal. Liver function tests should be obtained, since the alkaline phosphatase is usually markedly elevated in obstructive jaundice. CEA titers, although not specific, may be elevated in 90% of patients with pancreatic carcinomas.

A recent prospective study in 70 patients has shown that one of the most accurate, noninvasive initial tests for pancreatic carcinoma is an abdominal ultrasound examination. If this study is negative, pancreatic function tests (cholecystokinin-stimulated enzyme outputs) should then be performed. If either of these tests has given abnormal results, an endoscopic retrograde choledochopancreatogram (ERCP) is indicated. The above three examinations may provide the diagnosis with almost 90% accuracy. If the ERCP test cannot be performed, pancreatic arteriography should be considered. Other diagnostic tests that may be useful are hypotonic duodenography and CT scans. CT scans may not detect small lesions (<10 cm) but have a 64% to 85% accuracy rate in detecting larger pancreatic carcinomas. Transhepatic cholangiography may assist the surgeon in demonstrating the level of bile duct obstruction. Duodenal cytology lacks accuracy, as do pancreatic scintiscans. A liver biopsy may make the diagnosis when metastases are suspected. A tissue diagnosis may also be made by "skinny needle" aspiration cytology without laparotomy. This technique has diagnosed pancreatic carcinoma in 80% (14 of 18 patients) in whom cancer was suspected prior to biopsy.

Surgery is the treatment of choice for pancreatic carcinomas. However, 80% to 90% of patients have lymph node involvement, and 70% have liver metastases at the time of diagnosis. A Whipple procedure (radical pancreaticoduodenectomy) may be performed for carcinomas involving the head of the pancreas or of the ampulla of Vater. Cancers involving the body or tail of the pancreas are rarely operable, since they are usually not detected until far advanced. Contraindications to the Whipple procedure are the presence of distant metastases or invasion of the inferior vena cava or portal vein. There is a high mortality from this procedure, and most series reveal a 5-year survival of 10% or less. Postoperatively diabetes or steatorrhea may both occur. If the lesion is unresectable, a palliative bypass, including cholecystojejunostomy or choledochojejunostomy, may be performed. Metallic clips should mark the tumor and any local areas of extension for future radiation therapy postoperatively. Unfortunately, despite radical resection, 90% of patients with pancreatic carcinomas die in 1 year and only 2% usually survive for 5 years.

The other, rare pancreatic tumors may also be approached surgically. Islet cell cancers may be enucleated if benign, or resected with a margin of normal tissue if malignant. Cystadenocarcinomas should also be resected. Non-beta cell carcinomas may be resected primarily, but total gastrectomy is usually necessary for patients with severe Zollinger-Ellison syndrome.

Until recently radiation therapy was felt to have only a palliative role in carcinoma of the pancreas. The close proximity of the spinal cord, kidneys, liver, and surrounding bowel have all sharply limited the total radiation dose safely deliverable to the pancreatic region. However, when 23 patients with unresectable pancreatic carcinomas were given a split course of irradiation and total doses of 6000 rads in 8 to 10 weeks, 1-year survival of 34% was noted, with a median survival of 7½ months; 20% of those patients survived for 5 years. In another series, in 7 to 9 weeks 18 patients received 6300–6700 rads from a 45 meV Betatron, through three or four radiation fields, either with photons alone or with mixed photon-electron beams. Fifty-nine percent of these patients survived for 12 months, and 7 have no evidence of disease. Therefore radiation therapy may be able to provide long-term palliation in a limited number of patients with pancreatic carcinomas. Another radiation modality currently being studied is Iodine[125] seed implants in patients with unresectable but localized cancers. Trials of such high linear energy transfer (LET) radiation sources as fast neutrons are also being carried out.

No chemotherapeutic agents have given consistently good results or high response rates in pancreatic carcinomas. When 5-FU, 15 mg/kg, was given on the first three days of a 4000-rad radiotherapy course, however, survival was significantly increased over that of irradiated patients who had not received 5-FU (from 6.3 to 10 months). Patients with recurrent or metastatic islet cell tumors may receive palliation from streptozotocin. Retroperitoneal or epigastric pain secondary to locally extensive pancreatic carcinoma may also be palliated by a percutaneous celiac ganglion anesthetic block.

D.G.

Abrams H, McNeil B: Medical implications of computed tomography. N Engl J Med 298:310–318, 1978.
   An excellent review of CT scanning by organ site as well as an analysis of its benefits in patient management.
Brooks JR: Operative approach to pancreatic carcinoma. Semin Oncol 6:357–367, 1979.
   An excellent review of surgical management, results, and treatment complications, as well as surgical technique.
Brooks J, Culebras J: Cancer of the pancreas: Palliative operations, Whipple procedure or total pancreatectomy. Am J Surg 131:516–520, 1976.
   Authors conclude that total pancreatectomy is equally (or perhaps more) effective than the Whipple procedure for stages I and II carcinomas.
Carter S, Comis R: The integration of chemotherapy into a combined modality approach for cancer treatment: VI. Pancreatic adenocarcinoma. Cancer Treat Rev 2:193–214, 1975.
   Excellent review of all treatment modalities.
DiMagno E, Malegelada J, Taylor W, Go VLW: A prospective comparison of current diagnostic tests for pancreatic cancer. N Engl J Med 297:737–742, 1977.
   70 patients were studied. Recommended sequence of evaluation (89% accu-

racy) was first an ultrasound test, then a pancreatic function test (cholecystokinin-stimulated enzyme outputs) if ultrasound negative. If either was positive, endoscopic retrograde choledochopancreatography was performed.

Dobelbower RR Jr: The radiotherapy of pancreatic cancer. Semin Oncol 6:378–389, 1979.

Review of external beam and interstitial irradiation techniques, plus combined modality treatment.

Dobelbower RR Jr, Borgelt B, Suntharalingam N, Strubler K: Pancreatic carcinoma treated with high-dose, small-volume irradiation. Cancer 41:1087–1092, 1978.

45 MeV betatron irradiation was used, with either three or four field techniques consisting of mixed photon-electron beams. The median survival was 12 months in 18 patients. Seven patients were free of disease 11.5 to 57 months after diagnosis; results were comparable to those from radical resection.

Ferucci J, Eaton S: Radiology of the pancreas. N Engl J Med 288:506–510, 1973.

Excellent review of all procedures except CT scans.

The Gastrointestinal Tumor Study Group. A multi-institutional comparative trial of radiation therapy alone and in combination with 5-fluorouracil for locally unresectable pancreatic carcinoma. Ann Surg 189:205–208, 1979.

Median survival was significantly better for those receiving combined treatment (36–40 weeks) as compared to radiation therapy alone (20 weeks) in 89 patients studied.

Goldstein H, Zornoza J, Wallace S, et al: Percutaneous fine needle aspiration biopsy of pancreatic and other abdominal masses. Radiology 123:319–322, 1977.

Correct or presumptive diagnosis in 14 of 18 patients with suspected pancreatic carcinoma was made by "skinny needle" aspiration biopsy.

Haslam J, Cavanaugh P, Stroup S: Radiation therapy in the treatment of unresectable carcinoma of the pancreas. Cancer 32:1341–1345, 1973.

In 23 patients with unresectable cancers there was 34% survival at 12 months and a median 7.5 month survival.

Robbins AH, Gerzof SG, Pugatch RD: Newer imaging techniques for the diagnosis of pancreatic cancer. Semin Oncol 6:332–343, 1979.

CT, ultrasound, and needle biopsy techniques all discussed.

Rosch J, Keller FS, Bilbao MK: Radiologic diagnosis of pancreatic cancer. Semin Oncol 6:318–331, 1979.

Review of radiologic procedures.

Schein P, Kahan R, Gorden P, et al: Streptozotocin for malignant insulinomas and carcinoid tumors. Arch Intern Med 132:555–561, 1973.

In 4 patients with insulinomas there was a complete response to the drug.

Tepper J, Nardi G, Suit H: Carcinoma of the pancreas. Cancer 37:1519–1524, 1976.

Review of 145 patients treated at the Massachusetts General Hospital.

46. CARCINOID—PRIMARY OR REGIONAL

Carcinoid tumors, accounting for 1.5% of all malignancies, are found in 1 of every 300 appendectomy specimens. These neoplasms are one of the APUD (amine precursor uptake and decarboxylation) tumors. Carcinoids are the most common neoplasms of the appendix and small bowel, and in the rectum second in frequency only to adenomatous polyps. Most of these carcinoids are found incidentally during surgery for other conditions. The age at diagnosis for patients with carcinoids ranges from 14 to 88 years, with most cases occurring between 40 and 50. Patients with carcinoids have a 25% to 33% risk of developing other carcinomas, especially adenocarcinomas of the gastrointestinal tract. Coexistent neoplasms such as parathyroid adenomas, non-beta cell pancreatic islet tumors, and eosinophilic pituitary tumors have also been reported. Ninety percent of carcinoids are located in the gastrointestinal tract: most are found in the midgut, with a smaller number involving foregut structures. The remaining 10% are found in the lung (arising from bronchial epithelium) and in ovarian teratomas. The ileum is the primary site of involvement in 28% of cases, the rectum in 24%, appendix in 22%, lung in 8%, colon in 7%, stomach in 3%, and miscellaneous sites in the remaining 8%. Forty percent of carcinoids are multiple, since the enterochromaffin cells of origin are widespread throughout the gastrointestinal mucosa.

Carcinoids occur submucosally and spread either by direct invasion or through lymphatic or hematogenous routes. The rate of distant metastases varies with the site of origin. Three percent of appendiceal carcinoids metastasize. Metastases are present in 33% of ileal-jejunal and in 79% of ileocecal carcinoids. A large percentage of bronchial carcinoids metastasize early. An overall metastatic rate of 38% has been noted, but in only 18% was the carcinoid syndrome produced. Since vasoactive substances are inactivated by the liver (and probably the lung also), hepatic metastases must occur from gastrointestinal primaries to produce the carcinoid syndrome. The malignant carcinoid syndrome can occur without metastases from primary bronchial carcinoids or ovarian teratoma, since the tumor secretions enter the circulation and bypass the liver. Only 5% of patients with abdominal lymph node or peritoneal involvement alone (without hepatic metastases) experience the carcinoid syndrome.

Carcinoid tumors secrete a variety of substances: elevated serotonin, kinin, histamine, catecholamine, prostaglandin, insulin, ACTH, gastrin, glucagon, and parahormone levels have all been reported. The particular substances secreted by a tumor determine whether or not the carcinoid syndrome will occur. The classic carcinoid syndrome occurs most often in patients with midgut primary tumors and liver metastases. Early in the syndrome episodic palpitations, diarrhea, and abdominal cramps occur. Later, when the full carcinoid syndrome has developed, flushes occur due to secretion of the enzyme kallikrein, which leads to a release of bradykinin, producing vasodilation; cramping and diarrhea are due to 5-hydroxytryptamine (serotonin) release. The late effects of all these vasoactive substances on the endocardium may be right-sided congestive heart failure with pulmonary congestion, edema, ascites, and hepatomegaly. The carcinoid syndrome may be induced by emotional changes or by such foods as milk, cheese, and eggs. Late in the course, the mesentery may be shortened and fibrosed, producing bowel obstruction and retroperitoneal and endocardial fibrosis.

When carcinoids are located in the foregut (biliary tract, pancreas, stomach, or duodenum), histamine may be released rather than serotonin, producing an atypical syndrome with patchy flushing, lacrimation, facial edema, and peptic ulceration. Since foregut carcinoids usually secrete hydroxytryptophan rather than 5-HT, fewer episodes of such abdominal symptoms as diarrhea and cramping occur with neoplasms in this location. Foregut tumors may also elaborate other substances, such as insulin, glucagon, and gastrin, which by their effects may mask the carcinoid syndrome.

5-HTP, 5-HT, and histamine may all be secreted by bronchial carcinoids.

Neoplasms in this site may produce severe symptoms of tremulousness, disorientation, prolonged flushing, nausea and vomiting, diarrhea, hypotension, headaches, lacrimation, and pulmonary and facial edema.

In addition to the carcinoid syndrome, right lower quadrant abdominal pain, intestinal obstruction due to prolapse or intussusception, or gastrointestinal bleeding may also occur.

A careful history of complaints referable to the carcinoid syndrome should be obtained. In asymptomatic patients the diagnosis is usually made fortuitously during surgery for another condition. The physical examination should include estimation of liver size, the presence or absence of a hepatic friction rub, abdominal tenderness, masses, or hyperperistalsis. Any skin flushing should be noted, lymph node areas palpated, wheezing detected, and blood pressure obtained. The complete blood count and chemical screening panel may both be normal early in the course of patients with carcinoid tumors; however, the WBC and platelet counts may be elevated and a fever present during the carcinoid syndrome. Carcinoids that secrete serotonin (midgut location) have an associated elevation of urine 5-hydroxyindoleacetic acid (5-HIAA), usually greater than 20 to 30 mg/24 hours. The 24-hour urine values may be as high as 60 to 1000 mg. There is also an increased serotonin concentration in blood and platelets. False-positive 5-HIAA urine elevations may be caused by ingestion of serotonin-rich foods, such as bananas, or drugs (glyceryl guaiacolate). 5-HIAA in the urine may be slightly increased in patients with celiac disease, tropical sprue, or Whipple's disease. False-negative 5-HIAA determinations may be obtained in patients using compazine and thorazine. Foregut and bronchial carcinoids may elaborate greater quantities of 5-HTP than 5-HT (serotonin). However, both blood and urine 5-HTP and 5-HT concentrations may be increased secondary to metabolism of these two substances. In a patient in whom the carcinoid syndrome is suspected, epinephrine, 5 μg intradermally, may produce the characteristic flushing. Chest radiographs may reveal a bronchial mass or pulmonary metastases. A liver scan may demonstrate either hepatomegaly or multiple liver metastases. Ultrasound and CT scans may also aid in detecting hepatic metastases. A barium enema and upper GI series may reveal the primary neoplasm or demonstrate the characteristic late findings of retroperitoneal fibrosis and/or bowel obstruction. Gastroscopy may allow visualization and biopsy of a primary carcinoid in the stomach or duodenum. Arteriography often indirectly confirms the diagnosis when stellate vascular changes, vascular kinking, and delayed venous opacification secondary to bowel and retroperitoneal fibrosis are present. Bronchoscopic biopsy may be necessary to the diagnosis of bronchial carcinoids, while liver biopsy may confirm the presence of metastases.

The carcinoid syndrome can be mimicked be secreting medullary thyroid carcinomas, ovarian teratomas, and small cell carcinomas of the lung. Right lower quadrant abdominal pain may also occur in acute appendicitis, Crohn's disease, primary carcinoma, and lymphoma of the bowel. Systemic mastocytosis may also cause flushing, but the 24-hour urinary 5-HIAA determination will be normal in this condition.

The proper surgical procedure for patients with the carcinoid syndrome depends on the size, location, and degree of malignancy of the tumor. When the carcinoid syndrome is present, curative surgery is possible only for patients with bronchial carcinoids or ovarian teratomas, since neoplasms of gastrointestinal origin cause the syndrome only after hepatic metastases have occurred. Segmental bowel and mesenteric resections, palliative removal of enlarged, symptomatic tumor masses, or partial hepatectomy may be necessary in selected cases. The surgical risks are apparently increased in these cases, as there is a greater likelihood of development of postoperative adhesions and/or the short bowel syndrome than after surgery for other abdominal malignancies.

Surgery may precipitate a carcinoid crisis, so the use of preoperative serotonin antagonists should be considered to avoid this complication. Radiotherapy has only a palliative role in the treatment of carcinoid tumors. Little information is available on the radiation doses and treatment techniques necessary to control carcinoids.

Emergency relief of carcinoid crisis from serotonin release may be obtained by prednisone, 15 to 30 mg daily. Phenothiazines and/or antihistamines may decrease the associated flushing of an acute attack. Nausea, vomiting, and diarrhea may also be reduced less acutely by inhibiting serotonin synthesis with parachlorophenylalanine or by the use of serotonin antagonists Sansert or Periactin. Methyldopa may be necessary if severe hypotension occurs. Diarrhea should be controlled by the use of Lomotil and restriction of eggs, milk, and cheese in the diet.

Patients with carcinoid tumors may have a life expectancy of 10 or more years, although most patients with malignant carcinoids eventually die from carcinomatosis. The median survival from the first episode of flushing was 38 months in one series. If 24-hour 5-HIAA urinary excretion was 10 to 49 mg, a median survival of 29 months was noted. For those with 50 to 149 mg of 5-HIAA in 24 hours, the median survival was 21 months, while 13-month survivals were noted when 5-HIAA levels exceeded 150 mg in 24 hours.

D.G.

Davis Z, Moertel C, McIrath D: The malignant carcinoid syndrome. Surg Gynecol Obstet 137:637–644, 1973.
   In 94 patients survival varied inversely with the 24-hour 5-HIAA excretion.
Friesen S: APUD tumors of the gastrointestinal tract. Curr Probl Cancer 1:37–41, 1976.
   Fifty-page review of the entire subject.
Kowlessar O: The carcinoid syndrome. *In* MH Sleisinger and JS Fordtran (Eds), Gastrointestinal Disease: Pathophysiology, Diagnosis, and Management. Philadelphia, W.B. Saunders, 1978. Pp. 1190–1200.
   Excellent review.
Martin R: Management of carcinoid tumors. Cancer 26:547–551, 1970.
   In this analysis of 59 cases the most common sites of involvement were ileum, rectum, and appendix.

47. RENAL CARCINOMA—PRIMARY OR REGIONAL

Approximately 16,900 new renal cancers (2% of all malignancies) and 7900 deaths from this neoplasm were predicted for 1980. There is a 2 : 1 male preponderance. Most new cases of renal carcinoma occur in the fifth and sixth decades. The etiologic factors associated with renal carcinomas are not known. Eighty-five percent of renal cancers are renal cell carcinomas. These neoplasms spread by direct extension and through lymphatic and hematogenous routes. At diagnosis, approximately 33% of patients have distant metastases, while 50% have extension through the renal capsule. Spontaneous regressions occur in less than 1% of cases.

Approximately 15% of all renal neoplasms are tumors of the renal pelvis and ureters. Most are transitional cell carcinomas, but squamous carcinomas and

adenocarcinomas are occasionally noted. There is a high risk of multiple carcinomas in these cases, perhaps through (1) multicentric origin, (2) lymphatic
spread, or (3) direct extension.

The most common symptoms of renal carcinoma, occurring in 70% of patients,
is painless microscopic or gross hematuria. Chronic flank pain affects 50% of
patients. The pain may be acute if ureteral clots are passed. Fever is noted by
approximately 15% of patients. Weight loss, anorexia, nausea, and vomiting
may also occur. Polycythemia is found in 3% of patients. Anemia, hypertension,
and high-output cardiac failure (vascular shunts in a hypervascular tumor)
may all be noted. If the inferior vena cava is obstructed, lower extremity edema
may result. If the hepatic veins are obstructed by local extension of the tumor,
ascites may develop. Rarely, a left varicocele may form if a renal tumor has
obstructed the left renal and testicular veins.

In the evaluation of a patient with a suspected renal carcinoma, a history of
the above symptoms should be sought. The physical examination includes an
abdominal examination for hepatomegaly or a palpable flank mass, noting the
presence or absence of lower extremity edema, a blood pressure determination,
and a scrotal examination for a varicocele. A complete blood count, liver and
renal function tests, measurement of serum calcium (to rule out hypercalcemia), and erythrocyte sedimentation rate (elevated in 33% of patients) should
be done. A urinalysis and urine cytologic test should also be obtained. A chest
radiograph may reveal pulmonary metastases. If an intravenous urogram reveals a renal mass, infusion nephrotomography may further delineate the mass
by differentiation between a renal cyst and a solid tumor. Cysts and solid
tumors may also be identified by an ultrasound examination. If a cyst is present, needle puncture with cytologic examination of the aspirated fluid may be
carried out. Selective renal arteriograms are almost 100% accurate in differentiating renal neoplasms (neovascularity) from inflammatory lesions or benign renal cysts. Cystoscopy and retrograde ureteral studies should include a
brush biopsy of the renal pelvis if tumor is suspected. Washings from the renal
pelvis should also be obtained for cytologic examination.

The therapy of choice for renal carcinomas is radical nephrectomy, including
the regional lymph nodes and surrounding perirenal fat. If a bulky tumor is
causing flank pain and hemorrhage, a palliative nephrectomy should be considered, even when metastases are present. Reported 5-year survivals after
nephrectomy alone are approximately 40% but may be as high as 60% when
renal cell carcinomas are localized to the kidney. When vein involvement or
lymph node metastases are present, however, or when tumors have extended
through the renal capsule, only 25% to 30% of patients can be expected to
survive for 5 years. Five-year survivals for those with distant metastases is less
than 5%.

Radiation therapy has been used preoperatively in a prospective trial in 141
patients. In this study the renal area received a radiation dose of 3000 rads in 3
weeks, but no differences in 5-year survival were noted between the irradiated
group and those patients treated by nephrectomy alone. However, even though
no differences in survival were noted, more advanced carcinomas were resectable in the irradiated group. In several series, 4500 rads given postoperatively
in 4½ to 5 weeks have apparently produced improved survival, especially when
perinephric fat, vascular or lymphatic involvement were noted.

Nephroureterectomy and resection of a bladder cuff are recommended for
patients with carcinomas of the ureter or renal pelvis, due to the high risk of
multicentric involvement. There is no proved role for postoperative irradiation
in these cancers. A 30% to 40% 5-year survival may be expected. In patients
with ureteral cancers, one series demonstrated a 52% 5-year survival for papillary cancers without invasion but only a 17% survival invasion was present.

When the primary tumor was nonpapillary or had extended into veins or lymphatics, only 4% to 7% 5-year survivals were noted.

Follow-up examinations should include routine chest radiographs, blood counts, and chemical screening batteries. Intravenous urograms are recommended at 1- to 2-year intervals, and regular cystoscopies and cytologic examination of bladder washings should also be performed.

D.G.

Batata M, Whitmore W Jr, Hilaris B, et al: Primary carcinoma of the ureter: A prognostic study. Cancer 35:1636–1632, 1975.
In 41 patients 5-year survivals ranged from 91% for early lesions confined to the submucosa to 0% for patients with extraureteral extension.

Clayman RV, Williams RD, Fraley EE: Current concepts in cancer: The pursuit of the renal mass. N Engl J Med 300:72–74, 1979.
Discusses the diagnostic approach to the asymptomatic renal mass.

Holland J: Cancer of the kidney—natural history and staging. Cancer 35:1030–1042, 1973.
Good review article.

Robson C, Churchill B, Anderson W: The results of radical nephrectomy for renal cell carcinoma. Trans Am Assoc Genitourin Surg 60:122–126, 1968.
In 88 patients there was a 66% 5-year survival if the cancer was confined to the kidney, 42% if vein or nodes were involved.

Rubin P, Keller B, Cox C: Preoperative irradiation in renal cancer. Evaluation of radiation treatment plans. Am J Roentgenol 123:114–121, 1975.
Rationale given for preoperative radiation therapy trial.

Van der Werf Messing B: Carcinoma of the kidney. Cancer 1056–1061, 1973.
141 patients were studied. One-half received 3000 rads (preoperative radiation therapy) in 3 weeks. There were no significant differences in 5-year survivals between those having preoperative radiation therapy and those having nephrectomy alone. However, more large lesions in the radiation therapy group were resectable than in the surgery alone group.

Wagle D, Moore R, Murphy G: Primary carcinoma of the renal pelvis. Cancer 33:1642–1648, 1974.
Nephroureterectomy and resection of a bladder cuff is the recommended treatment.

48. BLADDER CANCER—PRIMARY OR REGIONAL

Carcinoma of the bladder accounts for 3% of all deaths due to malignancies, occurs primarily in the 50 to 70 age group, and has a 2.5 : 1 male predominance. Thirty-five thousand five hundred new cases of bladder cancer were predicted for the United States in 1980. Bladder cancer is related to heavy tobacco use, as well as to exposure to aniline dyes and other chemicals, and to chronic bladder irritation from cystitis, calculi, and schistosomiasis. Ninety percent of bladder cancers are transitional cell carcinomas, occurring primarily on the posterior and lateral vesical walls, less frequently at the trigone. The other 10% are usually squamous carcinomas.

Seventy-five percent of patients with bladder cancers have hematuria, which may be intermittent and is usually painless. Such urinary symptoms as dysuria, frequency, and urgency may also be present in 30% to 50% of patients. If ureteral obstruction and hydronephrosis are present, flank pain may occur. A pelvic mass may be present with an advanced bladder cancer and there may be painful osseous metastases.

The history should take into account these etiologic factors and symptoms. Physical examination should include careful rectal palpation for evidence of posterior extension of the bladder neoplasm or a coincidental prostate carcinoma. Bone tenderness should be elicited, the abdomen should be examined, and a careful palpation of lymph node areas, including the supraclavicular regions, should also be carried out. Urinalysis, urine cytologic examination, and urine culture should all be obtained. Sterile urine cultures with symptoms of cystitis are suspicious for bladder cancer in most patients over 40 to 50. An excretory urogram is important and may show ureteral dilatation and hydronephrosis, ureteral deviation secondary to large retroperitoneal lymph nodes, or a bladder mass. If a bladder tumor is suspected, cystoscopy should be performed; the entire bladder should be inspected and adequate biopsies or resection of a tumor performed. The bimanual examination, including rectal palpation, should also be done under anesthesia at the time of cystoscopy. Routine studies such as complete blood count, chemical screening battery, and chest radiographs should be obtained. Bone scan, bladder arteriogram with intravesical or paravesical air insufflation, and lymphangiograms are all optional studies. A lymphangiogram may fail to opacify the internal iliac and obturator lymph nodes, commonly first involved by metastatic bladder cancer.

The histologic grade of a bladder cancer should be noted, but the most important single prognostic factor is the depth of invasion into the bladder wall. The most common staging system is that of Jewett and Marshall. Stage 0—in situ carcinoma; A—submucosal invasion; B_1—superficial muscle invasion; B_2—deep muscle invasion; C—extension of tumor through bladder wall; D_1—extension to pelvic organs; D_2—distant metastases. It should be remembered that considerable clinical inaccuracy exists in staging and that a particular tumor may be either more deeply invasive or less extensive than estimated on clinical examination. Tumors with a B_2 or deeper level of invasion all have a poor prognosis. Lymph nodes are involved in at least 50% of patients with deep muscular invasion.

Considerations for choosing therapeutic options in bladder carcinoma include the stage and grade of the tumor, its location in the bladder, the general medical condition of the patient, and the presence of other genitourinary or gastrointestinal diseases. Low-grade, superficial bladder cancers $(0,A,B_1)$ may be managed either by transurethral resection or by intravesical installation of thiotepa if the tumors are widespread. In selected patients with a sharply localized lesion on the dome or lateral bladder wall, a segmental resection may be performed. After multiple recurrences, cystectomy or external beam irradiation should be considered, while diffuse involvement by in situ carcinoma is often managed by cystectomy. Radiation therapy for superficially invasive bladder carcinomas usually consists of 6000–7000 rads to the bladder, with adequate margins, in 6 to 7 weeks, using rotational or multiple field techniques. The entire pelvis is not irradiated. The bladder is treated empty. Five-year survivals of 40% to 70% have been reported for both radiotherapy and cystectomy for superficial or noninvasive bladder cancers, depending on case selection and the number of surgical procedures performed prior to definitive treatment.

Invasive bladder carcinomas (B_2,C) may be managed by cystectomy and ileal loop diversion, external beam irradiation, or combined cystectomy and radiation therapy. Cystectomy has an operative mortality of approximately 5% and a 20% acute morbidity rate. Curative radiation therapy for invasive carcinoma delivers 4500–5000 rads to the pelvis in 5 to 6 weeks, followed by a booster dose to the bladder itself, usually by a small rotational field over an additional 2 weeks, for a total dose to the bladder of 6500–7000 rads in 7 to 8 weeks. Five-year survivals of 8% to 30% for cystectomy and 10% to 25% for radiotherapy have been reported. Approximately 50% of patients undergoing curative radiotherapy will have transient acute dysuria, urinary frequency, and diarrhea, all of which are self-limited. However, late, severe complications such as bowel stenosis or obstruction and bladder contraction occur in 5% to 15% of irradiated patients.

Five-year survivals with combined radiotherapy and cystectomy appear superior to those obtained by either cystectomy or external beam irradiation alone. Radiation doses of 2000 rads in 1 week (400 rads × 5), 4000 rads in 4 weeks, 4500 rads in 4½ weeks, and 5000 rads in 5 weeks to the pelvis have all been used. In a retrospective comparison of 4000 rads in 4 weeks and 2000 rads in 1 week followed by delayed and immediate cystectomy, respectively, no differences in survival rates, complications, or local recurrences were noted between the two radiation regimens. When tumor stage is reduced by preoperative radiation, there is apparently an improved prognosis (Van der Werf Messing, 1975). In a randomized study, preoperative irradiation, 5000 rads in 5 weeks, and cystectomy were compared to full-dose external beam irradiation alone for stages B_2 and C bladder cancers, and the combined modality group had significantly increased survival (50%) over the radiation alone group (20%). Most patients with invasive bladder cancers are now treated by one of the above combined radiotherapy-cystectomy techniques.

D.G.

Cummings KB, Shipley WU, Einstein AB, Cutler SJ: Current concepts in the management of patients with deeply invasive bladder carcinoma. Semin Oncol 6:220–228, 1979.
Complete review.

Goffinet D, Schneider M, Glatstein E, et al: Bladder cancer: Results of radiation therapy in 384 patients. Radiology 117:149–153, 1975.
In this large series, relapse-free survivals were determined for clinical stage A to D carcinomas.

Miller L: Bladder cancer: Superiority of preoperative irradiation and cystectomy in clinical stages B2 and C. Cancer 39:973–980, 1977.
5000 rads in 5 weeks followed by cystectomy significantly improved survival over radiation therapy alone.

Van der Werf Messing B: Carcinoma of the bladder $T_3N_XM_0$ treated by preoperative irradiation followed by cystectomy. Cancer 36:718–722, 1975.
There was increased survival when the extent of tumor was diminished by preoperative radiation therapy.

Whitmore W, Batata M, Ghoneim M, et al: Radical cystectomy with or without prior irradiation in the treatment of bladder cancer. J Urol 118:184–187, 1977.
In 451 patients there was nonrandomized but better survival in invasive tumors when cystectomy and radiation therapy were combined.

Whitmore W Jr, Batata M, Hilaris B, et al: A comparative study of two preoperative radiation regimens with cystectomy for bladder cancer. Cancer 40:1077–1086, 1977.
Nonrandomized comparison of results of administration of 4000 rads in 4 weeks and 2000 rads in 1 week preoperatively to true pelvis. There were no differences in survival rates, complications, or recurrences.

Carcinoma of the prostate accounts for 17% of male cancers (36/100,000 population) and causes 10% of the deaths due to cancer (approximately 20,000 yearly). Only lung and colorectal cancers are more lethal than carcinoma of the prostate. The predicted number of new cases for 1980 was 66,000 with 21,500 deaths. Prostatic cancer, the most common malignancy in men over 50, has a median age of onset of 70 years. The neoplasms, primarily adenocarcinomas, have a marked variability in their biologic behavior. Eighty-five percent of nodules affect the posterior lobes of the gland, while 15% are located more anteriorly, near the urethra. As the carcinoma enlarges, the prostatic sulci are obliterated, and invasion of the seminal vesicles, bladder, and levator muscles might occur. Prostatic cancers are commonly found on routine physical examination or in tissue obtained from transurethral resections of the prostate. The etiology is unknown.

Carcinoma of the prostate may be asymptomatic but may also be associated with such urinary symptoms as hesitancy, dribbling, decreased force of the urinary stream, and, rarely, terminal hematuria. In advanced carcinomas there may be uremia from bilateral ureteral obstruction, bone pain from osseous metastases, signs of spinal cord compression, lower extremity edema from venous obstruction, or enlarged lymph nodes, including those in the supraclavicular region.

The history may elicit any or all of these symptoms. A careful rectal examination is performed, noting the size of the prostate; the location, size, consistency, and extent of any nodules; and whether or not a nodule obliterates the lateral sulci or extends into the seminal vesicles. The regional lymph node areas and the supraclavicular fossa should be palpated, the abdomen examined, the spine percussed to elicit tenderness, and the lower extremities evaluated for edema and symmetry of reflexes and motor strength.

A complete blood count, urinalysis, chemical screening battery, serum creatinine analysis, and acid phosphatase determination should all be obtained. Cystoscopy with careful inspection of the bladder and prostatic urethra and simultaneous biopsy of the prostate either by the transrectal or by the transperineal route are also important. Excretory urograms may reveal ureteral obstruction, prostatic hypertrophy, or ureteral deviation secondary to enlarged lymph nodes. The KUB radiograph may also show blastic vertebral or pelvic metastases. A chest radiograph should also be obtained. A routine part of the evaluation in patients with prostate cancers is a bone scan, to be followed by detailed radiographs of areas where any abnormal isotope uptake on the bone scan was noted.

Surgical staging with extraperitoneal biopsy of pelvic lymph nodes has also been performed (in a research setting). This procedure has provided important information on the relative incidence of lymph node metastases for the various clinical stages of prostate carcinoma (next paragraph). Lymphoceles or lower extremity or scrotal edema occur in approximately 10% of patients after these lymph node biopsy procedures. Lymphangiograms have also been performed prospectively in a research setting. A false-negative rate of 27% has been reported, while as many as 40% of the abnormal lymph nodes obtained by surgical staging procedures may not be detected by lymphangiograms. Nevertheless, a lymphangiogram may be useful in localizing lymph nodes for radiation therapy, in identifying patients with obvious metastases who might be spared a surgical lymph node biopsy (or biopsied by the thin needle aspiration technique), or in revealing involved para-aortic lymph nodes. If these lymph nodes are involved, cure is unlikely, and no further investigation need be performed. Lymphangiograms have a low yield in patients with small, low-grade cancers.

The prognosis for patients with prostatic carcinomas varies markedly with both size and local extent of the primary tumor and with the histopathologic grade. A common staging system identifies four stages of prostate cancer: stage A (5% of all carcinomas), occult cancer in which no palpable prostatic abnormality is present; stage B (10%), a palpable nodule within the confines of the gland; stage C (45% of prostate cancer at presentation), distortion or invasion of the prostatic capsule or the seminal vesicles; stage D (40% of cancers), distant metastases. In patients with stage B carcinoma, the pelvic lymph nodes are involved in 20% of patients, but metastases are present in the lymph nodes of 56% to 70% of patients with clinical stage C prostate cancers.

Two common histologic grading systems are used. In the first, grade I to IV are assigned in order of decreasing degrees of cellular differentiation. The other system (of Gleason) consists of three observations that combine to give a final numerical value: (1) a score for the major morphologic type of cancer present; (2) a score determined by the minor cellular pattern of the cancer; and (3) a score based upon the clinical extent of the carcinoma. With low Gleason scores of 2 to 6, only 0% to 17% of patients have involved lymph nodes, while those with Gleason scores of 7 to 10 have a 39% to 100% risk of having positive lymph nodes, respectively.

The standard treatment for the small number of patients (<10%) with operable stage B prostate cancers is radical prostatectomy, by either the perineal, retropubic, or suprapubic route. These patients should preferably be under 70 years of age, be in good general health, and have a 1- to 2-cm nodule entirely contained within the prostatic substance. In this select group, 5-year survivals of 70% to 92% and 10-year survivals of 50% to 70% have been obtained. The local recurrence rate is approximately 10% to 15%. Almost 100% of patients are impotent following radical prostatectomy, while a smaller number become incontinent. Surgery also has a role in palliating more advanced or recurrent prostate cancers; transurethral resections of the prostate are often necessary to restore satisfactory urinary function. Orchiectomy or trans-sphenoidal hypophysectomy may also be used sequentially for palliation in patients with metastatic disease.

External beam and interstitial irradiation have both been used to treat prostatic carcinoma. When external beam radiotherapy is used, 70% 5-year and 42% 10-year disease-free survivals have been obtained for those patients whose carcinomas were limited to the prostate gland. When patients with extracapsular extension were treated, 36% were disease-free at 5 years and 29% at 10 years, in a large series from the Stanford Medical Center. Approximately two-thirds of these patients retained their potency. Clinical prostatic recurrences were noted in 10% to 15% of the patients. External beam irradiation carries additional risk in patients with inflammatory bowel disease, those with chronic cystitis and a decreased bladder capacity, and those with prior pelvic surgery who have fixed bowel loops in the area to be irradiated. For patients with well-differentiated stage B carcinomas a lymphangiogram is probably not needed, as lymph nodes are rarely involved. In this instance, 7000–7500 rads are delivered to the prostate in 7 to 8 weeks, using bilateral arcs rather than 360° fields to decrease rectal morbidity. The patient is treated with a full bladder. For patients with larger, locally extensive, or poorly differentiated carcinomas, a lymphangiogram should be considered, and the pelvis may be irradiated in addition. The pelvis and prostate may be successfully irradiated by delivering 2600 rads to the pelvis through a four-field anteroposterior and lateral technique, in 2½ to 3 weeks, then irradiating only the prostate gland to an additional dose of 2000 rads in 2 weeks, and finally completing the pelvic irradiation by enlarging the fields and delivering another 2400 rads in 2½ weeks to that region. In this way the prostate receives 7000 rads in 7 weeks, while at the same time the pelvic radiation dose is 5000 rads. Postirradiation complications such as colorectal stenosis or obstruction or cystoproctitis occur in approximately 10% of irradiated patients. When the para-aortic (PA) lymph nodes are involved, external beam irradiation to the pelvis and PA regions does not appear to prolong survival. No improvement in either local control or survival was noted when estrogens were combined with external beam irradiation.

Interstitial, intraoperative ^{125}I seed implants of the prostate combined with a lymph node dissection have also been performed in a few centers. These low-dose rate sources, with a half-life of 60 days, have a very low energy (30 KeV). Approximately 15,000–20,000 rads are delivered to the prostate in 1 year by these implants. The short-term local control rates with this procedure appear excellent, averaging about 90%. There appears to be less postirradiation impotence with this technique than with external beam irradiation. With all the surgical and radiotherapeutic methods described here, metastases still occur in 70% to 80% of patients who have involved lymph nodes.

D.G.

Bagshaw M, Ray G, Pistenma D, et al: External beam radiation therapy of primary carcinoma of the prostate. Cancer 36:723–728, 1975.
There were relapse-free survivals of 70% at 5 years and 42% at 10 years for patients with cancer limited to the prostate and 36% and 29% at 5 and 10 years, respectively, for those with extracapsular extension.
Correa R Jr, Gibbons R, Cummings K, Mason J: Total prostatectomy for stage B carcinoma of the prostate. J Urol 117:328–329, 1977.
In 67 selected patients there was 92% 5-year and 62% 15-year survival with perineal prostatectomies.
Flocks R, O'Donoghue E, Milleman L, Culp D: Surgery of prostatic carcinoma. Cancer 36:705–717, 1975.
Review of surgical technique and therapeutic results.
Hilaris B, Whitmore W, Batata M, Barzell W: Behavioral patterns of prostate adenocarcinoma following an 125-I implant and pelvic node dissection. Int J Radiat Oncol Biol Phys 2:631–637, 1977.
Article covers 208 patients. Pelvic nodes were involved in 29% of patients with stage B and 59% of those with stage C cancers. Local control was excellent. Metastases were frequent when lymph nodes were involved.
Jewett H: The results of radical perineal prostatectomy. JAMA 210:14–15, 1969.
Long-term follow-up on a 103-patient surgical series.
Klein LA: Prostatic carcinoma. N Engl J Med 300:824–833, 1979.
A discussion of all aspects of management.
Liebner EJ, Stefani S, Uro-oncology Research Group: An evaluation of lymphography with nodal biopsy in localized carcinoma of the prostate. Cancer 45:728–734, 1980.
A retrospective study of 149 patients; overall accuracy was 79% to 86%.
Neglia W, Hussey D, Johnson D: Megavoltage radiation therapy for carcinoma of the prostate. Int J Radiat Oncol Biol Phys 2:873–882, 1977.
Local control was gained in 86.4% of patients. There was no improvement in either survival or local control from hormonal manipulation in addition to radiation therapy.

Testicular carcinoma causes approximately 1% of cancer deaths in males (2 or 3 per 100,000) and accounts for 4% to 10% of all male genitourinary malignancies. Testicular carcinomas are one of the most common malignant tumors in men between the ages of 20 and 34 and usually occur in the 15 to 44 age group. The etiology is uncertain, but the incidence of testicular carcinomas is increased in those with congenitally undescended testes.

Approximately 93% to 95% of testicular cancers arise from germ cells. Leydig cell tumors, which produce androgens, and Sertoli cell tumors, which secrete estrogens, are both rare. A commonly used classification of testicular carcinomas has five general categories: (1) seminoma, 40% of testicular carcinomas (60% are pure seminomas, 40% are mixed seminoma and carcinoma); (2) embryonal carcinoma (with or without seminoma), 30%; (3) teratoma (with or without seminoma), 9%; (4) teratocarcinoma, 20%; (5) choriocarcinoma, 1% of all testicular cancers.

The signs, symptoms, and evaluation of a testicular nodule are given in Part II, Chapter 30.

The history should include symptoms referable to a testicular mass or the presence or absence of retroperitoneal lymph node or distant metastases. Physical examination should include careful palpation of the scrotum and its contents; abdominal palpation to elicit hepatomegaly, an epigastric mass, or tenderness; examination of lymph nodes, including the supraclavicular regions; and noting the presence or absence of gynecomastia or lower extremity edema. A complete blood count, chemical screening panel, and chest radiograph are all routine examinations. An excretory urogram may show ureteral obstruction or dilatation, or renal displacement secondary to retroperitoneal masses. After the above tests are completed, an inguinal, not scrotal, orchiectomy should be performed to make the diagnosis of a testicular carcinoma. Lymphangiograms are important in follow-up, in treatment planning for radiation therapy, and in assessing the extent ot bulk disease prior to retroperitoneal lymph node dissection. Lymphangiograms have an approximate 90% accuracy rate when the para-aortic lymph nodes appear abnormal. There is an 18% to 25% false-negative rate when the lymphangiogram is interpreted as normal (no lymph node involvement). An inferior vena cavagram may reveal the presence of unopacified lymph nodes, and CT scans may demonstrate laterally placed bulky retroperitoneal masses not visualized by a lymphogram. Supraclavicular lymph node biopsies in patients with clinical stage II disease have revealed unsuspected involvement in 15% to 20% of patients.

Biochemical marker titers should be obtained in all cases. The alpha fetoprotein (AFP) titer is elevated in 66% of patients with pure or mixed embryonal carcinomas, while 40% to 60% of all patients with carcinomas have elevated human chorionic gonadotropin (HCG) titers. The beta subunit of HCG is elevated in choriocarcinomas. Neither marker is elevated in pure seminoma, while titers are uniformly high in patients with stages II and III testicular carcinomas. Marker determinations are probably not useful in the initial evaluation of patients with a testicular mass, as they are rarely elevated in the early stages of the disease. If elevated marker titers persist 1 month or more after orchiectomy, however, residual or metastatic carcinoma should be suspected. False-positive examinations are rare. The marker titers fall after carcinoma is resected or eradicated by radiotherapy or chemotherapy, but if these titers rise during the follow-up period, recurrence should be suspected.

There are three stages of increasing involvement by testicular carcinomas. In stage I the carcinoma is limited to the testis, while in stage II the retroperitoneal lymph nodes are involved. In stage III supradiaphragmatic metastases are present. Institutional variations in the definition of these stages exist. Five-year survivals for patients in the prechemotherapy era were as follows: seminoma, 90%; teratocarcinoma, 48%; embryonal carcinoma, 38%; and choriocarcinoma, 9%.

Treatment

Seminoma

Patients with stage I seminomas, with a negative lymphangiogram, normal serum marker determinations, and no evidence of supradiaphragmatic metastases, should be treated with a "hockey stick" radiotherapy field, which includes bilateral para-aortic lymph nodes and the ipsilateral iliac region to 3000–3500 rads in 3 to 4 weeks. Cure rates approaching 100% may be obtained by this treatment. If the retroperitoneal lymph nodes are involved, irradiation of the mediastinum and supraclavicular nodes produces similar excellent results. For those with metastatic seminoma or elevated markers, postirradiation chemotherapy should be considered.

Testicular Carcinomas

Patients with stage I testicular carcinomas have been treated either by surgery or radiation alone or by combined lymph node dissection and postoperative irradiation. When retroperitoneal lymph node dissections are performed, approximately 90% 5-year survivals are obtained if the retroperitoneal lymph node specimens are negative. With radiotherapy alone, 80% to 86% 5-year survivals have also been noted. In 4½ to 6 weeks 4500–5000 rads are delivered to the para-aortic lymph nodes. Severe postirradiation complications consist primarily of radiation enteritis, occurring in 10% or less of patients, but the risk increases in those with prior abdominal surgery. Eighty to 100% of the patients who undergo lymph node dissections experience retrograde ejaculations. They are also at risk for the usual postoperative complications. There is no apparent gain from using postoperative irradiation after lymph node dissection in patients with stage I testicular carcinomas.

The management of patients with stage II testicular carcinomas is controversial. The chance of controlling retroperitoneal lymph node metastases depends on both the number of involved lymph nodes and the size of the nodal masses. In selected patients with stage II carcinomas, Staubitz et al. [1974] reported 70% 5-year relapse-free survival in 20 patients treated only with retroperitoneal lymph node dissections. Sandwich treatment, in which a portion of the radiation therapy course, usually 2500–3000 rads, is given prior to lymph node dissection and is followed by completion of the radiotherapy postoperatively, results in 50% to 75% 5-year survivals. Similar results have been obtained for postlymphadenectomy irradiation. In a retrospective study from the MD Anderson Hospital, local irradiation reduced the risk of retroperitoneal lymph node recurrences following dissection from 55% to approximately 6%. In another series, 10 of 15 patients had local relapses following radiation alone if the para-aortic lymph nodes were larger than 2 cm; however, with nodes less than 2 cm, only 2 of 14 patients had a relapse in the retroperitoneum. In another study, patients with stage II testicular carcinomas were randomized to receive either a minimum radiation dose of 4000 rads in 4 weeks to the para-aortic lymph nodes without surgery or a sandwich treatment of 3000 rads in 3 weeks and retroperitoneal lymph node dissection, followed 10 days later by another 1500 rads to the para-aortic region. All patients in both groups had negative supraclavicular lymph node biopsies, and all received 4000 rads to the mediastinum and supraclavicular regions. There were no differences at 3 years in disease-free survival between the 2 groups (81%). When the retroperitoneal lymph nodes are involved but small, many authors recommend combined surgery and irradiation, with chemotherapy to be used if the dissection is incomplete. When bulky retroperitoneal adenopathy is present, chemotherapy and lymph node dissection are recommended, with consideration of radiation therapy if residual carcinoma exists after lymph node dissection.

D.G.

Anderson T, Waldmann TA, Javadpour N, Glatstein E: Testicular germ-cell neoplasms: Recent advances in diagnosis and therapy. Ann Intern Med 90:373–385, 1979.
Excellent review of NIH conference.
Buck A, Schamber D, Maier J, Lewis E: Supraclavicular lymph node biopsy and malignant testicular tumors. J Urol 107:619–621, 1972.
A series of consecutive supraclavicular node biopsies showed: clinical stage I, none positive in 15 patients; clinical stage II, 4 in 25 involved (16%).
Earle J, Bagshaw M, Kaplan H: Supervoltage radiotherapy of the testicular tumors. Am J Roentgenol 117:653–661, 1973.
Radiation therapy and "sandwich" XRT in a surgery series are discussed.
Einhorn L, Donohue J: Cis-diamminedichloroplatinum, vinblastine, and bleomycin combination chemotherapy in disseminated testicular cancer. Ann Intern Med 87:293–298, 1977.
Seventy-four percent complete remissions, 26% partial remissions in 50 patients with disseminated testicular cancer; 32 alive and disease-free at 6 to 30 months.
Fraley EE, Lange PH, Kennedy BJ: Germ-cell testicular cancer in adults. N Engl J Med 301:1370–1377, 1420–1426, 1979.
A comprehensive review of all aspects.
Hussey D, Luk K, Johnson D: The role of radiation therapy in the treatment of germinal cell tumors of the testis other than pure seminoma. Radiology 123:175–180, 1977.
In a series of 279 patients, postlymphadenectomy radiation therapy to the para-aortic region decreased local relapse frequency if lymph nodes were involved. Patients with positive nodes also have a high risk of developing distant metastases.
Javadpour N: Testicular germ cell tumors. Urol Digest 18:19–34, 1979.
Marks, staging and treatment are discussed.
Johnson D, Bracken R, Blight E: Prognosis for pathologic stage I non-seminomatous germ cell tumors of the testis managed by retroperitoneal lymphadenectomy. J Urol 116:63–65, 1976.
There was a 90.8% 5-year survival for 72 patients with pathologic stage I carcinomas managed only by lymphadenectomy.
Lange P, McIntire K, Waldmann T, et al: Serum alpha fetoprotein and human chorionic gonadotrophin in the diagnosis and management of non-seminomatous germ cell testicular cancer. N Engl J Med 295:1237–1240, 1976.
Review article.
Maier J, Mittemeyer B: Carcinoma of the testis. Cancer 39:981–986, 1977.
In a Walter Reed General Hospital randomized trial radiation therapy–surgery sandwich vs. radiation therapy alone for stage IIA carcinomas was given. All patients also received mediastinal irradiation. There were no differences in 3-year relapse-free survivals: 17 of 21 (81%) vs. 9 of 11 (82%).
Maier J, Schamber J: The role of lymphangiography in the diagnosis and treatment of malignant testicular tumors. Am J Roentgenol 114:482–491, 1972.

Histopathological confirmation of lymphangiographic findings were obtained in 69 patients· 42/45 (93%) accuracy with positive LAG. 18/24 (75%) accuracy when LAG negative.

Smithers D, Wallace E, Wallace D: Radiotherapy for patients with tumours of the testicle. Br J Urol 43:83–92, 1971.
Article discusses a radiotherapy series.

Staubitz W, Early K, Magoss I, Murphy G: Surgical management of testis tumor. J Urol 111:205–209, 1974.
In this discussion of pathologic staging there was a 70% 5-year survival in selected patients with stage II carcinomas (positive retroperitoneal nodes). There were excluded cases.

Tyrell C, Peckham M: The response of lymph node metastases of testicular carcinoma to radiation therapy. Br J Urol 48:363–370, 1976.
Of patients with large, involved retroperitoneal lymph nodes (>2 cm) 67% had relapses in these lymph nodes after radiation therapy. Smaller involved nodes were controlled by radiation therapy alone.

51. OVARIAN CARCINOMA—PRIMARY OR REGIONAL

Cancer of the ovary causes 20% of female genital malignancies. It is less common than cancer of the cervix and endometrium but causes greater mortality than these two neoplasms combined. The prediction for 1980 was 17,000 new cases and 11,200 deaths from ovarian cancer. The peak age is 40 to 65 (60% of cases). Of these cancers 80% to 90% are epithelial in origin. Serous cystadenocarcinomas are most common, followed by mucinous cystadenocarcinomas, endometrioid tumors, and undifferentiated cancers. Other tumors, such as clear cell carcinomas, endodermal sinus malignancies, and dysgerminomas, are less frequent. There is a slight familial tendency to develop ovarian carcinomas, and these neoplasms are more common in women of low parity and in those with such ovarian dysfunction as infertility or menstrual irregularities.

Most ovarian carcinomas are asymptomatic early in their course. Sensations of pelvic pressure and discomfort are experienced ultimately by 50% to 70% of patients, as is abdominal fullness. Gastrointestinal or urinary symptoms, or weight loss, also occur in 20% to 30% of patients. Menstrual irregularities are noted in approximately 15%. Late in the course, ascites, bowel obstruction, localized pain, or shortness of breath from pleural effusions may all be noted.

In the evaluation of a patient with suspected ovarian cancer, a family history of carcinoma of the ovary, menstrual irregularities, infertility, or any of the above symptoms are all suggestive of an ovarian malignancy. A careful physical examination, including palpation of regional and distant lymph nodes, breasts, and an abdominal examination, should be performed. Finally, a detailed pelvic examination should be carried out. In a menstruating woman with a cystic adnexal mass less than 3 to 4 cm in greatest dimension, a postmenstrual repeat examination should be performed, since such masses are usually follicular or luteal cysts. If the mass persists, a more complete evaluation should be performed (see next paragraph). A solid mass, larger than 5 to 10 cm and fixed, is highly suspect for carcinoma, while a palpable ovary in a postmenopausal woman also suggests carcinoma, since the normal ovaries in this age group are usually not palpable.

Complete blood counts, liver and renal function tests, and chest x-ray are routine examinations. Either ultrasound or CT scans may assist in differentiating solid from cystic ovarian masses. These examinations appear to be complementary, however: one does not provide additional information over the other. Cystoscopy and a proctoscopy should also be performed. Other radiologic examinations that should be considered are a barium enema and upper GI series in older women, to rule out either gastric or bowel malignancies, and excretory urography to note the course of the ureters and the presence or absence of ureteral obstruction. Lymphangiograms are positive in approximately 20% of patients with stage I and II ovarian cancers. If ascites is present, paracentesis may reveal malignant cells.

A pelvic examination under anesthesia with a fractional dilatation and curettage may also be important diagnostically. However, neither cul de sac cytology nor cervical Papanicolaou smears has been helpful in providing a diagnosis in most instances. Laparoscopy, with careful examination of the diaphragm, surface of the liver, and pelvis, should be considered prior to laparotomy. After the above evaluations, laparotomy is indicated. At the time of abdominal exploration, the para-aortic lymph nodes should be evaluated, the liver and diaphragm inspected, pelvic and abdominal washings obtained for cytology, the omentum biopsied or resected, and the tumor mass resected, if possible, with total abdominal hysterectomy and bilateral salpingo-oophorectomy.

The proper therapy for several stages of ovarian cancer is controversial. It should be remembered, however, that 70% of the tumors have extended beyond the ovary at the time of diagnosis. Ovarian cancer spreads intraperitoneally, with cells that have been shed by the neoplasm moving over the peritoneal surface and collecting centrally at the diaphragm. Six of seven patients with apparent stage I and II ovarian carcinomas had diaphragmatic involvement in one peritoneoscopy series. Since widespread peritoneal seeding may occur, large potentially morbid treatment volumes are necessary for adequate radiation therapy, and partially for this reason, chemotherapy has also been used with increasing frequency.

Important factors in prognosis for patients with ovarian cancers are the degree of histologic differentiation of the tumor, mass size, stage of disease, and completeness of resection (particularly well demonstrated by the Princess Margaret Hospital trial in Canada).

Stage I (limited to ovary). Total abdominal hysterectomy and bilateral salpingo-oophorectomy are recommended. With surgery alone, 5-year survivals of 50% to 80% have been achieved. Intraperitoneal ^{32}P or radiogold have been added, and external beam irradiation has also been used. The role of these modalities in addition to surgery is unclear, and randomized trials will be necessary to determine the value of external beam irradiation in stage I ovarian cancer. Many authors agree, however, that patients with poorly differentiated carcinomas should have pelvic irradiation, usually to 4000–5000 rads in 5 weeks. Ascitic fluid positive for cancer cells is not common in stage I ovarian carcinoma but may be managed by radiocolloid instillation, chemotherapy, or wide-field irradiation.

Stage II. Again, total abdominal hysterectomy and bilateral salpingo-oophorectomy are recommended. It is important to resect the mass completely, if possible, since the Princess Margaret Hospital trial demonstrated a 75% 5-year survival with complete resection versus 20% if the mass was not completely removed. Metallic marker clips should be applied to guide future radiotherapy if the tumor cannot be resected completely. With stage II ovarian carcinoma, surgery alone has resulted in 10% to 35% 5-year survivals, while the addition of postoperative irradiation has improved these figures to 25% to 70%. In patients with stage II carcinomas and positive lymphangiograms (asymptomatic stage III), excellent results have been obtained when the entire abdomen is treated by the moving strip technique, in which 2250 rads in 10 fractions are delivered from above the level of the diaphragm to the pelvis. Wide-field whole abdominal irradiation may also be used, protecting the liver and kidneys after 2000 rads, then limiting the bowel dose to 3000–4000 rads but giving booster radiation doses to the central abdomen (para-aortic region) and central liver to a total of 4000–4400 rads in 5 to 7 weeks. In the randomized, prospective Princess Margaret Hospital trial, moving strip abdominal irradiation was superior to pelvic irradiation and chlorambucil chemotherapy for patients with asymptomatic stage III ovarian carcinomas.

Stages III and IV. For intra-abdominal involvement or distant metastases, see Part IV, Chapter 74 on relapsing or metastatic disease.

Patients with dysgerminomas are usually less than 35 years old. These tumors, which are often unilateral, are quite radiosensitive, and 90% survival has been obtained in stage I_A patients with postoperative pelvic irradiation. In very selected, favorable groups, no treatment other than oophorectomy may be necessary. This group includes patients less than 35 years of age with neoplasm limited to one ovary, no capsular invasion or external ovarian excrescences, a normal lymphangiogram, and normal intraoperative cytologic washings. When these criteria are met, and when close follow-up is possible, a patient may be watched closely without other treatment in an attempt to preserve fertility and menstrual function.

D.G.

Bush R, Allt W, Beale F, et al: Treatment of epithelial carcinoma of the ovary: Operation, irradiation and chemotherapy. Am J Obstet Gynecol 127:692–704, 1977.
  In this prospective study of 279 patients completeness of pelvic surgery was one of the most important variables. Also, patients with Stages IB, II and "asymptomatic III" did well with XRT alone. Whole abdominal XRT was superior to chlorambucil in preventing extensions to that area.
Fazekas J, Maier J: Irradiation of ovarian carcinoma: A prospective comparison of the open field and moving strip techniques. Am J Roentgenol 120: 118–123, 1974.
  No significant differences were noted between the two techniques.
Fisher R, Young R: Advances in the staging and treatment of ovarian cancer. Cancer 39:967–972, 1977.
  Excellent review of the entire subject.
Fuks Z: External radiotherapy of ovarian cancer: Standard approaches and new frontiers. Semin Oncol 2:253–266, 1975.
  Complete review.
Krepart G, Smith J, Rutledge F, Delclos L: The treatment for dysgerminoma of the ovary. Cancer 41:986–990, 1978.
  Excellent results were obtained in 36 patients.
Kurman RJ, Norris HJ: Germ cell tumors of the ovary. Pathol Annu 13: 291–325, 1978.
  A good review.
Parker B, Castellino R, Fuks Z, Bagshaw M: The role of lymphography in patients with ovarian cancer. Cancer 34:100–105, 1974.
  Lymphography revealed 20% positive studies in patients with stages I and II carcinomas.
Pezner R, Stevens K Jr, Tong D, Allen C: Limited epithelial carcinoma of the ovary treated with curative intent by the intraperitoneal installation of radiocolloids. Cancer 42:2563–2571, 1978.
  Usual treatment was 15 m Ci ^{32}P intraperitoneally 4 to 6 weeks postlaparotomy in 104 patients. Excellent results occurred in stages I_A to II_A.

Rosenoff S, Young R, Anderson T, et al: Peritoneoscopy: A valuable tool for the initial staging and "second look" in ovarian carcinoma. Ann Intern Med 83:37–41, 1975.

Six of seven patients with stages I or II ovarian carcinoma had advanced disease at peritoneoscopy.

Walsh J, Rosenfield A, Schwartz P, et al: Prospective comparison of ultrasound and computed tomography in the evaluation of gynecologic pelvic masses. Am J Roentgenol 131:955–960, 1978.

US and CT scans are not complementary, since both give similar information. Perhaps one (but not both) should be used.

52. CARCINOMA OF THE CERVIX—PRIMARY OR REGIONAL

Cervical cancer is the fourth most frequent malignancy in women. Only carcinomas of the breast, colorectum and lung are more common. There were approximately 16,000 invasive cervical carcinomas predicted in 1979, with 7400 deaths. The number of invasive cancers is decreasing. Ninety percent of these neoplasms are squamous carcinomas, while the remainder are adenocarcinomas. Epidemiologic studies have shown a relationship between elevated herpes simplex virus II titers and cervix cancer. The risk of this malignancy is increased in lower socioeconomic groups, blacks, in those who have early marriages, begin sexual activity or have children early, in those with many sexual partners, and in prostitutes. Nuns and Jewish women have a decreased risk of developing cancer of the cervix.

Carcinoma of the cervix may be asymptomatic in its early stages but may be detected by a routine Papanicolaou smear. As the lesion enlarges, it may be associated with a foul vaginal discharge, vaginal bleeding, or localized pain. In advanced malignancies the bladder or bowel may be invaded, with symptoms referable to those organs. Anorexia and weight loss may also occur, while in far-advanced tumors, symptoms from uremia, bone pain from osseous metastases, lower extremity edema, and enlarged lymph nodes may all be noted.

In the evaluation of a patient with suspected cervical carcinoma, a history of any of these symptoms should be elicited. A physical examination should include evaluation of hepatic size, palpation of regional and supraclavicular lymph node areas, inspection of the lower extremities for edema, and a careful pelvic examination with Papanicolaou smear. A complete blood count and chemical screening panel are recommended.

If cytology shows a class V smear, a random cervical biopsy may miss a carcinoma, but biopsies directed through colposcopy are accurate in more than 95% of cases. This procedure provides a magnified examination of the transformation zone at the squamocolumnar junction (the site of many cervix cancers), as well as of the remainder of the cervix. Since colposcopy accurately defines the best area for biopsy, this procedure has decreased the need for cervical conization. If facilities for colposcopic examination are unavailable, the cervix may be painted with iodine and nonstaining areas biopsied (Schiller's test, in which cancer cells, which do not produce glycogen, do not stain with iodine). A cervical conization may be important if a lesion is not seen by colposcopy, if it is not seen in its entirety (or extends into the endocervical canal), if the histologic and cytologic results do not correspond, or when this procedure must be used to identify invasive carcinoma. A pelvic examination and endocervical curettage under anesthesia should be performed. Cystoscopy is advised if the lesion is clinically stage II_B or larger.

Indicated x-ray examinations are chest radiography, excretory urography, and lymphangiography, if there are no medical contraindications to performance of the latter two studies. The lymph nodes may contain metastatic carcinoma in 10% to 20% of patients with normal-appearing lymphangiograms, while "skinny needle" aspiration cytology biopsies of suspicious lymph nodes may confirm the diagnosis of metastatic carcinoma. A barium enema should be performed on symptomatic patients, although as a routine procedure it has yielded little. Staging laparotomies have been performed in a research setting but are not recommended for routine use. These surgical procedures have revealed para-aortic lymph node involvement in few patients with stage I neoplasms, in 20% of those with stage II lesions, in 40% with stage III, and in 50% with stage IV cancers.

Three types of carcinoma may be encountered: in situ cancer, which may evolve to invasive carcinoma; microinvasive cancer (up to 3 mm of invasion); and frankly invasive cancer, extending deeper than 3 mm into the cervix. Cervical carcinoma spreads by direct extension into surrounding organs, usually into the uterus or vagina initially and later into the adjacent rectum or bladder. These cancers also spread through the lymphatics, to the paracervical, obturator, or internal or external iliac lymph nodes, and later into the common iliac, para-aortic, or inguinal nodes. Hematogenous metastases also occur.

The only curative modalities for primary cervical cancers are surgery and radiation therapy. Carcinoma in situ is usually managed by total abdominal hysterectomy with resection of an adequate vaginal cuff. Almost 100% of patients may be cured by this procedure. In stage I cervical carcinoma, the neoplasm is confined to the cervix, and there is a low (0% to 5%) risk of para-aortic lymph node involvement. In stage I_A carcinoma in younger women, a total abdominal hysterectomy and vaginal cuff resection should be considered if 1 mm of invasion or less is present. Intracavitary irradiation, usually 8000–10,000 mg hours and 7000–8000 rads to points AR and AL from two insertions, may be equally effective. Five-year survivals of 95% to 100% have been produced with intracavitary irradiation only, with no local and less than 4% regional failures in a series from the M.D. Anderson Hospital. Invasive cervical carcinoma, stage I_B, may be managed by radical hysterectomy and lymph node dissection in younger women; however, two radium applications as just described and external beam radiation to bring the pelvic sidewall dose up to approximately 5000 rads in 5 weeks after the two intracavitary insertions is equally effective. Both methods produce 84% to 90% five-year survivals.

In stage II carcinomas, the risk of para-aortic node involvement is 15%. When the cancer involves the upper vagina (stage II_A), radical hysterectomy is performed rarely in selected young patients, but the preferred treatment for stages II_A and II_B (parametrial extension) is radiation therapy, ordinarily two radium placements and external beam irradiation as described above. Five-year survivals of 60% to 80% may be expected from carefully performed radiotherapy treatment. If the patient has a massive central neoplasm (barrel cervix), combined preoperative irradiation and hysterectomy offer the best chance for cure, with reported 5-year survivals of 70% to 90% in stages II_A and II_B.

In stage III carcinoma, in which the tumor has spread to the lower vagina or pelvic side wall, the risk of para-aortic lymph node involvement is 35% to 50%. These cancers are managed by radiation therapy, initially with external beam irradiation and reevaluation between 3000 rads in 3 weeks and 5000 rads in 5 weeks for intracavitary source placements, if suitable regression has taken place. Optimal 5-year survivals for this stage of cervical carcinoma are 35% to 50%. In stage IV, with extension out of the pelvis or into the bladder or rectum, palliative radiation is used, but an occasional selected patient may be controlled by pelvic exenteration.

Carcinoma in a cervical stump is at present a rare lesion. If it is localized, resection may be considered, or the lesion can be managed by external beam irradiation supplemented by intracavitary or interstitial radiotherapy. If cervical carcinoma occurs during pregnancy, carcinoma in situ may be treated by conization, followed by normal pregnancy and a vaginal delivery. However, if invasive carcinoma is present, a cesarean section should be performed and standard treatment given, based on the stage of disease, in the third trimester. In the first and second trimesters, treatment for invasive carcinoma should be carried out as indicated by the stage of the cancer, as the risk of allowing the pregnancy to come to term is too great with an invasive carcinoma.

The complications from a surgical approach to cervical cancer involve the usual postoperative risks of pulmonary embolism, infection, wound dehiscence, and hemorrhage. There is a 1% to 5% ureteric fistula rate, while urinary retention or lymphoceles may also occur. Morbidity from surgery is 5% to 15%. The possible acute morbidity from irradiation consists of anorexia, nausea and vomiting, diarrhea, and acute urinary symptoms or cystitis. In the postirradiation period, subcutaneous fibrosis, cystitis, bladder contraction and decreased volume, ureteral or bowel injury (proctosigmoiditis), or rectovaginal, vesicovaginal, or enterocutaneous fistulae and necrosis of the cervical vault may be encountered. Severe late complications after carefully performed radiation therapy occur in less than 10% of patients.

D.G.

Griffin T, Parker R, Taylor W: An evaluation of procedures used in staging carcinoma of the cervix. Am J Roentgenol 127:825–827, 1976.
  In 277 patients cystoscopy and CXR, BE, and proctoscopy would have changed the stage in only 1%, 1%, 1.4%, and 2.2%, respectively. Recommended procedures are lymphangiogram (high yield), chest radiograph, intravenous pyelogram (7.3% yield), and proctoscopy. Use barium enema only if patient symptomatic and cystoscopy with stage II_B or greater.
Hamberger A, Fletcher G, Wharton J: Results of treatment of early Stage I carcinoma of the uterine cervix with intracavitary radium alone. Cancer 41:980–985, 1978.
  151 patients with either Stage I_A or I_B (small volume) cancers showed no local recurrences and less than 4% regional failures with this treatment.
Hoskins W, Ford J Jr, Lutz M, Averette H: Radical hysterectomy and pelvic lymphadenectomy for the management of early invasive carcinoma of the cervix. Gynecol Oncol 4:278–290, 1976.
  In 224 patients operative mortality was 0.89% and fistula rate 1.3%. There was an 87% 5-year survival for patients with Stage I_B and II_A carcinomas.
Jampolis S, Andras E, Fletcher G: Analysis of sites and causes of failures of irradiation in invasive squamous cell carcinoma of the intact uterine cervix. Radiology 115:681–685, 1975.
  For Stage I there was 91% 5-year survival and only 2% central failures. Article describes radiotherapy results for all stages.
Lehman M, Park R, Barham E, et al: Pre-treatment lymphangiography in carcinoma of the uterine cervix. Gynecol Oncol 3:354–360, 1975.
  Lymphography accuracy (in patients who underwent exploratory operation) was: true negative, 94.1%; true positive, 57.1%.
Marcial V: Carcinoma of the cervix. Cancer 39:945–958, 1977.
  Excellent review article.
Nelson A, Fletcher G, Wharton J: Indications for adjunctive conservative extrafascial hysterectomy in selected cases of carcinoma of the uterine cervix. Am J Roentgenol 123:91–99, 1975.
  Article gives results of combined treatment for bulky cancers.

Richart RM: Current concepts in obstetrics and gynecology: The patient with an abnormal Pap smear—Screening techniques and management. N Engl J Med 302:332–334, 1980.
   An excellent summary of the approach to cervical intraepithelial neoplasia.
Stafl A, Mattingly R: Colposcopic diagnosis of cervical neoplasia. Obstet Gynecol 41:168–176, 1973.
   In 1410 patients who underwent colposcopy conization was needed afterward in only 5.6%, while the false negative rate of directed cervical biopsies was only 0.3%.

53. ENDOMETRIAL CARCINOMA—PRIMARY OR REGIONAL

Cancer of the endometrium occurs primarily between the ages of 50 and 70. Approximately 37,000 new cases were predicted for 1979, with 3300 deaths. There is now a 2:1 preponderance of cervix to corpus cancer, but this ratio has decreased in recent years. These neoplasms are usually adenocarcinomas, and most remain confined to the uterus. Adenosquamous carcinomas or sarcomas are other rare endometrial malignancies. A grading system exists for adenocarcinomas: grade I, well-differentiated, 60% of the tumors; grade II, 30%; grade III, poorly differentiated, 10%. Premalignant cystic hyperplasia of the endometrium, progressing to adenomatous hyperplasia, may result in carcinoma in situ and ultimately in invasive carcinoma.

Endometrial carcinoma usually arises in a milieu of disturbed estrogen balance. Patients usually have a history of abnormal menstrual bleeding, but this malignancy is rare in patients who have had an oophorectomy. Many patients also have diabetes mellitus and hypertension. The use of exogenous estrogens increases the risk of developing endometrial carcinoma approximately 4½ times. When the use of estrogens decreased in the general population, a similar decline in the incidence of endometrial carcinoma was also noted.

Symptoms of endometrial cancer are usually associated with abnormal postmenopausal vaginal bleeding. However, an enlarged uterus or pelvic extension may both result in low back pain in addition.

When endometrial carcinoma is suspected, the history should include the use of estrogens and any of the above symptoms, but especially abnormal bleeding in the postmenopausal period. Examination should include palpation of the abdomen and the regional lymph nodes. A pelvic examination with careful palpation for vaginal metastases is carried out, and intrauterine aspiration for cytology or an endometrial biopsy may also be performed. A complete blood count, liver and renal function tests, and chest x-ray are also indicated. A pelvic examination should also be performed under anesthesia, in which the uterine size is determined by sounding, the parametria examined, and the vagina again carefully palpated for metastases. The prognosis is decreased by an enlarged uterus and especially by vaginal metastases. A fractional cervical dilatation and curettage should be performed, to detect involvement of the cervix. At the time of the evaluation under anesthesia, cystoscopy may be performed. Excretory urography may reveal ureteral obstruction in advanced cases or deviation of the ureters by enlarged lymph nodes. A proctoscopic examination is indicated for patients with larger tumors. Lymphangiography is still an investigational procedure in endometrial carcinoma.

Most endometrial carcinomas are confined to the uterine corpus (90% of cases). The tumor grade is important, with 5-year survivals of 88% to 90% for those with grade I and 70% or less for grade III tumors. When there is no myometrial invasion, 92% 5-year survival is expected; but with superficial invasion, the 5-year survival decreases to 85%. A 5-year survival of only 59% is obtained when more than 50% of the wall is invaded. Lymph node metastases occur in fewer than 10% of patients with stage I carcinomas (confined to the uterus) but are present in 33% of those with stage II carcinomas (cervix involvement). Nodal metastases are also more common with less differentiated tumors. Uterine malignancies may spread to the vagina (few, if any, 5-year survivors) or parametria or may break through the uterine wall and seed widely in the peritoneum. Distant hematogenous metastases also may occur.

Treatment Recommendations
Surgery is the mainstay in treatment for endometrial carcinoma, but radiation therapy also plays a major role in poorly differentiated, invasive tumors and in more advanced stages of the disease.

Stage I (carcinoma confined to the uterus). For grade I tumors, total abdominal hysterectomy and bilateral salpingo-oophorectomy (TAH and BSO) should be performed. No further therapy is necessary if there is no myometrial invasion and no change in grade in the surgical specimen. In grade II cancers, preoperative irradiation has been found to decrease local recurrences. This therapy has also led to increased survival for both patients with grade III carcinomas and for those with enlarged uteri (stage I_B). If preoperative irradiation is not given, external beam irradiation to the pelvis (4500–5000 rads) may be delivered in approximately 5 to 6 weeks. Preoperative irradiation may be by Heyman capsules or tandem and colpostats to a dose of 3000–4000 rads, or the pelvis may receive 4000–5000 rads by external beam irradiation. All these techniques produce similar results. Patients with stage I carcinomas who are poor surgical candidates may be given intracavitary treatments to 3000 rads, if possible, followed by external beam irradiation, with pelvic side wall doses of 5000 rads in 5 weeks.

Stage II (cervical involvement). Intracavitary irradiation to approximately 3000 rads, with postinsertion pelvic irradiation to approximately 5000 rads followed by TAH and BSO are recommended.

Stage III (pelvic extension). External beam irradiation and intracavitary insertions are the usual treatment.

Stage IV (bladder or rectal extension or extrapelvic spread). Recommended treatment is external beam irradiation to 5500 or 6000 rads to the pelvis, with possible small field booster doses to areas of bulky tumor, and hormone treatment or chemotherapy.

In stage I endometrial carcinoma, approximately 80% to 85% 5-year survival is obtained. In stage II, 50% 5-year survivals are noted, but these decrease to 25% in stage III and to 0% to 8% for patients with stage IV carcinomas.

Surgical complications include the usual postoperative sequelae, but rectovaginal or vesicovaginal fistulae, or intestinal obstructions, may also occur in 2% to 8% of patients. Postirradiation complications of vulvitis; radiation necrosis of the vulva, vaginal wall, or apex; proctitis, vesicovaginal fistula; cystitis; or hematuria also arise in 2% to 8% of patients.

Uterine sarcomas are rare but devastating malignancies that metastasize widely. The major factor in local control is the initial bulk and local extent of the sarcoma. Recommended treatment is to resect the tumors by performing a TAH and BSO if possible, mark the residual neoplasm with metallic clips, and use postoperative pelvic irradiation to doses of 5000–5500 rads in 5 to 6 weeks. Adriamycin appears to be the most active chemotherapeutic agent.

D.G.

Jick H, Watkins R, Hunter J, et al: Replacement estrogens and endometrial cancer. N Engl J Med 300:218–222, 1979.
Decreased prescriptions for replacement estrogens were associated with a decreased incidence of endometrial carcinoma.

Keller D, Kempson R, Levine G, McLennan C: Management of the patient with early endometrial carcinoma. Cancer 33:1108–1116, 1974.
Postoperative XRT is recommended only for stage I patients with greater than 50% invasion of myometrium.

Morrow C, DiSaia P, Townsend D: Current management of endometrial carcinoma. Obstet Gynecol 43:399–405, 1973.
Excellent review article.

Morrow C, DiSaia P, Townsend D: The role of postoperative irradiation in the management of stage I adenocarcinoma of the endometrium. Am J Roentgenol 127:325–329, 1976.
Good literature review.

Salazar OM, Bonfiglio TA, Patten SF, et al: Uterine sarcomas. Natural history, treatment and prognosis. Cancer 42:1152–1160, 1978.
A retrospective review of 73 cases of uterine sarcomas.

Salazar OM, Bonfiglio TA, Patten SF, et al: Uterine sarcomas. Analysis of failures with special emphasis on the use of adjuvant radiation therapy. Cancer 42:1161–1170, 1978.
Analysis of 47 treatment failures: prognosis correlated with stage; adjuvant irradiation improved local control but not survival.

Salazar OM, Bonfiglio TA, Patten SF, et al: The management of clinical stage I endometrial carcinoma. Cancer 41:1016–1026, 1978.
Article stresses importance of tumor grade on survival and local recurrence.

Shanklin DR: Endometrial carcinoma: Diagnostic criteria, pathogenesis, natural history, and associations. Pathol Annu 13:233–287, 1978.
An excellent review.

Smith D, Prentice R, Thompson D, Herrman W: Association of exogenous estrogen and endometrial carcinoma. N Engl J Med 293:1164–1167, 1975.
An increased risk of endometrial carcinoma is noted in this study.

Wharam M, Phillips T, Bagshaw M: The role of radiation therapy in clinical stage I carcinoma of the endometrium. Int J Radiat Oncol Biol Phys 1:1081–1089, 1976.
Article gives results of preoperative XRT: in stage I with grade 2 histology, recurrences decreased; in stage I with grade 3 histology it resulted in improved survival as well as decreased recurrences.

54. BONE TUMORS—PRIMARY OR REGIONAL

Bone tumors are rare in adults but account for 3% of all childhood cancers (3/100,000 adolescents). There were 1900 new bone tumors predicted in the United States in 1980, with 1750 deaths. The risk of developing a bone tumor is increased in patients with preexisting Paget's disease, those with such benign tumors as exostoses and multiple enchondromatoses (Ollier's disease), in patients with chronic osteomyelitis, and in those who have received prior high-dose irradiation to bones. Osteosarcomas, fibrosarcomas, and chondrosarcomas have all been reported in patients who receive bone irradiation either by external beam or through the ingestion of radioactive isotopes, particularly radium.

The two histopathologic types of intrinsic bone tumors, osteosarcomas (30%) and Ewing's sarcoma (7%), are most common in patients under 20 years of age.

Other bone neoplasms include chondrosarcomas (13%), fibrosarcomas (4%), and such rare tumors as fibrous histiocytoma and reticulum cell sarcoma of bone. Myeloma, described in Part V, Chapter 87, accounts for 40% of all intrinsic bone tumors. Osseous metastases, occurring primarily in the pelvis and vertebrae, account for 60% of all bone neoplasms.

Bone tumors usually produce increasingly severe pain, characteristically worse at night. There may also be a mass and local tenderness, or a functional deficit, depending on the size, extent, and location of the tumor. A pathologic fracture may occur. Fever, anorexia, and weight loss are frequently noted with Ewing's sarcoma. If a bone tumor has metastasized, there may be bone pain, cough, or dyspnea.

In the evaluation of a patient with a suspected bone tumor, a careful history referable to the presence of the above symptoms or predisposing factors should be obtained. The regional lymph nodes should be palpated, any functional or neurologic deficits ascertained, and the symptomatic area carefully examined for a mass, tenderness, or limited joint mobility. A pathologic fracture may also be found. A complete blood count, chemical screening panel, and chest radiograph are indicated. The diagnostic procedure second only to biopsy in importance is a radiograph of the involved bone. The integrity of the bone, the nature of the lesion, and extension into surrounding tissues may all be revealed by a bone radiograph. The x-ray may also be used to select the biopsy site. Subperiosteal reaction, soft tissue extension or mass, and Codman's triangle are all indicative of a malignant process. Tomograms of the bone lesion may help to delineate the process further, and an arteriogram may reveal neovascularity and tumor extent. Xeroradiographs may be helpful in resolving finer bone detail than a routine x-ray. A bone scan is indicated when metastases are suspected, as these are usually multiple. A proper biopsy is also of critical importance. The area to be biopsied should be approached through as normal a region as possible, and the incision for biopsy should be placed so as not to compromise any later definitive surgical approach. An adequate and representative bone sample must be obtained, and the wound should be carefully closed in layers. Expert review of the histopathologic findings is mandatory, and correlations should be made between the biopsy specimen and the diagnostic radiographs.

Nonmalignant bone tumors (for example, giant cell tumor of bone) may be removed surgically and the resultant defect filled with bone grafts. Radiation therapy is not indicated for most benign tumors, except for unresectable lesions, because of the risk of delayed radiation carcinogenesis and possible late effects on normal tissues. However, eosinophilic granuloma may be managed by low radiation doses of 1000–2000 rads. In addition, 8 of 9 recurrent or unresectable giant cell tumors of bone were controlled for periods of 5 to 17 years by radiation doses of 3500 rads in 3 weeks in one series.

For malignant bone tumors, the primary principle of surgery is amputation of the entire bone for patients with osteosarcomas, chondrosarcomas, fibrosarcomas, and most malignant fibrous histiocytomas. The proximal joint should be included in the amputation specimen. For lesions of the foot, a below-the-knee amputation is usually required; while for tibial tumors, an above-the-knee amputation is performed. Patients with lesions of the distal femur should be considered for hip disarticulation, but when the proximal femur is involved, a hemipelvectomy is recommended. Palliative amputation may be considered when pathologic fracture is present, when a massive tumor is noted, or when either or both of these processes produce severe pain. Currently, en bloc bone resection in selected patients with osteosarcomas and replacement grafting is being studied in a research setting. En bloc resection may also be indicated for patients with low-grade chondrosarcomas.

The role of radiation therapy in bone tumors is to eradicate the neoplasm but also to preserve function. To do this, careful attention must be paid to the details of treatment, such as treating two radiation portals per day, diminishing the irradiated volume as the dose increases, sparing as much normal tissue as possible to preserve lymphatic drainage, and providing for careful immobilization during each radiation therapy treatment. In reticulum cell sarcoma of bone, a standard lymphoma work-up consisting of bone marrow biopsy, lymphangiogram, chest radiograph, and appropriate blood studies should be performed. The entire bone is irradiated to 4000–5000 rads in 4½ to 5½ weeks, when an additional 500–1000-rad booster dose is given to the involved area. With these techniques, a 47% 5-year survival has been obtained. In Ewing's sarcoma, 4000–4500 rads are delivered to the entire bone through multiple ports, all fields treated each day. The fields are then reduced, so that a final dose of 6000–6500 rads in 7 weeks is given to the area of initial involvement. Few patients with osteosarcoma are cured with radiation alone, even when 7000–10,000 rads (conventional 200-rad fractions) are delivered to the bone in 7 to 10 weeks. When higher doses were given under hypoxic conditions, local control was still difficult to obtain, and severe soft tissue morbidity ensued. Combining high dose per fraction irradiation (760 rad treatments at 5-day intervals) with an intra-arterial sensitizer infusion and systemic chemotherapy has produced a high local control rate in a limited number of patients whose osteosarcomas were either unresectable or required such mutilating procedures as hemipelvectomy or forequarter amputation.

In osteosarcoma and Ewing's sarcoma, survival *may* have been increased by combined modality treatment. The addition of chemotherapy has improved 5-year survival in Ewing's sarcoma from 0–20% to 52–75% after the use of combined modality therapy. These improved survivals were obtained by high-dose megavoltage irradiation of the involved bone and either V-CAD (vincristine, cyclophosphamide, and Adriamycin) or V-CAD plus Actinomycin D chemotherapy, respectively. Similarly, only 5% to 20% 5-year survivals were noted for patients with osteosarcomas prior to the use of adjuvant chemotherapy. Approximately 80% of these patients developed lung metastases by 1 year after amputation. Three-year survivals of 50% to 60% have recently been reported with either high-dose methotrexate and citrovorum factor rescue, or with Adriamycin alone, or with V-CAD or COMPADRI (cyclophosphamide, vincristine, methotrexate, L-PAM, Adriamycin), all in uncontrolled studies. In a series from the Mayo Clinic, however, the 3-year survival for patients with osteosarcomas who underwent surgery alone improved from 20% prior to 1972 to 50% in patients treated between 1972 and 1974. Therefore the improved survivals noted with adjuvant chemotherapy are less impressive than they initially appeared, and prospective controlled trials will be necessary to prove its value.

Elective lung irradiation, 2000 rads in 2 weeks, significantly decreased the rate of pulmonary relapse in a European study in which patients undergoing lung irradiation were compared to those randomly assigned to receive no pulmonary radiotherapy.

Malignant fibrous histiocytomas are rare tumors. In a series of 11 patients with primary bone involvement, 9 ultimately developed pulmonary metastases. The role and effectiveness of chemotherapy or radiotherapy in the treatment of this neoplasm are unclear at present.

Chondrosarcomas are also managed initially by surgery. Patients with grade I well-differentiated chondrosarcomas have 5-year survival rates of 90%, and few, if any, develop pulmonary metastases. With grade II tumors, 81% 5-year survivals have been noted, with a 10% risk for pulmonary metastasis. In grade III, however, 43% 5-year survivals were obtained, but 71% of the patients developed distant metastases. Five-year survivals of approximately 33% may be expected for patients with fibrosarcomas of bone, which are also managed primarily by radical surgery.

D.G.

Breur K, Cohen P, Schweisguth O, Hart A: Irradiation of the lungs as an adjuvant therapy in the treatment of osteosarcoma of the limbs. Eur J Cancer 14:461–471, 1978.
Forty-four patients received 2000 rads to the lungs in 2 weeks after radical treatment of the primary lesion; 42 patients at random did not receive lung radiation therapy. Pulmonary irradiation significantly decreased the rate of lung metastases.

Codwick G: Solitary malignant tumors of bone. Semin Roentgenol 1:293–313, 1966.
Article gives detailed analysis of basic radiographic patterns of destructive bone lesions.

Dahlin D, Unni K, Matsuno T: Malignant (fibrous) histiocytoma of bone— fact or fancy? Cancer 39:1508–1516, 1977.
Thirty-five lesions with this diagnosis were discovered from more than 1000 lesions initially interpreted as either fibrosarcoma (158) or osteosarcoma (962).

Evans H, Ayala A, Romsdahl M: Prognostic factors in chondrosarcoma of bone. Cancer 40:818–831, 1977.
Histopathology and survival of patients with chondrosarcoma were compared.

Goldenberg R, Campbell C, Bonfiglio M: Giant cell tumor of bone. An analysis of 218 cases. Am J Bone Joint Surg 52:619–664, 1970.
Extensive review—very large series.

Harwood A, Fornasier V, Rider W: Supervoltage irradiation in the management of giant cell tumor of bone. Radiology 125:223–226, 1977.
Nine patients with either unresectable or recurrent tumors underwent irradiation (3500 rads in 3 weeks); in 8 the tumors were controlled for 5 to 17 years.

Huvos A, Higinbotham N: Primary fibrosarcoma of bone. Cancer 35:837–847, 1975.
Amputations were performed in most of 133 patients with this condition; there was a 34% survival.

Jaffe N, Traggis D, Cassady J, et al: The role of high dose methotrexate with citrovorum factor "rescue" on the treatment of osteogenic sarcoma. Int J Radiat Oncol Biol Phys 2:261–266, 1977.
This report discusses results of combined radiation therapy, methotrexate with citrovorum rescue plus Adriamycin treatment in localized and metastatic osteosarcoma.

Mankin HJ: Current concepts in cancer: Advances in diagnosis and treatment of bone tumors. N Engl J Med 300:543–545, 1979.
A brief summary of the subject with good reference list.

Muggia F, Louie A: Five years of adjuvant treatment of osteosarcoma: More questions than answers. Cancer Treat Rep 62:301–305, 1978.
The title says it all. Chemotherapy may be only delaying metastases.

Pomeroy T, Johnson R: Combined modality therapy of Ewing's sarcoma. Cancer 35:36–47, 1975.
With this therapy there was 5-year survival in 43 patients without demonstrable metastases at diagnosis.

Price G, Jeffree G: Metastatic spread of osteosarcoma. Br J Cancer 28:515–524, 1973.
In this large series rates of local control by radiation therapy and survival are discussed in detail.

Rosen G, Caparros B, Mosende C, et al: Curability of Ewing's sarcoma and considerations for future therapeutic trials. Cancer 41:888–899, 1978.
This is an updated Memorial-Sloan Kettering series.

Rosen G, Huvos A, Mosende C, et al: Chemotherapy and thoracotomy for metastatic osteogenic sarcoma. Cancer 41:841–849, 1978.
Best treatment appears to be surgical resection of all pulmonary metastases, if possible, and combination chemotherapy.

Suit H: Role of therapeutic radiology in cancer of bone. Cancer 35:930–935, 1975.
This is a review of the results of radiation therapy in Ewing's, osteosarcoma, and rhabdomyosarcoma of bone.

Sutow W, Gehan E, Dyment P, et al: Multidrug adjuvant chemotherapy for osteosarcoma: Interim report of the SWOG studies. Cancer Treat Rep 62:265–269, 1978.
COMPADRI-I, COMPADRI-II, and COMPADRI-III results are compared. There were significantly more relapses in regimens II and III.

Taylor W, Ivins J, Dahlin D, et al: Trends and variability in survival from osteosarcoma. Mayo Clin Proc 53:695–700, 1978.
Survival with surgery alone increased from 25% at 3 years (1963–1972) to 50% in patients treated after 1972. These are similar to results obtained in adjuvant, uncontrolled chemotherapy studies.

Wang C: Treatment of primary reticulum cell sarcoma of bone by irradiation. N Engl J Med 278:1331–1332, 1968.
This short review showed a 47% 5-year survival rate with irradiation alone.

55. SOFT TISSUE SARCOMAS (STS)—PRIMARY OR REGIONAL

Soft tissue sarcomas (STS) are rare neoplasms, accounting for less than 0.5% of cancers. There were 4500 new cases predicted for 1980, with 1600 deaths. There are a number of different histopathologic subtypes of soft tissue sarcomas: (1) fibrosarcoma (19% of all STS); (2) fibrous histiocytoma (11%); (3) liposarcoma (18%); (4) rhabdomyosarcoma (19%, fifth most common tumor in the pediatric age group); (5) leiomyosarcoma (7%); (6) angiosarcoma (3%); (7) synovial sarcoma (7%); and other, less common tumors—alveolar soft part sarcoma, extraskeletal osteosarcoma and chondrosarcoma, malignant schwannoma, unclassified sarcomas, and malignant mesenchymoma. All these neoplasms tend to metastasize by the hematogenous route, and 11% of patients have evident metastases at the time of the initial diagnosis. However, rhabdomyosarcomas, synovial sarcomas, and malignant fibrous histiocytomas all may metastasize to lymph nodes. The etiology of these tumors is unknown, although neurofibrosarcomas may arise in patients with von Recklinghausen's disease and lymphangiosarcomas have been reported to occur in patients with chronic upper extremity lymphedema following mastectomy and/or postmastectomy irradiation.

Soft tissue sarcomas usually present as a progressively enlarging mass, commonly in the thigh. Local pain may result, and metastases may cause cough (lung metastases) or bowel or ureteral obstruction (retroperitoneal tumor). Occasionally the neoplasms are associated with paraneoplastic syndromes, producing an insulin-like substance with hypoglycemia.

In the evaluation of patients with suspected soft tissue neoplasms, a history of an enlarging mass, any of the symptoms just listed, or the existence of a paraneoplastic syndrome should be elicited. The examination should include not only the size and mobility of the mass and possible involvement of nerves, blood vessels, or surrounding joints, but also palpation of the regional lymph nodes. A chest radiograph is mandatory, as is a soft tissue radiograph of the area of involvement to demonstrate both the soft tissue abnormality and the underlying osseous structures. Specialized radiographic procedures such as tomograms, xeroradiograms, and arteriograms may all be indicated. CT scans of extremity soft tissue sarcomas are currently being studied as methods for detecting the nature of the mass (cystic vs. solid) and its local extension. An adequate biopsy is essential. A small lesion may be excised, while incisional or needle biopsies may be performed for larger lesions. Expert histopathologic interpretation is mandatory. After the evaluation is completed, the patient may then be staged. The most important determinants appear to be tumor histologic grade and size. For example, the following 5-year survivals have been obtained: 80% for patients with stage I sarcomas (localized, low-grade tumors); 60% for stage II; 30% for stage III; and 10% for those with stage IV high-grade, large tumors.

The most widely used and still standard therapy for soft tissue sarcomas is radical surgery. Amputation, radical resection of the entire involved muscle mass, and/or resection of any adjacent involved structures are recommended surgical procedures. Since these tumors may have a pseudocapsule, the clinically apparent area of involvement may be misleading. In a series of 653 patients managed primarily by radical surgery, local recurrences were noted in 29%, ranging from 26% of 116 patients with liposarcomas to 36% of 97 patients with fibrosarcomas. If the tumor is low-grade, localized, and completely resected (stage I), additional radiotherapy or chemotherapy may not be necessary. However, if the tumor is high-grade or more extensive, additional therapy may be needed, especially for patients with stage IV tumors or any with grade III features.

At present, combined modality therapy, including limited resection, is being studied. At least one preliminary randomized trial has shown that local control rates for limited surgery and postoperative radiation are comparable to those for radical amputations. The best example of what can be accomplished by combined modality treatment is the treatment of embryonal rhabdomyosarcomas in children, in which limited surgery, high-dose radiotherapy to the resection bed, and pulse-VAC (vincristine, actinomycin D, cyclophosphamide) chemotherapy have resulted in relapse-free survivals of over 90% at 1 to 2 years for patients with localized tumors. Survival has also been improved for patients with more advanced tumors. However, survival rates are lower for patients with alveolar rhabdomyosarcomas or for those of adult onset.

Following local resection, careful attention must be paid to the details of radiation therapy. A portion of the entire limb should be left unirradiated to maintain functional lymphatic drainage. The total radiation dose should be 6500–7000 rads in 6 to 8 weeks; multiple radiation portals should also be used, with all fields treated each day. Careful immobilization during each treatment is essential for optimal results. Shrinking techniques are used, in which approximately 5000 rads in 5 weeks are delivered initially to a large volume, including the original tumor site and a 5- to 7-cm margin of normal tissue. Following this, an additional 1000 rads are delivered to the area of surgical manipulation. After another reduction in field size, another 500–1000 rads are delivered to the tumor bed alone, using more generous fields if the tumor is high-grade histologically, for a total dose to this region of 6500–7000 rads. When these techniques are used, local control rates of 80% to 90% have been obtained.

D.G.

Cantin J, McNeer G, Chu F, Booker R: The problem of local recurrence after treatment of soft tissue sarcoma. Ann Surg 168:47–53, 1968.
653 patients were treated curatively at Memorial-Sloan Kettering. The local recurrence rate was 29%.

Hellman K, Ryall R, MacDonald E, et al: Comparison of radiotherapy with and without razoxane (ICRF 159) in the treatment of soft tissue sarcomas. Cancer 41:100–107, 1978.
The combination treatment resulted in fewer local recurrences than the radiation therapy alone.

Maurer H, Moon T, Donaldson M, et al: The Intergroup Rhabdomyosarcoma Study. Cancer 40:2015–2026, 1977.
In Group I 92% of patients were relapse free 1+ years; in group II 85% of patients were NED at 12 months. Results were lower but still good for groups III (69% NED) and IV (50% survival with median 41- to 44-week follow-up).

Pritchard D, Soule E, Taylor W, Ivins J: Fibrosarcoma—a clinicopathologic and statistical study of 199 tumors of the soft tissues of the extremities and trunk. Cancer 33:888–897, 1974.
Tumor grade was the most important criterion re survival: for grade I 80% at 10 years, and 35%, 28%, and 18% for grades 2, 3, and 4, respectively.

Reszel P, Soule E, Coventry M: Liposarcoma of the extremities and limb girdles. J Bone Joint Surg 48A:229–244, 1966.
Extensive clinicopathological review of 222 patients with liposarcoma.

Rosenberg S, Kent H, Costa J, et al: Prospective, randomized evaluation of the role of limb-sparing surgery, radiation therapy and adjuvant chemotherapy in the treatment of adult soft-tissue sarcomas. Surgery 84:62–69, 1978.
Limb-sparing surgery and radiation therapy may be as effective as radical amputation in achieving local control.

Russell W, Cohen J, Enzinger F, et al: A clinical and pathological staging system for soft tissue sarcomas. Cancer 40:1562–1570, 1977.
Thorough review of the new American Joint Committee staging system for soft tissue sarcomas.

Suit H, Russell W: Radiation therapy of soft tissue sarcomas. Cancer 36:759–764, 1975.
Review article.

Suit H, Russell W: Soft part tumors. Cancer 39:830–836, 1977.
Article discusses local control and relapse-free survival rates for 100 patients whose disease was staged by the new American Joint Committee classification.

Suit H, Russell W, Martin R: Sarcoma of soft tissue. Clinical and histopathologic parameters and response to treatment. Cancer 35:1478–1483, 1975.
Local control was obtained in 87 of 100 patients by using conservative surgery and radiation therapy. Survival by histological grade was: grade 1, 86%; grade 2, 51%; and grade 3, 17%.

PART IV. RELAPSING OR METASTATIC MALIGNANCY

For the patient with relapsing or metastatic malignancy, therapeutic management and prognosis may be far different than for the patient with localized disease. Therefore pathologic documentation of relapse or distant sites should be obtained whenever possible. Suggestive radiologic or scintiscan studies may prove falsely positive (for example, a solitary bone abnormality in a woman with primary breast cancer), or an assumed relapse may prove to be a second, potentially curable, primary (such as a solitary pulmonary nodule in the patient with colon carcinoma). Ancillary laboratory studies may add weight to the evidence of relapsing or metastatic disease, but rarely by themselves are they indications to initiate therapy.

Once pathologic documentation has been obtained, then it becomes important to assess the extent of disease and sites of involvement. Although staging designations are not generally available for relapsing or metastatic disease, the discipline implied by staging is nonetheless important in treatment planning and prognosis. This is particularly relevant when a curative approach is contemplated. For example, the application of aggressive local therapy alone may be inappropriate if disseminated disease is detected. Furthermore, even when metastatic disease is present, anticipation of potential morbidity in a given site may ameliorate this complication (such as pathologic fracture in metastatic breast cancer or cerebral metastases in small cell carcinoma of the lung). Aside from extent of disease and sites of involvement, attention should also be paid to such pertinent therapeutic and prognostic variables as histopathology, estrogen receptor protein, performance status, age, and menopausal status. With knowledge of such variables, the potential benefits of treatment and a therapeutic plan can be defined. In addition, careful staging and evaluation of relapsing or metastatic disease can assist in the interpretation of treatment results and subsequent management. For those patients with disease relapse, detailed information about prior treatment is pivotal: Was the initial extent of disease thoroughly evaluated, was the initial therapy adequate, what was the disease-free interval prior to relapse, should the initial diagnostic pathology be reviewed again, etc.?

A multidisciplinary approach (such as combined irradiation and chemotherapy) is often indicated in the treatment of patients with relapsing or metastatic disease. In such cases a detailed course of therapy should be carefully planned in advance. Because prior treatment may adversely influence results of salvage therapy and/or lead to excessive or unexpected host toxicity, such patients may require closer follow-up than those receiving initial treatment. Moreover, anticipation of disease and/or treatment complications may obviate undue morbidity from them (such as early onset Adriamycin cardiomyopathy in the patient with prior mediastinal irradiation).

When the intent of treatment is palliation rather than cure, one must thoroughly examine whether there is value in initiating treatment at all. Is the disease symptomatic? Is it progressive? Is there evidence that treatment may prolong survival? Is the treatment likely to prevent a morbid disease complication? Will treatment prolong a patient's relatively asymptomatic state, or will it produce undue host toxicity without affecting the course of disease? What approaches can be tolerated by the patient? Once treatment is initiated, one should not lose sight of the goal—palliation—in pursuit of the disease. On the other hand, hesitancy to initiate appropriately aggressive, and often morbid, therapy may become a self-fulfilling prophecy where inappropriately conservative approaches compromise not only palliation but survival.

C.P.

57. METASTASES FROM UNKNOWN PRIMARY SITES—RELAPSING OR METASTATIC

The patient who presents with metastatic disease is frequently a diagnostic and therapeutic challenge. As many as 3% to 4% of patients referred to a cancer center have metastases from unknown primary sites even after extensive evaluation. Such patients are usually 40 to 70 years of age and are equally distributed according to sex. Presenting manifestations of malignancy may be regional lymphadenopathy alone, or there may be visceral, bony, and/or subcutaneous disease with or without lymphadenopathy.

The most common regional presentation for metastatic cancer from an unknown primary site is cervical lymphadenopathy, accounting for more than one-third of all patients in one series. Regional supraclavicular or axillary lymph nodes are less frequently encountered, and inguinal adenopathy alone is unusual. The histopathology of such cervical lymph node metastases is squamous carcinoma in most cases; and at autopsy, more than 70% of cases have a primary tumor documented within the head and neck region, usually in the nasopharynx, tonsil, or base of tongue. Regional supraclavicular and axillary adenopathy, on the other hand, is associated with adenocarcinoma. Lung and gastrointestinal cancer are found most often at autopsy with supraclavicular metastases, while breast cancer (in women) is more common with axillary metastases. When squamous carcinoma is identified in cervical lymph nodes, an extensive search of the head and neck, including blind biopsies, is justified, so that therapy with "curative" intent can be delivered to all known disease. Several groups have emphasized that even when the primary site cannot be found, as many as 30% to 50% of patients are disease-free at 3 years after radical therapy. Relapses continue to be documented at 5 years, however, and it is uncertain how many of these patients are in fact "cured." The choice of therapy in this setting must be based on the clinical presentation, weighing what will give the greatest disease control and at the same time optimize the quality of life. Where it has been analyzed, both radical neck dissection and radical irradiation (5500 rads in 5 weeks to all tissues from the base of the skull to the clavicle, reaching to the midline) have given similar results in terms of local control and survival.

In contrast to cervical metastases, supraclavicular metastases connote a poor prognosis, with a median survival of 7 months in one study. Although unusual, axillary metastases of adenocarcinoma in a woman are usually treated in a like manner to primary breast cancer, and the results of therapy appear to be similar.

Visceral, bony, or subcutaneous metastases from an unknown primary site are most often adenocarcinoma or undifferentiated carcinoma. Sites of involvement vary in different series but include metastases to lung or pleura (20% to 40%), liver (10% to 60%), bone (10% to 20%), and subcutaneous tissue (10%). In general, radiologic studies are helpful in determining the extent of metastatic disease but not the primary site. Positive x-ray findings were documented in one study on chest x-ray (43%), bone survey (43%), intravenous pyelogram (9%), barium enema (6%), upper gastrointestinal series (10%), and mammogram (13%). The yield of radionuclide scans was highest for liver (35%), bone (78%), and brain (47%).

The purpose of such studies is to identify the primary site so that more specific therapy can be given (for example, endocrine maneuvers in breast cancer), or to provide information on the extent of disease so that specific problems can be anticipated (such as bowel obstruction). In spite of such extensive evaluations, the primary cancer is documented before death in less than 10% of patients. Nevertheless, the clinicians' working impression of the primary site is correct in up to 70% of cases later examined at autopsy. The primary malignancies most commonly found to present as visceral, bony, or subcutaneous metastases from an unknown primary site are lung (20% to 40%), pancreas (10% to 20%), stomach (7% to 10%), colorectal (4% to 7%), liver (10%), and kidney (3% to 6%). On the other hand, breast and prostate cancer are unusual causes.

The prognosis for such patients is poor, with a median survival of less than 7 months. Chemotherapy (usually 5-FU alone or in combination) has had little impact: objective responses were seen in only 12% of patients with metastatic adenocarcinoma in Moertel's [1972] series, and the median duration of response was 3.5 months. The survival of those patients who responded to therapy was better (median = 12 months) than for those who did not (median = 7 months), but this may simply reflect the biology of the disease and may not be an effect of chemotherapy. On the other hand, chemotherapy does offer symptomatic improvement and/or stabilization of disease in the majority of patients and may prolong survival in those who respond. Since the bulk of patients have lung and pancreatic adenocarcinomas, the choice of chemotherapy should be directed toward these diseases.

C.P.

Barrie JR, Knapper WH, Strong EW: Cervical nodal metastases of unknown origin. Am J Surg 120:466–470, 1970.
Overall survival was 30% at 3 years for 123 patients treated with curative intent (either radical neck dissection or radical irradiation).

Didolkar MS, Fanous N, Elias EG, Moore RH: Metastatic carcinomas from occult primary tumors: A study of 254 patients. Ann Surg 186:625–630, 1977.
Patients with metastatic disease in high or mid-cervical lymph nodes alone had significantly better survival (median of 21 months) when compared to those with other metastatic sites (median of 5 to 7 months).

Fitzpatrick PJ, Kotalik JF: Cervical metastases from an unknown primary tumor. Radiology 110:659–663, 1974.
Squamous carcinoma is the most common histology seen in cervical lymph nodes.

Fu KK, Stewart JR, Bagshaw MA: Cervical node metastases from occult primary sites. Rocky Mt Med J 70:31–35, 1973.
An analysis of 67 patients with cervical lymph node metastases.

Jesse RH, Perez CA, Fletcher GH: Cervical lymph node metastasis: Unknown primary cancer. Cancer 31:854–859, 1973.
Article presents an analysis of 210 patients who received definitive treatment—radiation therapy and/or surgery. At three years 48% were free of disease.

Moertel CG: Adenocarcinoma of unknown origin. Ann Intern Med 91:646–647, 1979.
A well-written editorial discussing the appropriate work-up and therapy of patients with adenocarcinoma of unknown origin.

Moertel CG, Reitemeier RJ, Schutt AJ, Hahn RG: Treatment of the patient with adenocarcinoma of unknown origin. Cancer 30:1469–1472, 1972.
Objective responses to chemotherapy (5-fluorouracil) occurred in 12% of 162 patients studied; median survival was 4 months.

Nystrom JS, Weiner JM, Heffelfinger-Juttner J, et al: Metastatic and histologic presentations in unknown primary cancer. Semin Oncol 4:53–58, 1977.
Article presents a multivariate analysis of 152 patients with metastases from an unknown primary cancer.

Richardson RG, Parker RG: Metastases from undetected primary cancers. West J Med 123:337–339, 1975.
The median survival for 86 patients referred for palliative irradiation was 3 months.

Westbrook KC, Gallagher HS: Breast carcinoma presenting as an axillary mass. Am J Surg 122:607–611, 1971.
Review of 18 patients with breast carcinoma.

58. MELANOMA—RELAPSING OR METASTATIC

More than half of all patients with melanoma will develop recurrent or metastatic disease following primary therapy. Initial local and/or regional relapse in skin, subcutaneous tissue, and lymph nodes accounts for the majority of these treatment failures. Other common sites of metastatic disease include lung, liver, bone, gastrointestinal tract, and central nervous system. In addition, melanoma may involve such organs as the kidneys, heart, adrenals, and spleen.

Several prognostic variables have been identified in metastatic melanoma: females survive longer than males stage for stage and treatment for treatment; the time to appearance of metastatic disease is shorter for head and neck primaries (1 year) than for lesions of the distal extremities (2 years); patients with skin or subcutaneous metastases alone have a longer survival than do those with visceral disease; central nervous system metastases connote an ominous prognosis, with a median survival of less than 3 months. An unusual feature of melanoma that can affect prognosis is the documented incidence of spontaneous regression that occurs in approximately 2.2/1000 melanoma patients. Although melanoma accounts for less than 1% of all malignancies, it accounts for 11% of the documented cases of spontaneous regression in malignancy. Sites of disease most frequently affected are the skin, subcutaneous tissue, lymph nodes, and lung. In most instances of spontaneous regression of melanoma, the patient is apparently cured.

The treatment of regionally metastatic melanoma is frequently difficult. If the disease recurs locally in the skin, with a small number of lesions, then the surgical principles for local control of primary melanoma may apply (usually requiring wide local excision with skin grafting). With multiple subcutaneous nodules, simple local excision can be performed. If there are multiple cutaneous metastases, however, then massive resectional surgery is probably not justified, since the patient will die of progressive metastatic disease in spite of surgery. Other therapies that have been used include local radiation therapy (in general, the results are poor, since this is a highly radioresistant tumor), local perfusion chemotherapy (of uncertain benefit), immunotherapy, and systemic chemotherapy.

Although immunotherapy is not known to be curative, it may provide effective and sometimes prolonged palliation of cutaneous metastases. In immunocompetent patients, the intralesional injection of live Calmette-Guérin bacillus (BCG) results in complete tumor regression in up to 90% of lesions. Furthermore, there may be concomitant regression of uninjected nodules located within the same lymphatic region in 15% to 20% of patients receiving intralesional BCG. The results of such therapy are usually transient, although Morton et al [1974] have reported 11 of 36 patients disease-free for 6 to 74 months; it is not known, however, whether intralesional BCG therapy prolongs survival. Intralesional BCG is ineffective in patients who are anergic to dinitrochlorobenzene (DNCB) and tuberculin skin tests; the local skin response is less frequently seen in patients with visceral metastases or "large" tumor burdens; BCG intralesional injection of subcutaneous nodules is much less effective than of cutaneous lesions; and nodal or visceral metastases do not respond. Other methods of local immunotherapy include the application of DNCB or the intralesional injection of smallpox or mumps vaccine. Intralesional BCG is associated with several toxicities, including local abscess formation, high fevers and shaking chills, systemic BCG infection, granulomatous hepatitis, and anaphylaxis.

Systemic chemotherapy is most effective in the palliation of metastatic melanoma involving skin, subcutaneous, and nodal sites. Objective response rates to DTIC are reported as high as 40% to 70% in these sites; however, the duration of response is usually short (<7 months). Whether the addition of immunotherapy (BCG by scarification) improves these results is not known. DTIC and the nitrosoureas (BCNU and methyl-CCNU) appear to be the most effective single agents in the treatment of metastatic melanoma (overall objective response rates of approximately 18%; and DTIC alone has a reported complete remission rate of 5%). Unfortunately, combination chemotherapy with DTIC plus a nitrosourea does not appear to improve the objective response rate or survival as compared to the single agents. Patients who respond to chemotherapy have a longer survival (median, 11 months) than those who do not (4 months). Metastatic sites that respond poorly to chemotherapy are those in bone and liver, whereas central nervous system metastases do not respond at all.

Approximately 10% of patients with metastatic melanoma have central nervous system (CNS) metastases at presentation, and more than 50% of patients have CNS metastases at autopsy. In one series, 25% of patients with positive brain scans were entirely asymptomatic and had no abnormalities on neurologic examination. Since chemotherapy is ineffective treatment for CNS metastases, such patients should receive palliative whole brain irradiation.

C.P.

Amer MH, Al-Sarraf M, Vaitkevicius VK: Clinical presentation, natural history and prognostic factors in advanced malignant melanoma. Surg Gynecol Obstet 149:687–692, 1979.
A retrospective analysis of 140 patients: disease-free interval greater than 6 months, performance status greater than or equal to 50, and metastases to skin or lymph nodes were associated with a more favorable prognosis at the onset of metastatic disease.

Carella RJ, Gelber R, Hendrickson F, et al: Value of radiation therapy in the management of patients with cerebral metastases from malignant melanoma: Radiation Therapy Oncology Group Brain Metastases study I and II. Cancer 45:679–683, 1980.

Symptomatic (76% of 54 evaluable patients) and functional (41% of 44) improvement was obtained with whole brain irradiation; median survival was 10 to 14 weeks.

Comis RL: DTIC (NSC-45388) in malignant melanoma: A perspective. Cancer Treat Rep 60:165–176, 1976.
DTIC is the most effective single agent in metastatic melanoma, with an objective response rate of 16% to 31%.

Costanza ME, Nathanson L, Schoenfeld D, et al: Results with methyl-CCNU and DTIC in metastatic melanoma. Cancer 40:1010–1015, 1977.
This prospective randomized trial showed no significant differences between methyl-CCNU, DTIC, or methyl-CCNU plus DTIC in terms of response or survival.

DeVita VT Jr, Fisher RI: Natural history of malignant melanoma as related to therapy. Cancer Treat Rep 60:153–157, 1976.
This excellent review emphasizes the importance of prognostic variables.

Einhorn LH, Burgess MA, Vallejos C, et al: Prognostic correlations and response to treatment in advanced metastatic malignant melanoma. Cancer Res 34:1995–2004, 1974.
In this analysis of 426 patients skin, subcutaneous, and lung metastases showed the most favorable responses to chemotherapy.

Goodnight JE, Morton DL: Immunotherapy for malignant disease. Ann Rev Med 29:231–283, 1978.
An excellent review with exhaustive references.

Gutterman JU, Mavligit GM, Reed R, et al: Bacillus Calmette-Guérin immunotherapy in combination with DTIC (NSC-45388) for the treatment of malignant melanoma. Cancer Treat Rep 60:177–182, 1976.
The objective response rate (27%) and median survival (approximately 12 months) for the use of DTIC plus BCG appear superior to DTIC alone; however, the DTIC plus BCG is compared to a historical DTIC group and not a concurrent control.

Morton DL, Eilber FR, Holmes EC, et al: BCG immunotherapy of malignant melanoma: Summary of a seven-year experience. Ann Surg 180:635–643, 1974.
This article describes the results of intralesional BCG therapy.

Nathanson L: Spontaneous regression of malignant melanoma: A review of the literature on incidence, clinical features, and possible mechanisms. Natl Cancer Inst Monogr 44:67–77, 1976.
Cutaneous metastases were the most common sites of regression, followed by metastases in nodal, pulmonary, and hepatic sites.

Shingleton WW, Siegler HF, Stocks LH, Downs RW Jr: Management of recurrent melanoma of the extremity. Cancer 35:574–579, 1975.
Article describes limb perfusion with L-Phenylalanine mustard (L-PAM). The 5-year survival was 28% in 43 patients.

59. BRAIN TUMORS—RELAPSING OR METASTATIC

While extraneural metastases from primary brain tumors are very rare, relapse within the central nervous system is the rule. The 5-year survival of patients with glioblastoma multiforme (astrocytoma, grade IV) is virtually zero, and it is only 20% for those with grade III astrocytomas. Progressive and/or recurrent brain disease rather than extraneural metastases accounts for these poor survival results.

The detection of relapsing primary brain tumors is frequently difficult. Patients may have residual neurologic deficits resulting from the brain tumor itself or its treatment. There may be complications of surgery or radiation therapy that simulate progressive disease such as reactive edema, transient radiation-induced encephalopathy, radiation necrosis, or pseudocyst formation. Cerebral infarct, hemorrhage, or seizures may occur and be entirely unrelated to progressive tumor. In addition, patients may have exacerbations of neurologic dysfunction with drug ingestion, fatigue, or changes in mood, or with a concomitant metabolic abnormality. And, rarely, such patients may develop a second neurologic disease. The history and physical examination provide sensitive indicators of neurologic function when compared to those obtained following primary therapy. Standard laboratory tests (skull films, EEG, brain scan, computed tomography, and angiography), however, are less reliable, since there may be distortion and/or loss of brain parenchyma and scarring as well as residual tumor. Again, these studies are most helpful when compared to post-primary treatment and serial examinations.

Relapsing brain tumors may be treated in a variety of ways. Radical surgery is reserved for those lesions that are accessible and apparently resectable. It is most effective when deterioration is secondary to increased intracranial pressure, particularly secondary to a cystic mass. Prognostic factors include the disease-free interval, histopathologic findings, and tumor site. Recurrent tumors are often found to be higher grade malignancies than at initial diagnosis (in one series, 43% of 37 low-grade astrocytomas), and such cases benefit little from surgery. The overall results of surgery in selected patients with recurrent tumors are good, with as many as 44% receiving palliation for a year or more. In contrast to surgery, radiation therapy may be delivered to any involved site, accessible or not, that has not received prior irradiation. If there has been no prior irradiation, then the principles of therapy are the same as for primary treatment. When there has been prior irradiation, retreatment must be individualized depending upon the initial doses received and the risks to normal tissues with retreatment.

Chemotherapy has been employed at initial relapse, following surgery and/or irradiation, and in addition to these two modalities in the treatment of recurrent brain tumors. Interpretation of chemotherapy results is often difficult because of the loose criteria applied and the concurrent use of corticosteroids, which may ameliorate symptoms and cerebral edema and even reduce tumor size. A drug response is usually defined as "unequivocal neurologic improvement plus findings of a 'better' brain scan." Unfortunately no objective size criteria are required to identify a "better" brain scan, and few reports to date have correlated drug therapy with computerized tomography of the brain. Furthermore, many studies evaluate drug results only in patients who survive two or more months, and therefore the impact of chemotherapy on survival cannot be assessed.

The most effective drugs identified to date are the nitrosoureas (BCNU, CCNU, and methyl-CCNU) and procarbazine. Responses to therapy are seen in approximately 40% to 50% of patients with median response durations of 6 to 9 months. Unfortunately, drug combinations do not appear to be better than single agents, and there are very few patients who have cross-over responses from one drug to another.

It is of interest that those drugs that are most effective in primary brain tumors are lipophilic and cell cycle–nonspecific. Whether it is necessary for the drug to be lipophilic in order to reach adequate therapeutic concentrations in all parts of the tumor is uncertain. There is extreme neovascularization in most brain tumors, and these blood vessels do not have the same tight capillary structure as normal vessels of the blood-brain barrier. It is at the tumor's periphery, however, where tumor cells may invade normal brain parenchyma, that some hypothesize the blood-brain barrier may be most effective in limiting therapeutic drug concentrations. Other parameters that must be considered in future chemotherapy studies include drug dose, route of administration, tumor cell uptake, metabolic fate of tumor cells, and washout or sink effect of the extracellular space and cerebrospinal fluid.

C.P.

Avellanosa AM, West CR, Tsukada Y, et al: Chemotherapy of nonirradiated malignant gliomas: Phase II. Study of the combination of methyl-CCNU, vincristine, and procarbazine. Cancer 44:839–846, 1979.
In this pilot study responses were seen in 9 of 28 previously unirradiated patients.
Levin VA, Crafts DC, Norman DM, et al: Criteria for evaluating patients undergoing chemotherapy for malignant brain tumors. J Neurosurg 47:329–335, 1977.
Neurological examination, radionuclide scintiscan of the brain, and computerized tomographic brain scan were of equal value in predicting response to therapy.
Pool LJ: The management of recurrent gliomas. Clin Neurosurg 15:265–287, 1968.
Article gives results of a series of 52 patients managed by surgery.
Shapiro WR: High-dose methotrexate in malignant gliomas. Cancer Treat Rep 61:753–756, 1977.
This article presents a report of therapy in six patients with no neurological benefit.
Vick NA, Khandekar JD, Bigner DD: Chemotherapy of brain tumors: The "blood-brain barrier" is not a factor. Arch Neurol 34:523–526, 1977.
An incisive editorial with good references.
Walker MD, Alexander E, Hunt WE, et al: Evaluation of mithramycin in the treatment of anaplastic gliomas. J Neurosurg 44:655–667, 1976.
This prospective randomized trial demonstrates no significant benefit of mithramycin as compared to supportive care.
Wilson CG, Gutin P, Boldrey EB, et al: Single-agent chemotherapy of brain tumors: A five-year review. Arch Neurol 33:739–744, 1976.
Response rates to chemotherapy were 38% to 52%, with median durations of 4 to 9 months; effective drugs included BCNU, CCNU, procarbazine, and imidazole carboxamide (BIC).

60. HEAD AND NECK CANCER—RELAPSING OR METASTATIC

With improving methods of initial local and regional control in head and neck cancer, the incidence of distant metastatic disease at relapse has increased. In 1923 Crile reported an incidence of 1% at autopsy, whereas more recent autopsy series report an incidence of 17% to 57%. More importantly, clinically apparent distant metastatic disease at relapse has been documented in 11% to 12% of patients who were initially treated with "curative" intent; and in half these patients, the primary region was free of recurrent disease at relapse. Nevertheless, the most difficult problem in the treatment of head and neck cancer remains the progression or recurrence of loco-regional disease (occurring in approximately 40% of patients treated with "curative" intent).

Both local recurrence and/or distant metastases are most likely to occur within the first 18 to 24 months; and both occur most frequently with large primaries (T_3 and T_4) and positive lymph nodes (N_2 and N_3). Lesions of the true vocal cord are most favorable for local control as well as for their low incidence of later metastatic disease (1.4%), whereas lesions of the nasopharynx and hypopharynx are difficult to control locally and have a high incidence of later metastatic disease (22.1% and 14.6% in one study). The prognosis for patients with recurrent and/or metastatic head and neck cancer is poor, with more than 90% of patients dead within the first 2 years following relapse.

Although progressive or recurrent loco-regional disease accounts for the majority of head and neck relapses, local therapeutic modalities are frequently unsuitable, since most patients have received aggressive surgery and irradiation as primary management. Radiation therapy of recurrent disease in a patient without prior irradiation follows the principles of primary therapy, whereas re-irradiation may be impossible where normal tissues have received doses in excess of 5000 rads. However, transient palliation may sometimes be achieved by local field therapy or tumor implantation. Likewise, surgery can sometimes be used to palliate local symptoms, although it must be remembered that patients with recurrent or progressive head and neck cancer have short survivals and usually cannot tolerate extensive reconstructions. Whatever local therapy is contemplated for recurrent loco-regional disease, it is important to rule out the presence of distant metastatic tumor that would be left untreated. The most common sites of distant metastases are lung, bone, and liver. Therefore chest x-ray, full-lung tomography (in selected cases), liver function tests, and bone and liver scans are recommended.

Systemic chemotherapy has been used in the treatment of progressive or recurrent loco-regional disease as well as in the treatment of distant metastases. The most effective drugs appear to be methotrexate, bleomycin, and *cis*-diamminedichloroplatinum (CDDP). Objective responses are reported in 25% to 50% of patients, with response durations of 2 to 6 months. Variables important in analyzing the results of therapy include tumor stage, site of primary (lesions of the oral cavity and oropharynx respond better than those of the nasopharynx or hypopharynx), prior therapy (both prior irradiation and chemotherapy adversely affect response), nutritional status, and performance status.

Methotrexate is the drug most extensively investigated to date. Intermittent methotrexate administration appears to be superior to continuous daily regimens. On the other hand, there is no convincing data that conventional dose therapy is superior to high-dose methotrexate with leukovorin rescue in terms of response or response duration. However, methotrexate toxicity (mucositis and hematologic depression) is ameliorated with the high-dose regimen utilizing leukovorin rescue. The standard dose schedule for methotrexate is 40 to 60 mg/M^2 intravenously once a week. Attention must be paid to renal function, hydration, and alkalinization. Patients with head and neck cancer are frequently malnourished and have low serum folate levels prior to chemotherapy. As a result, methotrexate's toxicity to normal tissues may be more pronounced than expected from the dose administered. Intra-arterial methotrexate or other drug perfusion studies have yielded response rates comparable to those with intravenous therapy. The intra-arterial route is technically difficult to administer and is associated with greater local morbidity.

Combination chemotherapy utilizing methotrexate, bleomycin, and/or *cis*-diamminedichloroplatinum has not been shown to date to be superior to the single agents alone in terms of response or response duration. Similarly, there is little cross-over responsiveness to sequential single agents.

Complications of relapsing head and neck cancer include local pain, inability to handle secretions, and inability to eat, with resulting inanition. Nasogastric tube feedings and intravenous hyperalimentation have been used successfully to increase body weight and improve wound healing following surgery.

C.P.

Bertino JR, Mosher MB, De Conti RC: Chemotherapy of cancer of the head and neck. Cancer 31:1141–1149, 1973.
This article reviews a study comparing intermittent conventional dose methotrexate with intermittent high dose methotrexate with leukovorin rescue.
Carter SK: The chemotherapy of head and neck cancer. Semin Oncol 4:413–424, 1977.
In this comprehensive review the most effective single agents are methotrexate and bleomycin.
Copeland EM, MacFadyen BV Jr, MacComb WS, et al: Intravenous hyperalimentation in patients with head and neck cancer. Cancer 35:606–611, 1975.
This article reports an effective means of achieving weight gain, improved wound healing, and recovery in malnourished, debilitated patients who might otherwise be denied treatments with "curative" intent.
Donegan WL: Regional infusion chemotherapy for cancer of the head and neck. Surg Annu 7:137–173, 1975.
A comprehensive review of the technique.
Goodwin WJ Jr, Chandler JR: Hypercalcemia in epidermoid carcinoma of the head and neck. Am J Surg 132:444–448, 1976.
Hypercalcemia was documented in 7.2% of 139 patients with advanced recurrent and/or metastatic head and neck cancer.
Merino OR, Lindberg RD, Fletcher GH: An analysis of distant metastases from squamous cell carcinoma of the upper respiratory and digestive tracts. Cancer 40:145–151, 1977.
Of 5019 patients treated with "curative" intent, 10.9% developed distant metastases; lung (52%) and bone (20.3%) were the most common sites.
Probert JC, Thompson RW, Bagshaw MA: Patterns of spread of distant metastases in head and neck cancer. Cancer 33:127–133, 1974.
Distant metastases found in 12% of 779 patients; nasopharyngeal lesions were most frequently associated with later metastatic disease.
Robson MC: Resection and immediate reconstruction for patients with "inoperable" recurrent head and neck cancer. Surg Clin North Am 56:111–123, 1976.
This article presents illustrative case reports.
Rozencweig M, Von Hoff DD, Muggia FM: Investigational chemotherapeutic agents in head and neck cancer. Semin Oncol 4:425–429, 1977.
A review of cis-diamminedichloroplatinum in the treatment of head and neck cancer.
Wittes RE, Cvitkovic E, Shah J, et al: Cis-dichlorodiammineplatinum (II) in the treatment of epidermoid carcinoma of the head and neck. Cancer Treat Rep 61:359–366, 1977.
Objective responses were identified in 8 of 26 patients with recurrent head and neck cancer.

61. THYROID CANCER—RELAPSING OR METASTATIC

As methods of detection and primary therapy have improved, the numbers of patients with locally unresectable or distant metastatic thyroid cancer at presentation have decreased (in one series from 7% prior to 1950 to 1% in 1970). Nevertheless, locally recurrent tumor or the development of distant metastatic disease following primary therapy remains a persistent problem in the long-term management of thyroid carcinoma. Differentiated thyroid cancers account for 80% to 90% of all thyroid malignancies (papillary and mixed papillary with follicular = 60% to 70%, follicular = 15% to 20%). It is in this group of patients that the survival curve is characterized by a slow continuous fall over more than 10 years (in one series, 10-year survival was 80% for papillary tumors and 40% for follicular), representing the late development of distant metastatic disease and subsequent death. Although some patients may survive for more than 5 or 10 years with documented distant metastases (particularly those with follicular tumors), the majority of such patients with metastatic differentiated thyroid cancer die of disease within 2 to 5 years.

Prognostic factors at primary presentation that appear to have a correlation with poor survival (and thus the development of metastatic disease) in papillary tumors include extent of capsular invasion, extraglandular extension, and age greater than 40 years; and in follicular tumors the degree of vascular invasion and histologic tumor grade are important. Of interest is that the presence of pathologically involved lymph nodes in these differentiated tumors at presentation does not adversely affect prognosis, and some even report improved survival. Approximately half of patients with relapsing papillary tumors will have local recurrences without evidence of distant metastases, whereas more than 75% of those with relapsing follicular tumors will have distant metastases. Sites of distant metastatic disease in both are most commonly lung, bone, pleura, and pericardium.

Unlike the survival curve of differentiated thyroid cancer, that for anaplastic carcinoma (comprising 10% to 15% of thyroid cancers) falls to approximately 20% within two years of primary therapy and remains relatively flat thereafter. This disease is characterized by rapid local progression as well as early dissemination to almost any organ (particularly lungs and bones). In the majority of patients, the cause of death is recurrent local disease unresponsive to therapy.

Medullary carcinoma of the thyroid (MCT) accounts for only 3% to 6% of thyroid malignancies. Relapse may be documented in 20% to 40% of patients, with most relapses detected within the first 8 years following primary therapy. The presence of involved lymph nodes has a correlation with relapse and thus poor survival in both MCT and anaplastic tumors. Other poor prognostic factors in MCT include age greater than 50 years and unilateral tumors (a negative family history). Half the relapses in MCT are local recurrences, whereas distant metastases alone are uncommon (18% in one series). Distant sites of disease are lungs, bone, and liver. The 10-year survivorship for patients with MCT is 60% to 80%.

Since the most common sites of relapse in thyroid cancer are recurrent neck disease and metastases to lungs and bone, special attention should be paid to these areas on physical examination and by serial chest x-ray and bone scans. In addition, detection of recurrent or distant metastatic thyroid cancer may be facilitated by several studies. As many as 50% to 80% of metastatic differentiated thyroid cancers will demonstrate uptake of radioiodine with prior thyroid ablation and discontinuance of replacement thyroxine for 2 to 4 months. Purely papillary tumors, anaplastic carcinoma, Hürthle cell tumors, and MCT will not take up radioiodine. Therefore, in selected patients, radioiodine total body scans can be performed at 6- to 12-month intervals to identify possible metastatic sites of uptake. In patients with MCT, abnormal calcitonin secretion may be documented prior to primary therapy and at relapse. Provocative tests of calcitonin secretion, utilizing glucagon, calcium, pentagastrin, or whiskey, may increase detection sensitivity and can be performed serially following primary therapy.

The treatment of relapsing thyroid cancer may include surgical excision of locally recurrent adenopathy, radioiodine (^{131}I) ablation of functioning differentiated metastases, palliative external irradiation for nonfunctioning metastases, and palliative chemotherapy, as well as no therapy with close observation in patients with indolent metastatic disease. Radioiodine therapy is effective only for metastases demonstrating ^{131}I uptake after thyroid ablation and discontinuance of thyroxine replacement for 2 to 4 months. The standard dose is 150 to 200 mCi given every 6 to 12 weeks for a total of 6 to 10 doses. Response to therapy may be judged by changes in tumor dimensions and by following the percent retention of ^{131}I at 5 days or the percentage of ^{131}I organically bound to plasma at 6 days. Toxicities of treatment may include bone marrow suppression and radiation pneumonitis, but in general therapy is well tolerated. Whether there is an increased incidence of leukemia or second malignancies as late complications of therapy is uncertain. Reported results of radioiodine therapy are difficult to interpret since most series are small, and those patients most likely to respond are those with indolent disease. In addition, thyroid hormone replacement may in itself be tumor-suppressive, and all patients receive this therapy following ^{131}I. Lung metastases are reported to respond better than bone metastases, resulting in better survival for those with pulmonary disease. Also, it appears that treated patients live longer than untreated patients with metastatic follicular cancer, although this is not well documented.

Experience with chemotherapy for relapsing thyroid cancer is fragmentary. Drugs that have been used with minimal benefit are 5-fluorouracil, methotrexate, actinomycin D, cyclophosphamide, and L-phenylalanine mustard. Single agent Adriamycin has been reported to produce objective responses in one-third of patients and may be of particular efficacy in MCT.

C.P.

Block MA: Management of carcinoma of the thyroid. Ann Surg 185:133–144, 1977.
An excellent review with extensive references.
Cady B, Sedgwick CE, Meissner WA, et al: Changing clinical, pathologic, therapeutic, and survival patterns in differentiated thyroid carcinoma. Ann Surg 184:541–553, 1976.
In this extensive analysis of 792 patients, a poor prognosis was correlated with older age, male sex, extraglandular extension, blood vessel invasion, major capsular involvement, and multifocal disease.
Chong GC, Beahrs OH, Sizemore GW, Woolner LH: Medullary carcinoma of the thyroid gland. Cancer 35:695–704, 1975.
In a study of 139 patients, 25% developed recurrent or metastatic disease.
Deftos LJ: Calcitonin in clinical medicine. Adv Intern med 23:159–193, 1978.
Article reviews medullary carcinoma of the thyroid with reference to calcitonin secretion.
Franssila KO: Prognosis in thyroid carcinoma. Cancer 36:1138–1146, 1975.
Ten-year survival rates were 80% for papillary, 40% for follicular, and 20% for anaplastic carcinoma of the thyroid.
Gottlieb JA, Hill CS: Chemotherapy of thyroid cancer with adriamycin: Experience with 30 patients. N Engl J Med 290:193–197, 1974.
Objective responses were documented in 11 patients.
Harness JK, Thompson NW, Sisson JC, Beierwaltes WH: Differentiated thy-

roid carcinomas: Treatment of distant metastases. Arch Surg 108:410–419, 1974.

Article presents a study of 36 patients treated with radioactive iodine.

Leeper RD: The effect of ^{131}I therapy on survival of patients with metastatic papillary or follicular thyroid carcinoma. J Clin Endocrinol Metab 36:1143–1152, 1973.

Response to treatment and survival was poor in patients with papillary carcinoma who were over 40 years of age.

Lo Gerfo P, Colacchio D, Stillman T, Feind C: Serum thyroglobulin and recurrent thyroid cancer. Lancet 1:881–882, 1977.

In a study of 30 patients who had previously undergone total thyroidectomy all 10 patients with recurrent mixed papillary carcinoma had elevated levels of serum thyroglobulin, whereas those without recurrent disease had undetectable levels.

Pochin EE: Radioiodine therapy of thyroid cancer. Semin Nucl Med 1:503–515, 1971.

An excellent clinical review.

Woolner LB: Thyroid carcinoma: Pathologic classification with data on prognosis. Semin Nucl Med 1:481–502, 1971.

Article presents an analysis of 1181 cases of thyroid carcinoma.

62. BREAST CANCER—RELAPSING OR METASTATIC

At least 50% of all women who undergo mastectomy with "curative" intent will later relapse with local and/or distant metastatic breast cancer. Variables of prognostic significance at the time of primary therapy include tumor size, location, histologic type and grade, and extent of lymph node involvement. The majority of relapses occur during the first 18 to 24 months following mastectomy, although relapses may be detected as long as 5 to more than 20 years after. With 1 to 3 positive axillary lymph nodes, approximately 50% of patients have relapsed at 5 years; with 4 or more nodes positive, 80% have relapsed; whereas with no nodes positive, only 18% have relapsed. Unfortunately, survival data closely correlate with treatment failure rates, since available therapies for relapsing breast cancer are not curative.

Approximately 10% to 20% of relapsing breast cancers will recur locally in the chest wall and/or ipsilateral regional lymph nodes without evidence of distant metastases. Chest wall disease presents the most difficult problem, since it may be progressive, leading to ulceration and serious local morbidity. Radiation therapy (5000 rads in 5 weeks) is an effective local modality, resulting in complete regression in two-thirds of patients with a median remission duration of 22 months in one series. Although a rare patient may be reported to have no subsequent evidence of metastatic disease, essentially all patients go on to develop distant metastases following such local therapy for recurrent breast cancer. In one study the median time from documented loco-regional recurrence to distant metastases was 15 months.

Frequent sites of distant metastatic breast cancer include bone, lung and/or pleura, lymph nodes, skin, and liver. In addition to the physical examination, laboratory investigations may include chest x-ray, bone survey and bone scan, liver scan, liver function tests, and alkaline phosphatase.

The cornerstone of palliative breast cancer therapy is endocrine manipulation. A favorable response to such therapy may be anticipated in patients with indolent disease, a long disease-free interval (>18 to 24 months), prior response to endocrine therapy, and soft tissue or osseous metastases. Those patients with an aggressive clinical course, short disease-free interval, and visceral metastases (liver, brain, or lymphangitic tumor spread in the lungs) are unlikely to respond to a hormonal therapy. It may require at least 6 to 8 weeks before a patient's response to endocrine therapy can be assessed. Recently it has been shown that the presence of estrogen receptor protein (ER) in tumor tissue also has a correlation with endocrine responsiveness. ER is found in the cytoplasm of estrogen target tissues, and it is the estrogen-ER complex that enters the cell nucleus and promotes estrogen-dependent tumor growth. It is thought that when the source of estrogen is removed or antagonized, then this sequence is broken and the estrogen-dependent tumor regresses. Approximately 50% to 65% of breast tumors have ER, with postmenopausal patients possessing a greater proportion and higher level of ER than premenopausal patients. In general, ER-negative patients have a shorter disease-free interval and survival than do ER-positive patients. The ER assay can be performed on primary or metastatic tumor tissue, and usually the assay results are similar (although some report a discordance of more than 30%). If possible, ER should be obtained in all cases of relapsing breast cancer (either initially loco-regional or distant metastatic), since it is most useful in excluding ER-negative patients from hormonal therapies (particularly ablative procedures).

Bilateral oophorectomy is the initial endocrine treatment of choice in premenopausal patients. Responses are seen in 30% to 50%, with an average response duration of 12 to 16 months. Responders survive significantly longer (20 to 30 months mean) than do nonresponders (9 to 10 months mean). Patients with regular menses, aged 46 to 50 years, and with lymph node, bone, soft tissue, and/or skin disease, respond most favorably. Radiation oophorectomy can be performed on those not suitable for surgery, but it may take 4 to 8 weeks before its effects are complete. For postmenopausal patients (>5 years after menopause), oral diethylstilbestrol 15 mg per day produces responses in 30% to 35% of patients. Similarly, the antiestrogen, tamoxifen, or androgens may be used in the perimenopausal or postmenopausal patient. Response and survival results of these additive therapies are comparable to oophorectomy in premenopausal patients.

Bilateral adrenalectomy or hypophysectomy results in responses in 40% to 60% of patients who have shown prior hormone responsiveness or have positive ER assays. Likewise, in those without prior hormone responsiveness or in those with ER-negative assays, response to adrenalectomy or hypophysectomy is seen in less than 10%. Again, responders survive longer (22 to 24 months mean) than do nonresponders (6 to 8 months mean). Both adrenalectomy and hypophysectomy appear to yield comparable results in terms of response, remission duration, and survival. With transsphenoidal hypophysectomy, patients who might not tolerate adrenalectomy can still undergo a comparable ablative procedure. Rarely do patients respond to hypophysectomy following adrenalectomy, however. "Medical" adrenalectomy with aminoglutethimide and dexamethasone or hydrocortisone replacement has been reported to produce similar response results to surgical adrenalectomy and may be useful in patients who cannot tolerate any surgical procedure.

Metastatic breast cancer is responsive to a variety of chemotherapeutic agents. The most effective single agents are cyclophosphamide, Adriamycin, methotrexate, and 5-FU, with objective response rates of 30% to 35%. Other frequently used single agents include the vinca alkaloids and L-phenylalanine mustard. Combination chemotherapy yields objective response rates of 50% to 70% (20% are complete remissions), with median remission durations of 8 to 10 months. The chemotherapy program most often utilized is cyclophosphamide, 100 mg/M^2 po qd (days 1 to 14); methotrexate, 60 mg/M^2 IV (days 1 and 8); and 5-FU, 700 mg/M^2 IV (days 1 and 8) (CMF), given every 28 days for at least 10 cycles (as reported by Canellos et al. [1976]). CMF and other combinations are most effective in patients with lung, soft tissue, and nodal metastases. Responders survive significantly longer (median of 18 months) than nonresponders (median of 4 months). In general, chemotherapy has been reserved for those patients failing hormonal therapies or for those with aggressive disease, short disease-free interval, visceral metastases, or ER-negative tumors. Whether results of therapy would be improved with earlier intervention is uncertain. Prospective studies combining both chemotherapy and endocrine maneuvers have not yielded significantly increased response rates, remission durations, or survivals when compared to sequential approaches.

Radiotherapy may provide effective palliation in 70% to 90% of patients with painful bony metastases as well as prevent collapse or fracture of pathologically involved weight-bearing bones. Because destructive bone disease is such a common problem, attention must be paid to the skeleton at all times, particularly when changes in therapy are considered. The usual dose is 4000 rads in 4 weeks to weight-bearing bones, whereas 2000–2500 rads in two weeks may provide adequate palliation for other bony sites. Neither hormone therapy nor chemotherapy effectively treats central nervous system metastases. Therefore irradiation must be used for effective palliation in this site (4000–5000 rads in 4 to 5 weeks to the whole brain).

C.P.

Ahmann DL, O'Connell MJ, Hahn RG, et al: An evaluation of early or delayed adjuvant chemotherapy in premenopausal patients with advanced breast cancer undergoing oophorectomy. N Engl J Med 297:356–360, 1977.
Progression-free survival was improved with the combined approach; survival, however, was similar in both groups.

Allegra JC, Barlock A, Huff KK, Lippman ME: Changes in multiple or sequential estrogen receptor determinations in breast cancer. Cancer 45:792–794, 1980.
Simultaneous estrogen receptor (ER) assays from different metastatic sites were concordant in 23 of 27 patients studied. Sequential ER assays showed significant reduction in median ER concentrations following hormonal therapy in 10 patients but no significant change in ER concentrations following chemotherapy in 19 patients.

Brunner KW, Sonntag RW, Alberto P, et al: Combined chemo- and hormonal therapy in advanced breast cancer. Cancer 39:2923–2933, 1977.
No significant improvement was seen in terms of response, remission duration, or survival when the combined approach was used as compared to use of chemotherapy alone.

Canellos GP, DeVita VT, Gold GL, et al: Combination chemotherapy for advanced breast cancer: Response and effect on survival. Ann Intern Med 84:389–392, 1976.
Objective responses were documented in 68% of 40 patients treated with cyclophosphamide, methotrexate, 5-fluorouracil, and prednisone.

Carbone PP, Davis TE: Medical treatment for advanced breast cancer. Semin Oncol 5:417–427, 1978.
A good review.

Carter SK: Integration of chemotherapy into combined modality treatment of solid tumors: VII. Adenocarcinoma of the breast. Cancer Treat Rev 3:141–174, 1976.

Article reviews single agent and combination chemotherapy data in advanced disease as well as the role of adjuvant therapy in primary management.

Chu FCH, Lin F-J, Kim JH, et al: Locally recurrent carcinoma of the breast: Results of radiation therapy. Cancer 37:2677–2681, 1976.
Complete disease control was obtained in 67% of 215 patients with a median interval free of local disease of 22 months.

Falkson G, Falkson HC, Glidewell O, et al: Improved remission rates and remission duration in young women with metastatic breast cancer following combined oophorectomy and chemotherapy: A study by Cancer and Leukemia Group B. Cancer 43:2215–2222, 1979.
The objective response rate (72% vs. 18% and 50%) and median remission duration (17 months vs. 5 and 8 months) were better for combined vs. sequential oophorectomy and chemotherapy, respectively.

Harvey HA, Santen RJ, Osterman J, et al: A comparative trial of transsphenoidal hypophysectomy and estrogen suppression with aminoglutethimide in advanced breast cancer. Cancer 43:2207–2214, 1979.
Although estrogen receptor data were not utilized for patient selection, both therapies appeared comparable in terms of response and remission duration.

Hayward JL, Carbone PP, Heuson J-C, et al: Assessment of response to therapy in advanced breast cancer: A project of the Programme on Clinical Oncology of the International Union Against Cancer, Geneva, Switzerland. Cancer 39:1289–1294, 1977.
Article gives specific guidelines for objectively assessing response to therapy in advanced breast cancer.

Legha SS, Buzdar AU, Smith TL, et al: Complete remissions in metastatic breast cancer treated with combination drug therapy. Ann Intern Med 91:847–852, 1979.
Median duration of remission was 17 months in 116 complete responders. Relapse occurred in initial site(s) of disease in 56 of 81 patients (69%); in 12 of 81 relapses (15%) the initial site of failure was the central nervous system.

Legha SS, Davis HL, Muggia FM: Hormonal therapy of breast cancer: New approaches and concepts. Ann Intern Med 88:69–77, 1978.
An excellent review of estrogen receptor data, the use of antiestrogens, and medical adrenalectomy.

McGuire WL: Hormone receptors: Their role in predicting prognosis and response to endocrine therapy. Semin Oncol 5:428–433, 1978.
Clinical correlations of estrogen and progesterone receptor data are presented.

63. SMALL CELL CARCINOMA OF THE LUNG—RELAPSING OR METASTATIC

More than 70% of all patients with small cell carcinoma have disseminated disease at presentation: either *limited* to one hemithorax and regional lymph nodes or *extensive*, with distant metastases. Like other lung cancers, metastases may be documented in lymph nodes, bone, liver, brain, and contralateral lung. While bone marrow involvement is uncommon in other lung cancers (<20%), it has been found in 40% to 50% of patients with small cell carcinoma and may be the only site of distant metastases.

In contrast to other lung cancers, small cell carcinoma is characterized by a rapid doubling time (mean of 33 days on chest x-ray compared to 92 to 187 days for other lung cancers), a high labeling index (median of 17 compared to less than 3 for adenocarcinoma and squamous carcinoma), and responsiveness to radiation therapy and chemotherapy. Variables that may influence results of therapy and survival include the extent of disease, performance status, and prior treatment with radiation or drugs. Age, sex, and immune status appear to be less important prognostic factors.

Although radiation therapy results in objective responses in at least 90% of patients with small cell carcinoma, this modality alone had no significant survival benefit when prospectively compared to no treatment for those patients with limited disease (median survival 3.3 months for treated patients and 3.2 months for untreated). Nevertheless, like other lung cancers, radiation therapy is an effective tool for palliation of local symptoms and complications such as pain, hemoptysis, bronchial obstruction, and superior vena cava obstruction.

Chemotherapy has become the cornerstone of treatment in small cell carcinoma. In contrast to experience with other lung cancers, multiple single agents have yielded objective responses in more than 20% of patients with extensive small cell carcinoma, and, more importantly, drug combinations have been reported to result in response rates of 60% to 80%. Active single agents include cyclophosphamide, isophosphamide, nitrogen mustard, Adriamycin, methotrexate, CCNU, procarbazine, hexamethylmelamine, VP 16-213, and vincristine. When prospectively compared to a placebo, cyclophosphamide was found to prolong survival significantly in patients with extensive disease (median of 4 months vs. 1 month). Adjuvant cyclophosphamide following radiation therapy has also been shown to improve survival of patients with limited disease over irradiation alone (median of 8.5 months vs. 5.5 months).

Combination chemotherapy programs have proved to be superior to single agents in terms of response and survival in the treatment of extensive small cell carcinoma. The use of three or four drugs in combination appears to achieve better results than two-drug regimens. In addition to the documented objective responses in more than 60% of patients, complete responses are obtained in up to 25% of all patients, and the median overall survival is more than 9 months. Preliminary results of recent combination chemotherapy programs appear even more promising, with complete responses in approximately two-thirds of those with limited disease and one-third of those with extensive disease, and median survivals of 15+ months and 10 months, respectively. Furthermore, it has been emphasized by several case reports that some patients receiving chemotherapy alone are long-term survivors and have probably been cured of their disease.

Because responses to chemotherapy may be very rapid and occur in such a high proportion of previously untreated patients, local problems such as superior vena caval obstruction have been successfully treated with drugs alone rather than with radiation therapy. Whether chemotherapy plus radiation therapy to bulk disease significantly improves response and survival results compared to chemotherapy alone remains unanswered. In one small prospective trial there appeared to be no significant benefit of irradiation in extensive disease. The utility of radiation therapy has recently been tested prospectively in limited disease. Objective remissions (92% vs. 87%) were similar, whereas median remission duration (205+ vs. 180+ days) and survival (14 vs. 11 months) were better with chemotherapy alone than with chemotherapy plus irradiation.

The brain is a common site for distant metastatic disease in small cell carcinoma. At least 10% of patients are found to have brain metastases at diagnosis, and at autopsy 30% to 40% have evidence of brain involvement. Drugs are generally ineffective in treating overt brain metastases, while radiation therapy is a highly effective modality. Because brain metastases are frequently found as the first site of clinical relapse (18% of patients in one series) and also have such a high incidence at autopsy, whole brain irradiation has been employed prophylactically to prevent central nervous system (CNS) relapse. In one prospective trial, prophylactic irradiation was shown to reduce significantly the incidence of clinical CNS disease (0 of 14) as compared to no prophylaxis (4 of 15), although the median survival of both groups was the same. In other words, prophylactic brain irradiation reduces the morbidity of CNS disease but does not appear to affect the overall survival. Lipophilic drugs such as the nitrosoureas and procarbazine have been used in combination as a potential means of CNS prophylaxis. The incidence of clinical CNS relapse appears to be reduced when this modality is used alone; however, the data are not as convincing as those for prophylactic irradiation.

C.P.

Bunn PA, Cohen MH, Ihde DC, et al: Advances in small cell bronchogenic carcinoma. Cancer Treat Rep 61:333–342, 1977.
An excellent review.

Bunn PA Jr, Nugent JL, Matthews MJ: Central nervous system metastases in small cell bronchogenic carcinoma. Semin Oncol 5:314–322, 1978.
This article reviews data of CNS prophylaxis; it also emphasizes that in addition to cerebral metastases, leptomeningeal and spinal metastases are being reported with increasing frequency.

Cohen MH: Small cell bronchogenic carcinoma: A prolonged remission following chemotherapy. JAMA 237:2528, 1977.
This case report suggests a probable "cure" with chemotherapy alone.

Greco FA, Einhorn LH, Richardson RL, Oldham RK: Small cell lung cancer: Progress and perspectives. Semin Oncol 5:323–335, 1978.
A thorough review of clinical trials in small cell carcinoma of the lung.

Greco FA, Richardson RL, Snell JD: Small cell lung cancer: Complete remission and improved survival. Am J Med 66:625–630, 1979.
Of 32 patients treated with combined chemotherapy and irradiation, 29 achieved complete remission and 14 remain relapse-free for a median of 16+ months.

Hansen HH, Dombernowsky P, Hansen HS, Rorth M: Chemotherapy versus chemotherapy plus radiotherapy in regional small-cell carcinoma of the lung—a randomized trial. Proc Am Assoc Cancer Res (Abstract) 20:277, 1979.
Median remission duration and survival were better with chemotherapy alone.

Jackson DV Jr, Richards F II, Cooper MR, et al: Prophylactic cranial irradiation in small cell carcinoma of the lung: A randomized study. JAMA 237:2730–2733, 1977.
Brain metastases occurred in none of 14 patients undergoing prophylactic irradiation and 4 of 15 with no prophylaxis ($p < 0.05$); in spite of prophylactic irradiation, median survival was not significantly different in the two groups, however.

Kane RC, Cohen MH, Broder LE, Bull MI: Superior vena caval obstruction due to small-cell anaplastic lung carcinoma: Response to chemotherapy. JAMA 235:1717–1718, 1976.
Chemotherapy alone was effective in relieving superior vena cava obstruction in 7 of 7 patients treated.

Livingston RB, Moore TN, Heilbrun L, et al: Small-cell carcinoma of the lung: Combined chemotherapy and radiation. A Southwest Oncology Group study. Ann Intern Med 88:194–199, 1978.
In a study of 358 patients objective responses were achieved in 75% of 108 with limited disease and in 56% with extensive disease.

Muggia FM, Krezuski SK, Hansen HH: Cell kinetic studies in patients with small cell carcinoma of the lung. Cancer 34:1683–1690, 1974.
An in vivo study of 12 patients receiving tritiated thymidine in which the median labelling index was 16.7% was used.
Weiss RB: Small-cell carcinoma of the lung: Therapeutic management. Ann Intern Med 88:522–531, 1978.
Article presents a discussion of the roles of radiotherapy, chemotherapy, and combined modality approaches.
Williams C, Alexander M, Glatstein EJ, Daniels JR: Role of radiation therapy in combination with chemotherapy in extensive oat cell cancer of the lung: A randomized study. Cancer Treat Rep 61:1427–1431, 1977.
Involved field irradiation did not significantly improve response or survival in 12 patients receiving combined therapy as compared to 13 receiving chemotherapy alone.

64. NON-SMALL CELL CARCINOMAS OF THE LUNG—RELAPSING OR METASTATIC

More than three-quarters of all patients with lung cancer are found to have unresectable disease at presentation, either limited (in one hemithorax) or extensive (with distant metastases). Of the non-small cell lung cancers, epidermoid carcinoma most commonly grows by direct invasion and presents with limited disease, whereas adenocarcinoma and large cell carcinoma are more often found to have distant metastases. Sites of clinically apparent distant metastatic spread include lymph nodes, contralateral thorax, bone, liver, and brain. In one series palpable lymphadenopathy was present in 30% to 40% of patients at presentation, contralateral lung involvement in 30% to 40%, distant bone metastases in 16% of patients with epidermoid and 30% to 40% with adenocarcinoma and large cell, liver involvement in 8% with epidermoid and up to 20% with adenocarcinoma and large cell, and brain metastases in 10% to 20% of patients. At autopsy, metastases may also be documented in the adrenals, kidneys, and pancreas.

In addition to disease extent and sites of metastatic disease, performance status, age, and tumor histopathology are important prognostic variables. Whether treatment itself significantly improves survival in unresectable non-small cell lung cancer has been tested in several prospective clinical trials. For patients with limited disease, irradiation has been shown to be significantly superior to placebo in terms of survival, but only for those patients with epidermoid carcinoma. In the study by Roswit et al. [1968] the median survival was increased from 112 to 142 days. More importantly, several radiation therapy centers have subsequently reported 3% to 9% 5-year survival results in patients with unresectable limited disease receiving radical irradiation. In spite of its sometimes meager survival benefit, radiation therapy does provide important palliation. Progressive intrathoracic disease may result in atelectasis and infection secondary to bronchial obstruction, hemoptysis, and pain due to local invasion of ribs or the brachial plexus, as well as superior vena cava obstruction. With irradiation most patients will have transient symptomatic improvement, and objective tumor responses can be seen in 30% to 50% of patients. The usual radiation dose is 5000 rads in 5 weeks to the involved regions.

Like radiation therapy in limited disease, single agent chemotherapy of extensive non-small cell lung cancer has been shown to be superior to placebo, in terms of survival, but only for those patients with epidermoid carcinoma. Using nitrogen mustard, Green et al. [1969] reported an approximate 3-month improvement in median survival as compared to survival with placebo. Unlike the case with irradiation, however, there are no long-term survivors with non-small cell cancer who have received chemotherapy alone. Although chemotherapy, like radiation therapy, results in little survival benefit for most patients with non-small cell lung cancer, it may provide symptomatic palliation. Several single agents have been reported to yield objective responses in 15% to 30% of patients, including nitrogen mustard, cyclophosphamide, methotrexate, Adriamycin, CCNU, methyl-CCNU, procarbazine, bleomycin, and 5-fluorouracil. Epidermoid carcinoma is most responsive, large cell carcinoma is least responsive; and response to chemotherapy is correlated with patient performance status. In responding patients with extensive disease, the median remission duration is 12 to 20 weeks and the median survival 10 to 30 weeks.

Although combination chemotherapy programs have been extensively tested, few have reported significantly improved survival results over survival with single agents. Objective response data also show little advantage of combination chemotherapy over single agent treatment, although some recent reports are encouraging (Butler et al, 1979).

C.P.

Butler TP, Macdonald JS, Smith FP, et al: 5-Fluorouracil, adriamycin, and mitomycin-C (FAM) chemotherapy for adenocarcinoma of the lung. Cancer 43:1183–1188, 1979.
Article details the objective response in 9 of 25 patients with a median remission duration of 7 months.

Green RA, Humphrey E, Close H, Patno ME: Alkylating agents in bronchogenic carcinoma. Am J Med 46:516–525, 1969.
Median survival was significantly longer for patients with squamous carcinoma receiving nitrogen mustard, and for those with small cell carcinoma treated with cyclophosphamide, when compared to those receiving a placebo.

Lanzotti VJ, Thomas DR, Boyle LE, et al: Survival with inoperable lung cancer: An integration of prognostic variables based on simple clinical criteria. Cancer 39:303–313, 1977.
In an analysis of 316 patients with disseminated disease, symptom status, age, weight loss, and metastases to the liver, opposite hemithorax, brain, and bone were prognostic variables.

Livingston RB: Combination chemotherapy of bronchogenic carcinoma: I. Non-oat cell. Cancer Treat Rev 4:153–165, 1977.
A comprehensive review.

Muggia FM, Chervu LR: Lung cancer: Diagnosis in metastatic sites. Semin Oncol 1:217–228, 1974.
A good review of diagnostic procedures.

Perez CA: Radiation therapy in the management of carcinoma of the lung. Cancer 39:901–916, 1977.
A good review.

Roswit B, Patno ME, Rapp R, et al: The survival of patients with inoperable lung cancer: A large-scale randomized study of radiation therapy versus placebo. Radiology 90:688–697, 1968.
Irradiation was significantly superior to placebo use (survival median of 142 days vs 112 days) for patients with unresectable regional disease.

Sarna GP, Lowitz BB, Haskell CM, et al: Chemo-immunotherapy for unresectable bronchogenic carcinoma. Cancer Treat Rep 62:681–687, 1978.

In a randomized study of 79 patients no significant improvement in response rate or survival was found with the addition of immunotherapy.

Selawry OS: The role of chemotherapy in the treatment of lung cancer. Semin Oncol 1:259–272, 1974.

A good review of single agent chemotherapy results.

Selawry O, Krant M, Scotto J, et al: Methotrexate compared with placebo in lung cancer. Cancer 40:4–8, 1977.

The objective response to methotrexate was dose-related: 21% of 48 patients showed a response with 0.6 mg/kg IM methotrexate twice weekly, 11% of 37 showed a response with 0.2 mg/kg IM methotrexate twice weekly, and 6% of 32 responded to the placebo.

Zubrod CG, Selawry O: The treatment of lung cancer. Adv Intern Med 23:451–467, 1978.

A comprehensive review with recommendations for management according to histology.

65. ESOPHAGEAL CANCER—RELAPSING OR METASTATIC

Although 40% of patients with carcinoma of the esophagus have disease limited to the esophagus at presentation, only 5% of all patients will be cured of their disease. Recurrent tumor presents the most frequent and difficult problem, resulting in esophageal obstruction, tracheoesophageal or bronchoesophageal fistulae, and/or destruction of vital adjacent organs. One-third of patients will develop distant metastatic disease, usually in liver, lung, or bone; however, it is rare for this distant disease to be the cause of death. Most patients die of cardiopulmonary complications as a direct result of locally progressive tumor.

Even at diagnosis more than two-thirds of patients with esophageal carcinoma are malnourished. Inability to swallow food and saliva can lead to starvation and/or aspiration pneumonitis; and for the patient with recurrent or metastatic disease, relief of dysphagia should be the major goal of palliation. Treatments that have been used to restore swallowing include irradiation, dilation and intubation, esophageal bypass, and surgical resection. Patients with recurrent or metastatic carcinoma usually survive less than 6 months. Therefore, palliative methods should not require lengthy in-hospital procedures, if possible. Irradiation may be useful in those who have not received it as primary therapy; however, relief of dysphagia may only be transient (a median of 3 months in one series of selected patients). Intubation of the esophagus can provide effective palliation of esophageal obstruction but is not applicable to patients with cervical esophageal lesions. Both traction and pulsion methods have been evaluated, and it appears that pulsion intubation is less morbid and equally effective. Nutritional status can be improved, aspiration of food and/or saliva can be eliminated, and esophagorespiratory fistulae can be bypassed. The main risk of pulsion intubation is that of perforating the esophagus during the procedure. Surgical methods of relieving esophageal obstruction secondary to recurrent tumor are usually limited to bypass procedures. Rarely is resection indicated. Although surgery may be effective, it frequently requires prolonged hospitalization in patients with very limited survival.

There has been little experience with chemotherapy in esophageal carcinoma. Drugs that have been tested to some degree include cyclophosphamide, 5-FU, methotrexate, bleomycin, CCNU, and Adriamycin. All have demonstrated limited activity with only brief response. Because most patients will have received prior or concurrent irradiation to the esophagus, mucositis has been a common toxicity, particularly with bleomycin and Adriamycin. There is no combination chemotherapy experience in carcinoma of the esophagus.

C.P.

Haffejee AA, Angorn IB: Oral alimentation following intubation for esophageal carcinoma. Ann Surg 186:759–761, 1977.
All 15 patients had evidence of protein-calorie malnutrition prior to intubation; within 3 weeks all were in positive nitrogen balance.

Hegarty MM, Angorn IB, Bryer JV, et al: Palliation of malignant esophagorespiratory fistulae by permanent indwelling prosthetic tube. Ann Surg 185:88–91, 1977.
Article discusses utility of pulsion intubation. In the series discussed 36 of 48 patients received effective palliation.

Kolaric K, Maricic Z, Roth A, Dujmovic I: Adriamycin alone and in combination with radiotherapy in the treatment of inoperable esophageal cancer. Tumori 63:485–491, 1977.
Objective responses were seen in 6 of 18 patients when Adriamycin was given alone; median duration was 3.2 months.

Ravry M, Moertel CG, Schutt AJ, et al: Treatment of advanced squamous cell carcinoma of the gastrointestinal tract with bleomycin (NSC-125066). Cancer Chemother Rep 57:493–495, 1973.
None of 14 patients with esophageal carcinoma had an objective response.

Steiger Z, Nickel WO, Wilson RF, Arbulu A: Improved surgical palliation of advanced carcinoma of the esophagus. Am J Surg 135:782–784, 1978.
Article describes palliative bypass of the esophagus in 54 patients.

Wara WM, Mauch PM, Thomas AN, Phillips TL: Palliation for carcinoma of the esophagus. Radiology 121:717–720, 1976.
In an analysis of 169 patients median survival was 7 months and median duration of palliation with irradiation was 3 months.

66. STOMACH CANCER—RELAPSING OR METASTATIC

Following "curative" surgical resection for stomach cancer, local recurrence and regional lymph node relapse are the most common sites of failure. Distant metastases are documented in approximately 25% of cases at relapse; however, it is rare to find no evidence of local failure as well. Unlike other gastrointestinal malignancies, stomach cancer has a high frequency of peritoneal dissemination and commonly involves the ovaries. Other sites of distant metastatic spread include the liver, lungs, pleura, bones, brain, adrenals, and genitourinary tract.

Nearly one-third of all patients with stomach cancer have documented liver metastases at diagnosis. In contrast to colorectal cancer, in which case palliative surgical resection of the primary is indicated even in the presence of distant metastases, major surgical procedures are of little palliative benefit in disseminated stomach cancer, in which local obstruction is a late manifestation. For locally recurrent disease, however, irradiation may sometimes be of benefit. As pointed out by Moertel et al [1969] in locally unresectable stomach cancer, the addition of concurrent 5-fluorouracil to local irradiation significantly improved the results of therapy in terms of survival as compared to irradiation alone (13 months with concurrent 5-FU plus irradiation; 5.9 months with irradiation alone).

Treatment of relapsing or metastatic stomach cancer rests primarily, however, on chemotherapy. Several single agents have proved to be active, including 5-FU, mitomycin C, BCNU and Adriamycin. Both 5-FU and BCNU have objective response rates of approximately 20% with remission durations of 4 to 5 months. The response rates for mitomycin C and Adriamycin are slightly higher (25% to 30%), but the response duration for mitomycin C is very brief (<3 months).

Many variables may influence response to chemotherapy of advanced stomach cancer. Sites favorable to response include intra-abdominal tumor, liver metastases, and skin nodules, whereas lung metastases and peripheral adenopathy respond poorly. Males have higher response rates than females, and patients with a good performance status at initiation of chemotherapy respond better. Lower grade malignancies and patients who have a longer disease-free interval from diagnosis to first recurrence also respond better.

Encouraging information is beginning to accumulate regarding the utility of combination chemotherapy in stomach cancer. In two randomized studies comparing a nitrosourea plus 5-FU to either single agent alone, the combination was superior in terms of response (approximately 40% for the combination versus 20% for 5-FU and 8% for methyl-CCNU). And in one study the combination regimen of BCNU plus 5-FU also had significantly superior survival (26.5% at 18 months for the combination vs. 7% at 18 months for 5-FU alone). Another drug combination that looks promising is 5-FU plus Adriamycin plus mitomycin C (FAM). This drug program has resulted in objective responses in half the patients treated, with a median response duration of 9.5 months. The median survival of the responders was 13.5 months as compared to 2.5 months for nonresponders.

Unlike advanced colorectal cancer, for which combination chemotherapy has yielded superior response rates without significantly improving survival over single agent therapy alone, combination chemotherapy of advanced stomach cancer appears to have significantly improved not only response but survival as compared to single agent treatment alone.

C.P.

Carter SK, Comis RL: Gastric cancer: Current status of treatment. J Natl Cancer Inst 58:567–578, 1977.
A comprehensive review.
Cedermark BJ, Blumenson LE, Pickren JW, Elias EG: The significance of metastases to the adrenal gland from carcinoma of the stomach and esophagus. Surg Gynecol Obstet 145:41–48, 1977.
Article outlines sites and incidence of metastases as found at autopsy.
Kovach JS, Moertel CG, Schutt AJ, et al: A controlled study of combined 1,3-bis-(2-chloroethyl)-1-nitrosourea and 5-fluorouracil therapy for advanced gastric and pancreatic cancer. Cancer 33:563–567, 1974.
Using BCNU plus 5-FU resulted in a 41.3% response rate in 34 patients with stomach carcinoma, and survival was significantly superior to that occurring when 5-FU was used alone (26.5% at 18 months vs. 7%).
Macdonald JS, Woolley PV, Smythe T, et al: 5-Fluorouracil, adriamycin and mitomycin-C (FAM) combination chemotherapy in the treatment of advanced gastric cancer. Cancer 44:42–47, 1979.
Objective partial regressions were seen in 18 of 36 patients; median remission duration was 9.5 months and median survival was 13.5 months for responders.
Moertel CG, Childs DS Jr, Reitemeier RJ, et al: Combined 5-fluorouracil and supervoltage radiation therapy of locally unresectable gastrointestinal cancer. Lancet 2:865–867, 1969.

The use of concurrent 5-FU and irradiation resulted in significantly improved survival as compared to use of radiation therapy alone.

Moertel CG, Mittelman JA, Bakemeier RF, et al: Sequential and combination chemotherapy of advanced gastric cancer. Cancer 38:678–682, 1976.

Response was 40% with 5-FU plus methyl CCNU; performance status and sites of disease were significant variables.

O'Connell MJ, Moertel CG, Lavin PT: Adriamycin (*A*), 5-fluorouracil + mitomycin C + cytosine arabinoside (*FMC*), and 5-fluorouracil + adriamycin + methyl CCNU (*FAMe*) in advanced gastric carcinoma. Proc Am Soc Clin Oncol (Abstract) 19:343, 1978.

With all 3 regimens, response rates were approximately 25% in 55 previously untreated patients.

67. COLORECTAL CANCER—RELAPSING OR METASTATIC

Only 40% of all patients with colorectal cancer will be cured of their disease following primary surgical resection, although 75% are thought to be "curable" at presentation. Regional lymph node recurrence is documented in the majority of patients at relapse and is the only site of failure in 50% to 60%. Distant metastatic disease, on the other hand, is uncommon as the only site of failure in rectal cancer and is seen in only 25% of patients with colon carcinoma. However, approximately half of all patients at relapse will have evidence of distant metastatic disease, usually with concurrent regional lymph node relapse. Sites of distant metastatic disease include liver, lung, pleura, bone, brain, and ovaries. Relapse after "curative" resection is usually documented within 3 years following surgery, and fewer than 5% of patients relapse after 5 years.

Pathologic stage at presentation is the most important factor in predicting relapse following primary therapy. For Duke's A lesions the relapse rate is approximately 20% to 40%; Duke's B, 40% to 60%; and Duke's C, 80% to 90%. Overall median survival from the documentation of relapsing or metastatic disease is approximately 10 months and varies according to the sites of relapse. In one study, patients who suffered a relapse in regional lymph nodes only had a median survival of 23.7 months for colon cancer and 12.5 months for rectal cancer. By contrast, patients with liver metastases alone had a median survival of 10 months; and if both regional lymph nodes and distant metastases were documented at relapse, then the median survival was 5 months for colon cancer and 9 months for rectal cancer.

Following "curative" primary resection, what methods are best for detecting disease relapse? In many studies, symptoms appear to be the most sensitive indicator. Such complaints as abdominal discomfort, change in bowel habits, and loss of weight must be evaluated fully. The physical examination may reveal hepatomegaly, lower abdominal fullness or discomfort, or, more likely, no specific abnormality. Laboratory studies should include blood counts, liver function tests, and stool guaiac. A chest x-ray and/or liver scan may demonstrate focal lesions. Less than 10% of cancers will recur in the bowel suture line, so sigmoidoscopy, colonoscopy, and barium enema may have limited benefit, except in demonstrating areas of extrinsic compression. The carcinoembryonic antigen (CEA) test has been advocated by many as a useful screening study for relapsing colorectal cancer. It is probably more useful as a confirmatory test of other abnormal findings than as a first indicator of recurrent disease, however. If relapsing colorectal cancer is suspected, then pathologic documentation should be obtained, if possible. As pointed out by the retrospective analysis of patients with prior colon cancer and a solitary pulmonary nodule, more than half had a second primary malignancy and not relapsing colon cancer.

At initial diagnosis, approximately 15% to 25% of patients will have liver metastases or other evidence of incurable colorectal cancer. In spite of this extensive disease, such patients should still be considered for palliative resection of the primary lesion or diverting colostomy. In one series the operative mortality was 6% and the median survival for those surviving palliative surgery was 9 months. Problems of chronic blood loss and local bowel obstruction were relieved in most patients.

Treatment of relapsing colorectal cancer is usually limited to palliative regional irradiation and/or chemotherapy. Because of the high incidence of regional lymph node recurrence, either alone or with distant metastatic disease, regional irradiation is frequently employed to palliate local symptoms. The usual dose is 4500–5000 rads in 5 to 6 weeks. Although a vast literature is available on the chemotherapy of advanced colorectal cancer, few drugs are effective in treating this disease. 5-Fluorouracil is the standard single agent, yielding objective responses in approximately 20% of patients. Responses to chemotherapy are frequently difficult to document, because abdominal disease may not be easily measured; and this may account for the widely varied response rates reported with 5-FU, ranging from 0–80%. In addition, such factors as age, performance status, sites of disease, and prior therapy may influence treatment results. Necessary dose, route of administration, and drug schedule remain somewhat controversial, although it appears that intensive therapy (producing mild toxicity) is needed for maximal benefit. A commonly used regimen is 5-FU, 13.5 mg/kg/day intravenously for 5 consecutive days, repeated at 5-week intervals. The drug dose is modified or discontinued if toxicity (stomatitis, dermatitis, diarrhea, and/or leukopenia) develops during the 5-day loading course. In addition to an objective response rate of 20%, the median survival of responders to 5-FU (17 months) is significantly better than that for nonresponders (7 months). Even though the objective response rate is low, approximately half of all patients treated receive some symptomatic benefit from 5-FU therapy.

Other single agent drugs with some efficacy in colorectal cancer include the nitrosoureas (particularly methyl-CCNU) and mitomycin C. Responses are seen in 10% to 15% of previously untreated patients, and remission durations average 2 to 3 months. Whether combination chemotherapy can improve response or remission duration is unsettled. Moertel reported a 43.5% response rate to 5-FU + methyl-CCNU + vincristine, as compared to 19.5% with 5-FU alone. Other groups, however, have been unable to confirm these high response rates with combination therapy. Even in Moertel's series [1975], however, there was no significant difference in survival between those receiving the combination program and those receiving 5-FU alone.

Another approach that has been used in selected patients with liver metastases is intra-arterial hepatic perfusion. It is uncertain whether this method provides any advantage over intravenous 5-FU. It will be discussed in more detail in Part VI, Chapter 92.

C.P.

Ansfield F, Klotz J, Nealon T, et al: A phase III study comparing the clinical utility of four regimens of 5-fluorouracil: A preliminary report. Cancer 39:34–40, 1977.
Loading course 5-FU produced significantly better response and response duration than other regimens; survival was also improved (p > 0.08).

Cahan WG, Castro EB, Hajdu SI: The significance of a solitary lung shadow in patients with colon carcinoma. Cancer 33:414–421, 1974.

Of 54 patients analyzed, 25 had metastatic colon cancer and 29 had primary lung cancer.

Cedermark BJ, Schultz SS, Bakshi S, et al: The value of liver scan in the follow-up study of patients with adenocarcinoma of the colon and rectum. Surg Gynecol Obstet 144:745–748, 1977.

In a prospective study of 70 patients scans were accurate in predicting hepatic metastases in 78% of patients who later had laparotomy confirmation.

Gunderson LL, Sosin H: Areas of failure found at reoperation (second or symptomatic look) following "curative surgery" for adenocarcinoma of the rectum: Clinicopathologic correlation and implications for adjuvant therapy. Cancer 34:1278–1292, 1974.

Local and/or regional relapse alone was documented in 48% of 75 patients, without evidence of distant metastases.

Lokich JJ, Skarin AT, Mayer RJ, Frei E III: Lack of effectiveness of combined 5-fluorouracil and methyl-CCNU therapy in advanced colorectal cancer. Cancer 40:2792–2796, 1977.

Article emphasizes lack of response and survival benefit when this combination chemotherapy regimen is used as compared to 5-FU alone or supportive care.

Moertel CG, Schutt AJ, Hahn RG, Reitemeier RJ: Therapy of advanced colorectal cancer with a combination of 5-fluorouracil, methyl-1, 3-cis(2-chlorethyl)-1-nitrosourea, and vincristine. J Natl Cancer Inst 54:69–71, 1975.

A response rate of 43.5% was achieved with the combination regimen as prospectively compared to 5-FU alone (19.5%) in 80 patients.

Shani A, O'Connell MJ, Moertel CG, et al: Serial plasma carcinoembryonic antigen measurements in the management of metastatic colorectal carcinoma. Ann Intern Med 88:627–630, 1978.

CEA titers did not correlate with response, remission duration, or survival in 263 patients studied.

Silverman DT, Murray JL, Smart CR, et al: Estimated median survival times of patients with colorectal cancer based on experience with 9,745 patients. Am J Surg 133:289–297, 1977.

Sites and extent of metastatic disease are important variables in determining prognosis.

Sugarbaker PH, Zamcheck N, Moore FD: Assessment of serial carcinoembryonic antigen (CEA) assays in postoperative detection of recurrent colorectal cancer. Cancer 38:2310–2315, 1976.

Rising CEA titers may be helpful in assessing recurrence of disease but was the first indicator of disease progression in only 4 of 12 patients studied.

Takaki HS, Ujiki GT, Shields TS: Palliative resections in the treatment of primary colorectal cancer. Am J Surg 133:548–550, 1977.

Of 78 patients, the operative mortality was 6.4% and the overall median survival was 9.1 months.

Wooley PV III, Macdonald JS, Schein PS: Chemotherapy of colorectal carcinoma. Semin Oncol 3:415–420, 1976.

Reviews single agent, combination chemotherapy, and adjuvant chemotherapy data.

Zamcheck N: The present status of carcinoembryonic antigen (CEA) in diagnosis, detection of recurrence, prognosis, and evaluation of therapy of colonic and pancreatic cancer. Clin Gastroenterol 5:625–638, 1976.

An excellent review.

At diagnosis virtually all patients with pancreatic carcinoma have metastatic disease involving regional lymph nodes and/or distant sites. Symptoms are initially vague and poorly localized. Anorexia, weight loss, and abdominal discomfort may be the only complaints. Fewer than one-quarter of patients will present with epigastric pain that radiates to the back. Obstructive jaundice is seen in more than 75% of patients during the course of their illness and is frequently a presenting complaint. Except for jaundice, however, the physical examination may be entirely unremarkable. Other findings that may be present are an upper abdominal mass, hepatomegaly, and/or a palpable supraclavicular lymph node.

Sites of metastatic disease include regional lymph nodes, liver, lungs, peritoneum, duodenum, adrenals, and other intra-abdominal organs. Metastases may also be documented in brain, bone, and subcutaneous tissue. Local tumor extension is a difficult problem in many cases because of progressive obstructive jaundice, duodenal occlusion with ulceration and hemorrhage, occlusion of blood vessels (including the splenic vein and splenic mesenteric artery), and pancreatic cyst formation. Unfortunately bypass procedures carry a high mortality rate (approximately 30%) in distant metastatic disease, so that surgery is not indicated prophylactically as it is in metastatic colon cancer. Radiation therapy provides limited palliation for locally advanced disease (see Part III, Chapter 45).

Chemotherapy has been used to palliate both local symptoms and distant metastatic disease. To date, studies have been hampered by the lack of objective parameters to assess response to treatment. In spite of widespread metastatic disease, the only measurable tumor may be present on liver scan. Locally extensive disease can be documented by ultrasound or computerized tomography, but changes of prior surgery, cyst formation, or edema may make interpretation of data more difficult. Indirect measures such as serum carcinoembryonic antigen and alpha fetoprotein are not reliable indicators of chemotherapy effectiveness.

Drugs that have been used as single agents in the therapy of advanced pancreatic cancer include 5-fluorouracil, mitomycin C, streptozotocin, the nitrosoureas, and the alkylating agents. Objective response rates range from 10% to 30% for 5-FU, mitomycin C, and streptozotocin. Remissions are brief, lasting only 2 to 4 months; and survival is no more prolonged than with supportive care alone. Combination chemotherapy appears to be superior to single agent treatment in terms of response and duration of remission, although information regarding this is limited. One study compared 5-FU or BCNU alone to 5-FU plus BCNU and found twice as many responses to the combination (33% versus 16% for 5-FU and 0% for BCNU); however, there was no significant improvement in survival with the combination. Other regimens combining 5-FU with mitomycin C, streptozotocin, and/or Adriamycin have reported objective response rates of 12% to 50%, with median remission duration of 5 to 7+ months. Responders are surviving longer (7.5+ months median) than nonresponders (3 months median), but the data require longer follow-up.

It is clear that chemotherapy offers only limited palliative benefit to patients with advanced pancreatic cancer. Progressive hepatic metastases, biliary obstruction, and liver failure are the usual causes of death. However, locally advanced disease frequently causes severe pain due to invasion of the splanchnic nerves and blood vessels. In addition to oral and parenteral pain medications, other measures that may provide relief include percutaneous splanchnic nerve block of the involved thoracic dorsal roots and bilateral thoracic cordotomy or rhizotomy. Because of bilateral radiating pain, most patients will not receive pain relief from a unilateral cordotomy. Another common problem is anorexia and progressive cachexia. Although overt pancreatic exocrine insufficiency is unusual, patients frequently benefit from pancreatic enzyme supplementation in addition to medium chain triglycerides and a high calorie diet. In addition, approximately 20% of patients will develop diabetes mellitus and require insulin therapy.

C.P.

Haller D, Woolley P, Levin B, et al: Fluorouracil (F), adriamycin (A) and mitomycin-C (M), FAM, for advanced colorectal and pancreatic cancer. Proc Am Soc Clin Oncol (Abstract) 19:342, 1978.

The objective responses seen in 6 of 14 patients with pancreatic cancer had a median duration of 5+ months.

Kovach JS, Moertel CG, Schutt AJ, et al: A controlled study of combined 1,3-bis-(2-chloroethyl)-1-nitrosourea and 5-fluorouracil therapy for advanced gastric and pancreatic cancer. Cancer 33:563–567, 1974.

Objective responses in advanced pancreatic cancer were better with BCNU plus 5-FU (33%) as compared to either drug alone (<16%); however, overall survival was not improved (median of 6 months).

Macdonald JS, Widerlite L, Schein PS: Biology, diagnosis, and chemotherapeutic management of pancreatic malignancy. Adv Pharmacol Chemother 14:107–142, 1977.

A comprehensive discussion.

Macdonald JS, Widerlite L, Schein PS: Current diagnosis and management of pancreatic carcinoma. J Natl Cancer Inst 56:1093–1099, 1976.

A very good review.

Moertel CG, Douglas HO Jr, Hanley J, Carbone PP: Treatment of advanced adenocarcinoma of the pancreas with combinations of streptozotocin plus 5-fluorouracil and streptozotocin plus cyclophosphamide. Cancer 40:605–608, 1977.

An objective response was seen in 12% of patients on either regimen; the median response duration was 5.5 to 9 months.

Smith FP, Schein PS: Chemotherapy of pancreatic cancer. Semin Oncol 6:368–377, 1979.

An excellent review.

Wiggans RG, Woolley PV III, Macdonald JS, et al: Phase II trial of streptozotocin, mitomycin-C and 5-fluorouracil (SMF) in the treatment of advanced pancreatic cancer. Cancer 41:387–391, 1978.

Of 23 previously untreated patients, 10 had an objective response with a median duration of 7+ months and median survival of 7.5+ months.

---

69. CARCINOID—RELAPSING OR METASTATIC

Approximately one-third of all patients with carcinoid will have metastatic disease identified at diagnosis, but fewer than 20% will have carcinoid syndrome. The presence of metastatic disease has a correlation with the size of the primary tumor: tumors smaller than 1 cm are rarely found to be metastatic, whereas those larger than 2 cm are almost always associated with metastases. Sites of metastatic disease include regional lymph nodes, liver, lungs, bone, skin, and other intra-abdominal organs. Physical findings of advanced disease may include hepatomegaly, abdominal and/or pelvic masses, and peripheral lymphadenopathy. An elevated level of 5-HIAA (5-hydroxyindole acetic acid) in the urine may confirm the presence of metastatic disease but does not necessarily connote the symptomatic presence of carcinoid syndrome. Furthermore, metastatic carcinoid is not necessarily associated with 5-HIAA elevation or the presence of carcinoid syndrome.

The carcinoid syndrome is almost always found in association with metastatic liver disease, although it is occasionally seen in primary bronchial carcinoid and teratomas of the ovary and testis. It may include cutaneous flushing, hypotension, diarrhea, cardiac lesions, asthma, pellagra-like cutaneous lesions, and arthropathy. The symptoms and signs of carcinoid syndrome result from the release of bioamines and/or hormones from the tumor. The manifestations of carcinoid syndrome as well as the histologic features of primary and metastatic lesions differ according to their site of origin. Bronchial and gastric carcinoids are associated with severe, prolonged cutaneous flushing; are argyrophilic by histochemistry; and secrete 5-hydroxytryptophan and histamine. Mid-gut (ileal) carcinoids produce brief episodes of flushing, are argentaffin-positive and not argyrophilic, and secrete serotonin. Rectal carcinoids do not produce carcinoid syndrome, are unreactive by histochemistry, and do not secrete bioamines.

The most common symptom of carcinoid syndrome is cutaneous flushing, which occurs in 60% to 80% of patients. It may be precipitated by physical exertion, emotion, eating, defecation, changes in posture, manipulation of tumor masses, or alcohol consumption. There may also be associated hypotension, which can sometimes be severe. Both are thought to be secondary to the tumor release of kallikrein (bradykinin) and exacerbated by serotonin, histamine, and catecholamines. Phenothiazines and phenoxybenzamine can sometimes ameliorate flushing; hypotension is not reversed, but exacerbated, by the usual vasoconstrictors and responds to angiotension. Explosive watery diarrhea is also seen frequently and may be present in the absence of cutaneous flushing. It is probably caused by 5-hydroxytryptophan tumor release and is improved by serotonin antagonists such as methysergide, parachlorophenylalanine, and alpha-methyldopa, in addition to opiates and other symptomatic measures.

Right-sided cardiac lesions involving the valve cusps, endomyocardium, papillary muscles, and chordae may be found in up to 50% of patients with carcinoid syndrome. They are found in those patients with the longest history of metastatic carcinoid and the highest levels of 5-HIAA. Right heart failure, cardiac arrhythmias, and conduction disturbances are also documented frequently. 5-Hydroxytryptophan is thought to be the causative bioamine. Asthma is relatively unusual and most often seen with primary bronchial lesions. It is probably evoked by bradykinin and may be relieved by the usual bronchodilators. Niacin deficiency is a concomitant disturbance of carcinoid syndrome, since up to 60% of the ingested tryptophan may be diverted for serotonin synthesis. Therefore all patients with carcinoid syndrome should receive adequate dietary niacin supplementation.

Metastatic carcinoid is a relatively indolent neoplasm, even when extensive liver disease is present. The median survival for all patients is approximately 2 years, with 20% of patients surviving longer than 5 years. Because there may be a long natural history, palliative therapy must be carefully planned. Not all patients will require initiation of treatment when metastatic disease is first documented. Surgery is useful to bypass or resect areas of potential mechanical obstruction as well as to remove bulk disease, including hepatic metastases limited to one lobe. There are increased anesthetic risks in such patients due to tumor release of bioamines; however, these can usually be anticipated and avoided. The role of radiation therapy remains to be defined. It has been used for local tumor control in selected patients. In addition one series reports "cure" of metastatic carcinoid utilizing whole abdominal irradiation. Drugs that have been shown to produce objective tumor responses include 5-FU, streptozotocin, cyclophosphamide, and Adriamycin. The responses are generally transient, and there is no firm evidence that chemotherapy improves survival.

C.P.

Davis Z, Moertel CG, McIlrath DC: The malignant carcinoid syndrome. Surg Gynecol Obstet 137:637–644, 1973.
An excellent retrospective analysis of 91 patients with carcinoid syndrome.
Gaitan-Gaitan A, Rider WD, Bush RS: Carcinoid tumor-cure by irradiation. Int J Radiat Oncol Biol Phys 1:9–13, 1975.
Of 10 patients treated with whole abdominal irradiation, 5 are free of disease 18 months to 11 years later.
Jager RM, Polk HC Jr: Carcinoid apudomas. Curr Probl Cancer 1:3–53, 1977.
An excellent comprehensive review.
Legha SS, Valdivieso M, Nelson RS, et al: Chemotherapy for metastatic carcinoid tumors: Experiences with 32 patients and a review of the literature. Cancer Treat Rep 61:1699–1703, 1977.
Responses were found in 5 of 7 patients receiving Adriamycin combination chemotherapy programs.
Mariani G, Strober W, Keiser H, Waldmann TA: Pathophysiology of hypoalbuminemia associated with carcinoid tumor. Cancer 38:854–860, 1976.
Hypoalbuminemia was found to be secondary to decreased hepatic synthesis and increased loss from the gut.

70. RENAL CELL CARCINOMA—RELAPSING OR METASTATIC

Renal cell carcinoma has been termed the "internist's malignancy," since it presents so frequently with systemic manifestations, even when initially localized to the kidney. They may be toxic (fever, cachexia, fatigue, weight loss), hematologic (anemia, erythrocytosis, leukemoid reaction, eosinophilia, thrombocytosis), humoral (erythrocytosis, hypercalcemia, galactorrhea, hypertension, Cushing's syndrome), vascular (A-V fistulae, thrombophlebitis, inferior vena caval occlusion secondary to tumor), immune (glomerulonephritis, amyloidosis), and/or idiopathic (hepatopathy). Even though these systemic symptoms may occur early, metastatic disease leads to the diagnosis in up to 25% of patients, and another 10% to 25% will be found to have distant metastases during initial evaluation. Common sites of metastatic disease at presentation include lymph nodes, lung, bone, skin, liver, and extradural and/or central nervous system tumor. In addition, renal cell carcinoma may also be found in unusual metastatic sites such as the larynx, gallbladder, vagina, breast, and ear.

In order to adequately assess the extent of disease, all patients should have a thorough physical examination with attention paid to the presence of lymphadenopathy, skin nodules, bony discomfort, and neurologic dysfunction. Laboratory studies that may be useful include blood counts, liver and renal function tests, serum calcium, urinalysis, chest x-ray, intravenous pyelogram, and bone scan. Any areas of increased uptake on bone scan should be evaluated with x-rays, since bony lesions are usually lytic and often lead to pathologic fractures. Elevation of peripheral venous renin has been reported to be associated with high-grade lesions and advanced stage, whereas serum erythropoietin levels may be increased but do not necessarily correlate with disease extent.

In general the prognosis for patients with metastatic renal cell carcinoma is poor, with an overall survival of less than one year. However, the disease may be associated with rare spontaneous regressions, prolonged periods of stable or slowly progressive tumor, delayed occurrence of metastatic disease following primary therapy (with disease-free intervals of 30 years or more), the presence of a solitary metastasis at diagnosis or relapse, and hormone responsiveness.

Approximately 2% to 4% of patients with renal cell carcinoma will be found to have a solitary metastasis at diagnosis or relapse. Unlike patients with widespread metastatic disease, these patients may have prolonged survival, with eradication of the solitary metastasis. In one series 60% were alive at 3 years and 35% at 5 years. However, because of the unpredictable natural history of these tumors, it is unlikely that even the 5-year survivors are cured. In the presence of a solitary metastasis at diagnosis, surgical removal of the primary (nephrectomy) and of the solitary metastasis should be attempted whenever possible. Radiation therapy is a poor alternative in this setting, since renal cell carcinoma is a radioresistant tumor and it is difficult to achieve a sterilizing dose.

When widespread metastatic disease is present at diagnosis, nephrectomy should be considered only for palliation of local symptoms such as flank pain and intractable hematuria. Although there are anecdotal reports of generalized metastatic tumor regressions following nephrectomy, these are poorly documented and occur rarely, if at all. Radiation therapy may be used to treat lytic bone lesions or to palliate local symptoms. The response to therapy is usually slow and frequently incomplete. At least 4000 rads in 4 to 5 weeks need to be delivered in most instances.

Hormones have been used with some success in the management of patients with metastatic renal cell carcinoma. Both progestins and androgens are reported to be effective, with response rates of 10% to 15%. In some series, however, objective responses are rarely demonstrated, and most responses are merely subjective improvement or disease stability. Few chemotherapeutic agents have shown activity in renal cell carcinoma. Vinblastine has been reported to produce objective responses in 10% to 25% of patients, although the series are small.

C.P.

Bloom HJG: Hormone-induced and spontaneous regression of metastatic renal cancer. Cancer 32:1066–1071, 1973.
Objective regressions were seen in 16% of 80 patients treated with progestins or androgens.

Cronin RE, Kaehny WD, Miller PD, et al: Renal cell carcinoma: Unusual systemic manifestations. Medicine 55:291–311, 1976.
A comprehensive review.

Forbes GS, McLeod RA, Hattery RR: Radiographic manifestations of bone metastases from renal carcinoma. Am J Roentgenol 129:61–66, 1977.
A retrospective analysis of 167 patients with bone metastases.

Holland JM: Cancer of the kidney—natural history and staging. Cancer 32:1030–1042, 1973.
An excellent review.

Hrushesky WJ, Murphy GP: Current status of the therapy of advanced renal carcinoma. J Surg Oncol 9:277–288, 1977.
A complete review.

Lokich JJ, Harrison JH: Renal cell carcinoma: Natural history and chemotherapeutic experience. J Urol 114:371–374, 1975.

In this retrospective analysis of 84 patients 57% had distant metastatic disease when first seen.

Marcove RC, Searfoss RC, Whitmore WF, Grabstald H: Cryosurgery in the treatment of bone metastases from renal cell carcinoma. Clin Orthop 127:220–227, 1977.

This report describes the technique in 12 patients; 10 achieved good local bone control.

Sufrin G, Mirand EA, Moore RH, et al: Hormones in renal cancer. J Urol 117:433–438, 1977.

Peripheral vein renin elevation was associated with high grade tumors and an advanced stage.

Talley RW: Chemotherapy of adenocarcinoma of the kidney. Cancer 32:1062–1065, 1973.

Objective responses were limited to patients given progestins (7 of 61 patients) and to 2 of 15 patients who responded to vinblastine.

Tolia BM, Whitmore WF Jr: Solitary metastasis from renal cell carcinoma. J Urol 114:836–838, 1975.

This retrospective study of 19 patients represents 3.2% of all patients with renal cell carcinoma at diagnosis.

71. BLADDER CANCER—RELAPSING OR METASTATIC

More than three-quarters of all patients with bladder cancer will have disease limited to the bladder at diagnosis. Following initial therapy, tumor may be found to recur locally as a result of inadequate primary therapy or new tumor formation, and distant metastatic disease may be identified with or without local recurrence. Histologic grade, the presence of muscular invasion, and a history of prior bladder recurrence all connote a poor prognosis. In general, most primary treatment failures occur within the first two years. Because local recurrences are so commonly identified, all patients must be followed closely with urine cytologies, cystoscopic examinations, and random bladder biopsies when indicated. Serum levels of carcinoembryonic antigen (CEA) have also been reported to be useful in the detection of recurrent disease. Metastatic disease may be documented regionally, in para-aortic and/or inguinal lymph nodes, or in such metastatic sites as bone, lung, and liver.

With local bladder recurrence, the goals of palliative therapy include relief of symptoms and preservation of bladder function. Typical symptoms include frequency, dysuria, strangury, and hematuria. Intravesical therapy may be effective in controlling superficial neoplasms or reducing the bulk of infiltrative lesions. Approaches include hydrostatic pressure procedures; instillation of formalin, phenol, or silver nitrate; cytotoxic chemotherapy, and hyperthermia or cryothermia. Instillation procedures must take into account the presence of ureteral reflux and the potential of myelosuppression through mucosal absorption of cytotoxic agents. Transurethral procedures may also be used to surgically remove superficial growths or bulk tumor of infiltrative lesions. Partial cystectomy may provide effective palliation if focal disease only is present, whereas total cystectomy should be considered only if local measures fail to control symptoms. With locally invasive lesions or regional disease, radiation therapy may be delivered to those patients who have had no prior irradiation. In these cases the principles of primary treatment planning apply.

Distant metastatic disease in bone, lung, and/or liver may be present with or without concurrent local tumor recurrence, and frequently it may be difficult to identify measurable mass lesions to evaluate chemotherapeutic effectiveness. Studies that may aid in defining disease extent are chest x-ray, intravenous pyelogram, bone scan, liver scan, and computerized tomography or ultrasound of the abdomen and pelvis. Serum CEA levels have been reported to correlate with disease activity and response to therapy. Unfortunately experience with chemotherapy is limited to date. Single agents with reported objective response rates of 20% to 40% include methotrexate, 5-fluorouracil, cyclophosphamide, Adriamycin, mitomycin C, and *cis*-diamminedichloroplatinum (CDDP). In general, remissions are very brief, lasting only 2 to 3 months. Several combination chemotherapy programs have also been reported, demonstrating some improvement in objective remission rates and remission durations. None, however, have shown any significant impact on survival.

Radiation therapy may be used to palliate locally painful metastatic lesions, such as those in bone. The usual dose is 3000 rads in 2 weeks. One metastatic complication that may not justify palliative measures is ureteral obstruction. Relieving ureteral obstruction to prolong life in the face of severe local bladder symptoms or the presence of painful distant metastases is false palliation and should not be advised.

C.P.

Banks MD, Pontes JE, Izbicki RM, Pierce JM Jr: Topical instillation of doxorubicin hydrochloride in the treatment of recurring superficial transitional cell carcinoma of the bladder. J Urol 118:757–760, 1977.
Of 13 patients treated, 8 had complete regressions with a median duration of 10 months.

Carter SK: Chemotherapy and genitourinary oncology: I. Bladder cancer. Cancer Treat Rev 5:85–93, 1978.
Article reviews single agent and combination chemotherapy programs.

Culp DA: Palliative treatment of the patient with disseminated carcinoma of the bladder. Semin Oncol 6:249–253, 1979.
An excellent review of the palliative management of incurable bladder cancer.

Gilbert HA, Logan JL, Kagan AR, et al: The natural history of papillary transitional cell carcinoma of the bladder and its treatment in an unselected population on the basis of histologic grading. J Urol 119:488–492, 1978.
In a retrospective review of 365 patients survival correlated with histological grade.

Hahn RG: Bladder cancer treatment considerations for metastatic disease. Semin Oncol 6:236–239, 1979.
A brief summary of chemotherapy data.

Lessing JA: Bladder cancer: Early diagnosis and evaluation of biologic potential. A review of newer methods. J Urol 120:1–5, 1978.
Urine cytology, cytogenetics, immunological aspects, and biological markers in bladder cancer are discussed.

Merrin C, Cartagena R, Wajsman Z, et al: Chemotherapy of bladder carcinoma with cyclophosphamide and adriamycin. J Urol 114:884–887, 1975.
Objective responses were seen in 11 of 21 patients given cyclophosphamide, in 1 of 10 given Adriamycin, and in 9 of 18 given cyclophosphamide plus Adriamycin.

Sternberg JJ, Bracken RB, Handel PB, Johnson DE: Combination chemotherapy (CISCA) for advanced urinary tract carcinoma: A preliminary report. JAMA 238:2282–2287, 1977.
Of 10 patients who could be evaluated, 9 had objective responses.

Stewart BH, Novick AC: Current perspectives on palliative therapy in cancer of the bladder. Cancer Res 37:2781–2788, 1977.

An excellent summary of palliative approaches.

Yagoda A, Watson RC, Gonzalez-Vitale JC, et al: *Cis*-dichlorodiam-mineplatinum (II) in advanced bladder cancer. Cancer Treat Rep 60:917–923, 1976.

Partial remissions were obtained in 8 of 14 patients who had no prior chemotherapy; median remission duration was 3 months.

Yagoda A, Watson RC, Kemeny N, et al: Diamminedichloride platinum II and cyclophosphamide in the treatment of advanced urothelial cancer. Cancer 41:2121–2130, 1978.

Partial remissions were seen in 47% of patients, with a median response duration of 7 months.

72. PROSTATE CANCER—RELAPSING OR METASTATIC

Distant metastatic disease is documented in up to 40% of patients with prostate cancer at presentation. Osteoblastic bone lesions involving the pelvis, spine, femurs, and/or ribs are the most common sites. Lung, liver, and brain metastases may be found later in the course of the disease but are rarely presenting manifestations. Most patients with stage D prostate cancer have asymptomatic distant metastases at diagnosis and present to their physicians with complaints referable to the prostate. In addition to the physical examination, studies that may be useful in defining disease extent include serum alkaline phosphatase, serum acid phosphatase, CBC, platelets, liver and renal function tests, chest x-ray, intravenous pyelogram, metastatic bone survey, and bone scan.

The serum acid phosphatase (prostatic fraction) is elevated in more than 60% of patients with stage D disease, and with radioimmunoassay the yield may be as high as 92%. Not only is the enzyme level helpful in assessing initial disease activity, but it can also be used to follow response to treatment. Acid phosphatase elevation is not limited to patients with metastatic bone disease, but rather it correlates with disease extent whether those metastases involve soft tissue or bone. Acid phosphatase can also be measured in bone marrow; however, its presence is not diagnostic of metastatic disease in that site, since bone marrow acid phosphatase may be elevated in a variety of benign conditions.

A bone scan is the most sensitive indicator of metastatic bone disease, and its diagnostic utility is greatest in the patient with a normal metastatic bone survey. Unfortunately the abnormalities identified by bone scan are not specific for prostate cancer. Thus it may be necessary to biopsy suspicious bone lesions to document metastatic disease. In occasional patients with widespread osteoblastic lesions on x-ray, the bone scan will, paradoxically, be "negative" as the result of generalized increased uptake.

Following primary therapy of local or regional prostate cancer, relapse is most commonly documented in distant bony sites with or without concurrent regional recurrence. Relapse correlates with advanced clinical stage, a large prostate, the presence of regional nodal involvement, and poorly differentiated tumors. The probability of relapse is <20% for stage A, 30% to 40% for stage B, and 60% for stage C at 5 years. Once metastatic or relapsing disease has been documented, the overall median survival without therapy is approximately 12 months. Unfortunately there is no known curative treatment for advanced prostate cancer, so the therapeutic goal must be limited to palliation.

Hormonal manipulations remain the cornerstone of metastatic prostate cancer treatment. In a series of prospective trials, it has been demonstrated that bilateral orchiectomy and/or diethylstilbestrol (DES) confer no overall survival advantage as compared to a placebo. In contrast to the placebo, however, both are effective in relieving symptoms of metastatic disease in the majority of patients and achieving objective remissions in 20% to 30%. The recommended approach to palliative hormonal therapy is to withhold treatment until the patient's symptoms or general condition warrants it. Castration is usually the first maneuver, followed by DES (1–3 mg po qd) when there is evidence of disease progression. There is no advantage to combining castration with DES therapy and no evidence that higher doses of DES are more effective. In fact it has been clearly shown that 5 mg DES per day carries an increased risk of cardiovascular death. Other ablative procedures, such as adrenalectomy and hypophysectomy, have been used in small series of patients with few objective responses documented but good symptomatic relief in some cases.

Chemotherapy has not been widely tested in metastatic prostate cancer. Responses to therapy are difficult to assess, since most patients have only osteoblastic bone lesions with or without an elevated acid phosphatase. Few have measurable soft tissue masses, palpable lymph nodes, and/or liver or lung disease. The criteria that have been applied for an objective response include 50% reduction in a measurable mass, decrease in acid phosphatase to normal, recalcification of lytic bone lesions, no progression or new disease, and no fall in weight or performance status. Drugs with some efficacy are cyclophosphamide, Adriamycin, 5-fluorouracil, and estramustine phosphate. All have reported objective responses of 10% to 20%. Remission durations are generally less than 6 months. A promising new drug is *cis*-diamminedichloroplatinum, yielding objective regressions in 13 of 45 patients treated in one study, with a mean remission duration of 6 months.

Palliative radiation therapy plays an important role in metastatic prostate cancer management. Symptoms of pelvic pain, hematuria, urethral obstruction and/or leg edema may respond to local irradiation (5000 rads) in the majority of patients. Likewise, distant bone pain may be relieved by radiation therapy (3000 rads in 2 weeks) to the whole bone or to a vertebral column segment. Radiation therapy can also be used to prevent the gynecomastia that results from DES by prophylactically treating the breasts with 1000 rads prior to orchiectomy or DES initiation. If the radiation is delivered after DES has been started, it may not be effective, since glandular hyperplasia is already present.

C.P.

Barzell W, Bean MA, Hilaris BS, Whitmore WF Jr: Prostatic adenocarcinoma: Relationship of grade and local extent to the pattern of metastases. J Urol 118:278–282, 1977.
An excellent analysis of 100 patients treated with local irradiation and lymphadenectomy.
Bhanalaph T, Varkarakis MJ, Murphy GP: Current status of bilateral adrenalectomy for advanced prostatic carcinoma. Ann Surg 179:17–23, 1974.
Of 16 patients who had relapsed after orchiectomy or estrogen therapy, 1 had objective response and 10 had subjective improvement.
Boehme WM, Augspurger RR, Wallner SF, Donohue RE: Lack of usefulness of bone marrow enzymes and calcium in staging patients with prostatic cancer. Cancer 41:1433–1439, 1978.
Levels of acid phosphatase and calcium varied with aspiration technique.
Byar DP: The Veterans Administration Cooperative Urological Research Group's studies of cancer of the prostate. Cancer 32:1126–1130, 1973.

Article provides a review of prospective trials in which placebo, orchiectomy, diethylstilbesterol, or combined therapy in metastatic prostate cancer were compared.

Foti AG, Cooper JF, Herschman H, Malvaez RR: Detection of prostatic cancer by solid-phase radioimmunoassay of serum prostatic acid phosphatase. N Engl J Med 297:1357–1361, 1977.

The radioimmunoassay detected elevated levels in 92% of patients with stage IV disease as compared to 60% when the standard enzyme assay was used.

Merrin CE, Beckley S: Treatment of estrogen-resistant stage D carcinoma of prostate with cis-diamminedichloroplatinum. Urology 13:267–272, 1979.

Objective regressions were identified in 13 of 45 patients, with a mean remission duration of 6 months.

Mittelman A, Shukla SK, Murphy GP: Extended therapy of stage D carcinoma of the prostate with oral estramustine phosphate. J Urol 115:409–412, 1976.

Of 44 patients who could be evaluated, 8 had an objective response and nausea was the only major toxicity.

Osmond JD III, Pendergrass HP, Potsaid MS: Accuracy of ^{99m}TC-diphosphonate bone scans and roentgenograms in the detection of prostate, breast and lung carcinoma metastases. Am J Roentgenol Radium Ther Nucl Med 125:972–977, 1975.

In an analysis of 87 patients with prostate cancer 20 had positive scans and negative x-rays and 3 had negative scans and positive x-rays.

Scott WW, Gibbons RP, Johnson DE, et al: The continued evaluation of the effects of chemotherapy in patients with advanced carcinoma of the prostate. J Urol 116:211–213, 1976.

Of 74 patients receiving 5-FU or cyclophosphamide, 7 had objective remissions and 24 showed stability of the disease.

Torti FM, Carter SK: The chemotherapy of prostatic adenocarcinoma. Ann Intern Med 92:681–689, 1980.

An excellent review with extensive references.

73. TESTIS CANCER—RELAPSING OR METASTATIC

Unlike seminoma, germ cell tumors of the testis frequently present with supradiaphragmatic disease or relapse after regional therapy. The 5-year survival rates ("cure" rates) for seminoma (S) contrast sharply with those for non-seminomatous (NS) tumors: stage I = 100% (S), 85% (NS); stage II = 90% (S), 35% (NS); stage III = 75% (S), <20% (NS). Although the relapse sites for regional disease are similar for both histologies (retroperitoneal lymph nodes, mediastinum, lungs, supraclavicular lymph nodes, liver, bones, and brain), only seminoma is highly radiosensitive, rarely recurs in a previously treated field, and is approachable with radiation therapy alone when recurrent or metastatic. In addition, of patients with seminoma, approximately one-third who do relapse will be found to have nonseminomatous histologic findings at relapse.

Staging studies that may be useful in determining disease extent at relapse include stereo chest x-ray and full lung tomograms when indicated, intravenous pyelogram, abdominal ultrasound or computerized tomography, lymphogram, liver function tests, and liver, bone, and brain scans. Gallium^{67} scanning can be used to locate metastatic seminoma but has no value in detecting non-seminomatous metastases. The serum alpha fetoprotein and/or human chorionic gonadotropin (beta subunit HCG) are elevated in up to 85% of patients with metastatic disease. Persistent or new-onset elevations following regional therapy have a correlation with the presence of undetected metastases; therefore pretherapy and serial posttherapy levels are essential in follow-up management. In the setting of bulky abdominal disease at presentation, clinically unsuspected supraclavicular lymph node metastases may be detected in 10% to 15% of patients subjected to node biopsy.

Following aggressive regional therapy, relapse correlates with such factors as initial stage, bulk or abdominal disease, histology (particularly choriocarcinoma), a scrotal orchiectomy, and the presence of serum tumor markers. Combination chemotherapy is the treatment of choice for all patients with relapsing or metastatic nonseminomatous tumors. Some of the single agents that have demonstrated activity include actinomycin D, chlorambucil, cyclophosphamide, methotrexate, vinblastine, bleomycin, Adriamycin, and *cis*-diamminedichloroplatinum (CDDP). Both actinomycin D and mithramycin as single agents yield complete response rates of 10% to 25%, and up to half of all complete responders are long-term survivors and apparently cured. Recently the complete response rate has been dramatically improved using combination chemotherapy that includes CDDP, bleomycin, and vinblastine (the "Einhorn regimen"). This toxic regimen has achieved complete remissions in 33 of 47 evaluable patients (70%) treated at Indiana University. Although the results remain preliminary, thus far 80% of complete responders remain disease-free for 21+ to 45+ months. In previous chemotherapy series, most relapses following complete remission have occurred within 2 years after discontinuing drug therapy. Therefore these data suggest the potential for cure in a high proportion of patients. Response to chemotherapy does not appear to be adversely influenced by histology, prior irradiation, or chemotherapy. However, patients with bulky disease have fewer complete remissions, and those with prior therapy have more drug-related toxicity.

The roles of surgery and radiation therapy in metastatic or relapsing testis cancer are not well defined. Several reports have emphasized that surgical removal of residual bulky abdominal disease or pulmonary nodules following combination chemotherapy can assist in achieving complete remission. Furthermore, it has been documented that some mass lesions, stable during otherwise successful chemotherapy, are benign teratomas rather than malignant metastases; and that the presence of one benign lesion does not preclude the presence of a malignant one at another site. This apparent transformation of a malignant tumor to a benign one has been attributed to the following hypotheses: chemotherapy kills only the malignant cells, leaving the differentiated cells to form a teratoma; treatment induces the malignant cells to differentiate and form a teratoma; transformation is a process of benign evolution.

Guidelines for combination chemotherapy, developed by Einhorn [1979], include the following: (1) goal of treatment should be complete remission in all patients; (2) maximum benefit is usually achieved with 3 or 4 courses of chemotherapy; (3) surgical excision of residual disease at the conclusion of chemotherapy should be considered, if feasible; and (4) potential drug-related toxicities, particularly in those with prior radiation or chemotherapy, should be anticipated and treated promptly.

C.P.

Buck AS, Schamber DT, Maier JG, Lewis EL: Supraclavicular node biopsy and malignant testicular tumors. J Urol 107:619–621, 1972.
Of 23 patients with clinical stage II disease, 3 had positive node biopsies.

D'Aoust JC, Prestayko AW, Einhorn LH, et al: Cisplatin, bleomycin, and vinblastine combination therapy of testicular tumors: An analysis. Med Pediatr Oncol 6:195–205, 1979.
Article provides an analysis of prognostic variables in 86 patients with testicular tumors.

Donohue JP, Einhorn LH, Perez JM: Improved management of non-seminomatous testis tumors. Cancer 42:2903–2908, 1978.
Article discusses the role of surgery following combination chemotherapy.

Einhorn LH, Donohue JP: Combination chemotherapy in disseminated testicular cancer: The Indiana University experience. Semin Oncol 6:87–93, 1979.
Article provides a summary of the experience with CDDP plus vinblastine plus bleomycin in 47 patients.

Hong WK, Wittes RE, Hajdu ST, et al: The evolution of mature teratoma from malignant testicular tumors. Cancer 40:2987–2992, 1977.
A description of 12 cases.

Johnson DE, Appelt G, Samuels ML, Luna M: Metastases from testicular carcinoma: Study of 78 autopsied cases. Urology 8:234–239, 1976.
The metastatic disease in 6 of 19 patients dying of seminoma proved to have a nonseminomatous histology.

Krikorian JG, Daniels JR, Brown BW Jr, Hu MSJ: Variables for predicting serious toxicity (vinblastine dose, performance status, and prior therapeutic experience): Chemotherapy for metastatic testicular cancer with cis-dichlorodiammineplatinum (II), vinblastine, and bleomycin. Cancer Treat Rep 62:1455–1463, 1978.
The seriousness of toxicity correlated with the dose of vinblastine in 14 patients studied.

Lange PH, Fraley EE: Serum alpha-fetoprotein and human chorionic gonadotropin in the treatment of patients with testicular tumors. Urol Clin North Am 4:393–406, 1977.
Elevated levels of fetoprotein and gonadotropin may be detected in 85% of patients with metastatic disease; postorchiectomy persistent or new-onset elevation correlates with the presence of metastases.

Merrin C, Takita H, Weber R, et al: Combination radical surgery and multiple sequential chemotherapy for the treatment of advanced carcinoma of the testis (stage III). Cancer 37:20–29, 1976.
Of 16 patients who underwent surgery following chemotherapy, 8 were found to have benign tumors.

Quivery JM, Fu KK, Herzog KA, et al: Malignant tumors of the testis: Analysis of treatment results and sites and causes of failure. Cancer 39:1247–1253, 1977.
In an analysis of 150 patients sites of relapse following initial therapy were the lung and supraclavicular and mediastinal lymph nodes.

Williams C: Current dilemmas in the management of non-seminomatous germ cell tumors of the testis. Cancer Treat Rev 4:275–297, 1977.
An excellent review of all aspects of management.

Yagoda A, Vugrin D: Theoretical considerations in the treatment of seminoma. Semin Oncol 6:74–81, 1979.
Report discusses primary and relapse management, including the role of chemotherapy.

74. OVARIAN CARCINOMA—RELAPSING OR METASTATIC

Approximately 60% of women who have ovarian carcinoma have advanced disease (stage III or IV) at presentation. In addition, at least one-third of those with initially localized disease will develop recurrence. Unlike the case with many other solid tumors, hematogenous dissemination is infrequent and occurs late, while metastatic spread over the peritoneal surface is common and occurs early. The true incidence of retroperitoneal lymph node involvement is not known, but lymphography suggests that it is at least 50% in advanced disease and up to 10% in stage I or II disease.

Documentation of all known metastatic tumor is important in the treatment of advanced or recurrent ovarian cancer, since assessing response to therapy can be difficult. In addition to physical and pelvic examinations, standard staging procedures include chest x-ray, intravenous pyelogram, barium enema, and cytologic examinations of all fluids (ascites, pleural effusions). Lymphography can assess retroperitoneal lymph nodes and be used to follow disease activity with therapy. Peritoneoscopy can identify peritoneal metastases (particularly over the dome of the diaphragm), sometimes providing the only followable disease. Laboratory studies are frequently of little value, although liver function tests (especially alkaline phosphatase) and carcinoembryonic antigen (CEA) may provide indicators of disease activity.

The 5-year survival of patients with advanced ovarian carcinoma is less than 10%. Serous cystadenocarcinoma is the most common tumor in advanced disease, although all other histologic types can be seen as well. In addition, the more anaplastic the tumor (high-grade), regardless of its histologic type, the more likely it is to be of advanced stage. As in localized ovarian cancer, the histologic grade of stage III or IV disease is an important prognostic variable.

In general, surgery and/or radiation therapy is of little benefit in advanced disease, where tumor may involve the entire peritoneal surface or disseminate to extra-abdominal sites. Palliative surgery is frequently performed to remove bulk disease in the pelvis; however, more radical surgery, such as lymph node dissection and pelvic exenteration, does not improve survival. Whole abdominal plus pelvic irradiation has been used in stage III disease, but only in patients with minimal residual disease.

Alkylating agent chemotherapy has been used more extensively than any other class of drugs in advanced ovarian carcinoma. L-phenylalanine mustard (melphalan, L-PAM) has been the drug most commonly used. Response rates to single alkylating agents range from 35% to 65%, with 5% to 15% of all patients still responding two years after initiation of therapy. Factors that influence response or duration of response include prior therapy, disease bulk, histologic type, and grade of tumor. Although the overall 5-year survival of those treated with single agent chemotherapy is less than 10%, it is clear that chemotherapy can be of benefit. In a double-blind randomized study of placebo versus chlorambucil, the median survival of untreated patients was 9.3 months as compared to 33.5 months for treated patients. Similarly, responders to chemotherapy survive longer than nonresponders, with as many as 6% of all patients with advanced disease remaining disease-free for periods in excess of 5 years.

Many other drugs have demonstrated activity in advanced ovarian cancer, but none have proved superior to alkylating agents. These drugs include 5-fluorouracil, methotrexate, hexamethylmelamine, Adriamycin, and *cis*-diamminedichloroplatinum. Recently, combination chemotherapy programs utilizing alkylating agents plus other drugs have yielded significantly better response rates and median survivals than single alkylating agent therapy. One prospective study had a complete response rate of 33% with Hexa-CAF (hexamethylmelamine, cyclophosphamide, methotrexate, and 5-FU) versus 16% with melphalan. The median survival was 29 months with Hexa-CAF and only 17 months with melphalan. Response and survival were improved in those patients with minimal residual disease.

Second-look peritoneoscopy and subsequent laparotomy have been advocated for patients who have clinical complete tumor regressions, in order to assess completeness of response, the need to continue, change, or discontinue therapy, and the possibility of removing bulk tumor. The recommended interval of therapy prior to such restaging procedures is at least 10 to 12 months of chemotherapy. The need to discontinue alkylating agent therapy in complete responders has been emphasized recently by the reported increased risk of acute myelogenous leukemia.

For patients who do not achieve complete remission, the terminal phase of ovarian carcinoma is frequently protracted. Local tumor growth throughout the peritoneal cavity progresses, causing nausea, vomiting, abdominal distension with ascites, dyspnea, and intermittent partial small bowel obstruction. Symptomatic measures may include paracentesis, diuretics, low residue diet, parenteral hyperalimentation, and nasogastric suctioning. Intraperitoneal administration of radioactive isotopes or alkylating agents is of no value; and surgery for small bowel obstruction is usually futile, since tumor involves the bowel diffusely.

C.P.

Masterson JG: Discussion of Burns BC Jr, Rutledge FN, Smith JP, et al: Management of ovarian carcinoma: Surgery, irradiation, and chemotherapy. Am J Obstet Gynecol 98:374–386, 1967.
Article provides a description of a prospective trial in which a placebo was compared with chlorambucil for advanced ovarian carcinoma.

Ozols RF, Garvin AJ, Costa J, et al: Histologic grade in advanced ovarian cancer. Cancer Treat Rep 63:255–263, 1979.
Both chemotherapy response and survival were adversely affected by increasing histological grade of disease.

Parker BR, Castellino RA, Fuks ZY, Bagshaw MA: The role of lymphography in patients with ovarian cancer. Cancer 34:100–105, 1974.
Authors correlate lymphography findings with clinical stage.

Reimer RR, Hoover R, Fraumeni JF, Young RC: Acute leukemia after alkylating-agent therapy of ovarian cancer. N Engl J Med 297:177–181, 1977.
Report points out the increased risk of acute nonlymphocytic leukemia in patients receiving alkylating agents.

Rosenoff SH, Young RC, Anderson T, et al: Peritoneoscopy: A valuable staging tool in ovarian carcinoma. Ann Intern Med 83:37–41, 1975.
Article demonstrates that diaphragmatic metastases are common and that second-look peritoneoscopy can assist in evaluation of clinical complete responders.

Smith JP, Delgado G, Rutledge F: Second-look operation in ovarian carcinoma. Cancer 38:1438–1442, 1976.
Report analyzes benefits of second-look surgery in clinical complete responders and emphasizes the need for careful sampling of peritoneum.

Webb MJ, Malkasian GD, Jorgensen EO: Factors influencing ovarian cancer survival after chemotherapy. Obstet Gynecol 44:564–570, 1974.
Type of surgery, grade of malignancy, and initial leukocytosis were found to influence survival.

Young RC: Chemotherapy of ovarian cancer: Past and present. Semin Oncol 2:267–276, 1975.
Excellent review of chemotherapy for ovarian cancer.

Young RC: Ovarian carcinoma: An optimistic epilogue. Cancer Treat Rep 63:333–337, 1979.
This editorial reviews recent advances in therapy and emphasizes the need for careful initial staging and assessment of response.

Young RC, Chabner BA, Hubbard SP, et al: Advanced ovarian adenocarcinoma: A prospective trial of melphalan (L-PAM) versus combination chemotherapy. N Engl J Med 299:1261–1266, 1978.
Complete response (33% vs. 16%) and median survival (29 vs. 17 months) were significantly better when the drug combination was used than for melphalan alone.

75. CARCINOMA OF THE CERVIX—RELAPSING OR METASTATIC

Distant metastatic squamous carcinoma of the cervix is unusual at diagnosis, occurring in less than 5% to 10% of patients, and even at relapse, distant disease is not a common problem. When it does occur, metastatic sites include distant lymph nodes, lungs, liver, and bone. On the other hand, recurrent or persistent pelvic tumor is the major cause of failure after primary therapy and is coexistent in the majority of patients with distant metastatic disease as well. Some factors that are thought to influence the incidence of primary treatment failure include stage at diagnosis, bulky tumor, presence of pelvic infection, kind of primary therapy, and lack of response to radiation therapy. Most patients relapse during the first three years following treatment, and the time to relapse varies inversely with stage. Since there are few methods of effective salvage, prognosis is poor in this group of patients, with the majority surviving less than 1 year.

Evaluation of disease extent in patients with recurrent or persistent squamous carcinoma of the cervix is often difficult. In addition to the pelvic examination and Papanicolaou smear, ultrasound or computerized tomography of the abdomen and pelvis may reveal tumor masses. An intravenous pyelogram is a sensitive indicator of recurrent disease when ureteral obstruction is detected, since benign causes, such as radiation-induced stricture, are rare. A barium enema may demonstrate narrowing or deviation of the rectosigmoid, although these changes may be secondary to prior treatment. Distant metastatic studies include a complete physical examination, chest x-ray, and bone scan. Any bony abnormalities on scan should be evaluated with x-rays, since bone lesions are usually lytic and may lead to pathologic fracture. Laboratory studies may include blood counts, liver function tests, and renal function tests. The carcinoembryonic antigen has been reported to be elevated with disease recurrence.

Treatment at relapse depends upon prior therapy, extent of disease, and the patient's general physical condition. In the few cases in which recurrence consists of small, centrally located tumors, surgical resection may be possible. It is frequently difficult to define disease extent accurately without surgical exploration, however, because of prior surgery and/or radiation therapy. Factors that may influence surgical outcome include age, general health, obesity, prior irradiation, initial disease-free interval, the presence of ureteral obstruction, the location of pelvic recurrence, and the clinical estimate of resectability. The salvage rate may be as high as 50% to 60% for small central recurrences treated with radical hysterectomy, and even 30% to 50% for those selected patients with more extensive disease who undergo pelvic exenteration. However, most patients with recurrent or persistent squamous carcinoma are not candidates for surgical salvage, because there is fixation of tumor to the lateral pelvic wall, para-aortic lymph nodes are involved with tumor, or there is intraperitoneal or distant metastatic disease. Some patients who have had no prior radiation therapy may benefit from pelvic irradiation. The principles of primary treatment apply; however, efficacy may be compromised and morbidity increased because of postoperative changes in pelvic anatomy and the sites of recurrent disease.

There has been limited experience with chemotherapy in squamous carcinoma of the cervix. Single agents with reported objective response rates of 10% to 25% include cyclophosphamide, chlorambucil, melphalan, 5-FU, methotrexate, vincristine, Adriamycin, bleomycin, mitomycin C, methyl-CCNU, and hexamethylmelamine. Drug treatment and evaluation is made difficult by the presence of such factors as pelvic scarring and fixation, decreased tissue vascularity, ureteral obstruction, and limited bone marrow reserve following pelvic irradiation. Tumor regressions are often limited to areas without prior radiation therapy, whereas pelvic disease within the radiated field is less responsive, presumably due to poor chemotherapy perfusion. Several reports of combination chemotherapy have shown promise in terms of objective response rates (50% to 80%), but median remission durations remain brief (<7 months in most series).

C.P.

Baker LH, Opipari MI, Wilson H, et al: Mitomycin C, vincristine, and bleomycin therapy for advanced cervical cancer. Obstet Gynecol 52:146–150, 1978.
   A prospective study of 130 patients. Objective response was seen in 30 of 50 patients (60%) who received a twice-weekly bleomycin/vincristine schedule plus mitomycin C every 6 weeks.
Blythe JG, Ptacek JJ, Buchsbaum HJ, Latourette HB: Bony metastases from carcinoma of cervix: Occurrence, diagnosis, and treatment. Cancer 36:475–484, 1975.
   A retrospective study of 55 patients.
Conroy JF, Lewis GC, Brady LW, et al: Low dose bleomycin and methotrexate in cervical cancer. Cancer 37:660–664, 1976.
   Objective responses were seen in 12 of 20 patients; median duration was 7 months.
Creasman WT, Rutledge F: Preoperative evaluation of patients with recurrent carcinoma of the cervix. Gynecol Oncol 1:111–118, 1972.
   Article discusses criteria for and end results of pelvic exenteration.
Donaldson E, van Nagell JR Jr, Wood EG, et al: Carcinoembryonic antigen in patients treated with radiation therapy for invasive squamous cell carcinoma of the uterine cervix. Am J Roentgenol 127:829–831, 1976.
   Elevated CEA levels preceded clinical detection of recurrent disease in 5 patients studied serially.
Jampolis S, Andras J, Fletcher GH: Analysis of sites and causes of failures of irradiation in invasive squamous cell carcinoma of the intact uterine cervix. Radiology 115:681–685, 1975.
   In a review of 916 patients local recurrence was due to the presence of massive disease.

Lifshitz SG, Buchsbaum HJ: Spread of cervical carcinoma. Obstet Gynecol Annu 6:341–354, 1977.
Article reviews lymphatic and vascular dissemination of cervical carcinoma.

Miyamoto T, Takabe Y, Watanabe M, Terasima T: Effectiveness of a sequential combination of bleomycin and mitomycin-C on an advanced cervical cancer. Cancer 41:403–414, 1978.
Objective remissions were documented in 14 of 15 patients; 12 (80%) had complete responses.

Peeples WJ, Inalsingh CHA, Hazra TA, Graft D: The occurrence of metastasis outside the abdomen and retroperitoneal space in invasive carcinoma of the cervix. Gynecol Oncol 4:307–310, 1976.
In only 29 of 644 patients with invasive carcinoma were distant metastases detected.

Van Dyke AH, van Nagell JR Jr: The prognostic significance of ureteral obstruction in patients with recurrent carcinoma of the cervix uteri. Surg Gynecol Obstet 141:371–373, 1975.
Of 110 patients with recurrent cervical cancer, 46 had some evidence of ureteral obstruction and only 2 were long-term survivors following surgical resection.

76. ENDOMETRIAL CARCINOMA—RELAPSING OR METASTATIC

Fewer than 5% of women with endometrial carcinoma have distant metastases at diagnosis, yet the 5-year survival for all patients is only 60% to 75%. Local recurrence in the pelvis, involving the vagina, bladder, ureters, regional lymph nodes and peritoneum, is the major cause of primary treatment failure. Distant metastatic disease is most commonly documented in lung, bone, and liver. Local recurrence and/or distant relapse is usually detected within the first 3 years following primary therapy. Prognostic variables at initial diagnosis include clinical stage, tumor differentiation, uterine size, and myometrial invasion.

Documenting the extent of recurrent disease may be very difficult because of prior surgery and/or irradiation to the pelvis. In addition to the physical examination, a chest x-ray and intravenous pyelogram may provide useful information. Ultrasound and computerized tomography of the abdomen may demonstrate retroperitoneal and/or pelvic abnormalities. Laboratory studies are relatively nonspecific. Renal function tests may be normal even in the presence of unilateral ureteral obstruction. The serum carcinoembryonic antigen has been reported to be elevated at relapse but is not diagnostic.

Approximately one-third of those patients who have local recurrence following initial surgery alone may be salvaged with radiation therapy. The usual dose to the pelvis is 5000 rads in 5 weeks. Those patients who have local recurrence following combined surgical and irradiation approaches, or who relapse with distant metastatic disease, may benefit from palliative systemic therapy. Progestational agents are most often used in this setting: either hydroxyprogesterone caproate (Delalutin), 1 to 3 gm/week IM; medroxyprogesterone (Provera), 200 to 800 mg po daily or IM each week; or Depo-provera, 400 to 800 mg IM each month. An initial loading course of intramuscular Provera, 1 gm for 2 consecutive weeks, is usually administered in addition. Progestational therapy must be continued for at least 8 to 12 weeks before a response to treatment can be assessed. The overall objective response rate is approximately

30%. Patients with well-differentiated tumors respond more often, approximately 50% of the time, than do those with poorly differentiated tumors, whose response rate is only 15%. The average response duration is almost two years; and in one study responders survived a median of 26 months, with 30% surviving 5 years. By contrast, the median survival of nonresponders was only 4 months.

Other than tumor differentiation, few factors influence response to therapy. A long disease-free interval prior to relapse, a slow-growing tumor, and age less than 50 years are reported to give improved response. However, these variables are also characteristic of well-differentiated endometrial tumors and thus tumor responsiveness. There are few data available, to date, on the utility of progesterone receptors in endometrial cancer. Early reports suggest that the presence of receptors correlates with well-differentiated tumors and thus with improved response to progestational agents. Factors that do not appear to influence response are sites of disease and kinds of prior therapy. The mechanism of action for gestagens is not known. There appears to be a direct cytotoxic effect as well as the induction of cellular differentiation. Serial endometrial biopsies have demonstrated a decrease in cellular atypia and pleomorphism with progesterone administration, and in vitro studies have shown similar findings of differentiation.

There is little experience with cytotoxic agents in the treatment of endometrial cancer. The single agents that have been reported to produce objective regressions in 20% to 30% of patients include 5-FU, cyclophosphamide, cytembena, and Adriamycin. In most studies response durations are not defined. These drugs have also been used in combination with or without the addition of progestational agents. Early reports appear encouraging, with 50% to 100% of patients achieving objective tumor regressions. It remains to be documented whether there is also improved duration of remission and survival.

C.P.

Bruckner HW, Deppe G: Combination chemotherapy of advanced endometrial adenocarcinoma with adriamycin, cyclophosphamide, 5-fluorouracil, and medroxyprogesterone acetate. Obstet Gynecol 50:10s–12s, 1977.
Objective responses were documented in 7 of 7 patients treated with this drug combination.

Horton J, Begg CB, Arseneault J, et al: Comparison of adriamycin with cyclophosphamide in patients with advanced endometrial cancer. Cancer Treat Rep 62:159–161, 1978.
Objective responses were seen in 4 of 21 patients treated with adriamycin and in none who received cyclophosphamide.

Ishiwata I, Udagawa Y, Okumura H, Nozawa S: Effects of progesterone on human endometrial carcinoma cells in vivo and in vitro. J Natl Cancer Inst 60:947–954, 1978.
Article discusses progesterone-induced cellular differentiation in vitro. When nude BALB/c mice were pretreated with progesterone, tumors were well differentiated; without pretreatment, tumors were undifferentiated.

Kohorn EI: Gestagens and endometrial carcinoma. Gynecol Oncol 4:398–411, 1976.
A good review of therapy for endometrial carcinoma.

Malkasian GD Jr: Carcinoma of the endometrium: Effect of stage and grade on survival. Cancer 41:996–1001, 1978.
Article provides a retrospective analysis of prognostic variables in 523 patients.

Muggia FM, Chia G, Reed LJ, Romney SL: Doxorubicin-cyclophosphamide: Effective chemotherapy for advanced endometrial adenocarcinoma. Am J Obstet Gynecol 128:314–319, 1977.

Of 8 patients who could be evaluated, 5 achieved objective remissions with a median duration of 10 months.

Reifenstein EC Jr: Hydroxyprogesterone caproate therapy in advanced endometrial cancer. Cancer 27:485–502, 1971.
Article provides a comprehensive retrospective analysis of 314 patients treated with hydroxyprogesterone caproate.

Salazar OM, Feldstein ML, DePapp EW, et al: Endometrial carcinoma: Analysis of failures with special emphasis on the use of initial preoperative external pelvic radiation. Int J Radiat Oncol Biol Phys 2:1101–1107, 1977.
Article provides an analysis of 75 patients with endometrial carcinoma for whom therapy was not successful.

van Nagell JR Jr, Donaldson ES, Wood EG, et al: The prognostic significance of carcinoembryonic antigen in the plasma and tumors of patients with endometrial adenocarcinoma. Am J Obstet Gynecol 128:308–313, 1977.
CEA elevation correlated with uterine size, histological differentiation, and stage of disease in the 60 patients with endometrial adenocarcinoma studied.

77. OSTEOGENIC SARCOMA—RELAPSING OR METASTATIC

Pulmonary metastases are the most common type of relapsing disease in patients with osteogenic sarcoma. More than two-thirds of all patients have disease limited to the lung at relapse, whereas fewer than 10% have relapses with extrapulmonary metastases alone. Although extrapulmonary sites are uncommon at first relapse, most patients will be found to have extrapulmonary metastases at autopsy, involving such sites as bone, lymph nodes, liver, and brain. Factors known to influence prognosis, and thus the development of metastatic disease, include pathologic type, extent of disease, site of primary, duration of symptoms prior to diagnosis, tumor size, presence of Paget's disease, and age. The most favorable histologic type is parosteal osteogenic sarcoma, whereas osteogenic sarcoma arising in Paget's disease has a very poor prognosis. Axial skeleton lesions have a poorer prognosis than those arising in the extremities, and adults have a shorter survival than children with the disease.

Most retrospective studies prior to the use of adjuvant chemotherapy reported a median disease-free interval of approximately 6 to 10 months and a survival of 3 to 6 months following the documentation of pulmonary metastases. Currently the median disease-free interval is at least 18 months with the use of adjuvant chemotherapy. The probability of development of relapsing disease after primary therapy changed with the introduction of adjuvant chemotherapy. In retrospective studies approximately 80% of patients relapsed within the first 2 years, whereas that figure is currently 50% to 60% within 3 years. Whether this improvement represents selection and/or the influence of adjuvant chemotherapy is yet to be determined.

Since the lung is the most common site of relapsing disease, chest x-ray, full-lung tomograms, and computerized tomography are important studies in detecting relapse. Serum alkaline phosphatase and bone scan may also be useful.

The approach to treatment of metastatic osteogenic sarcoma is evolving rapidly. Prior to the introduction of chemotherapy, surgical resection of pulmonary nodules was reported to be effective salvage therapy in some selected patients. Criteria for selection included the number of nodules and their technical resectability, the initial disease-free interval, and the tumor doubling time as calculated by sequential chest x-rays. Few patients were eligible for this approach, and in one study less than half survived 2 years.

Few effective single agents have been identified in the treatment of metastatic osteogenic sarcoma. Adriamycin has a reported response rate of 22%, and high-dose methotrexate with folinic acid rescue, 40%; cis-diamminedichloroplatinum also appears promising, but experience with it is limited. Combination chemotherapy programs utilizing these drugs along with DTIC, vincristine, and/or cyclophosphamide have yielded response rates of 40% to 50%. Although remissions are usually brief, the median survival of responders may be as long as 9 months. Variables associated with improved drug responses include an initial long disease-free interval and the presence of pulmonary or liver metastases. Bone metastases, on the other hand, respond poorly.

Recently, aggressive investigational approaches that use combination chemotherapy and surgical resection of pulmonary nodules have been described. Early reports suggest that such combined modality therapy may improve survival. Guidelines include the following: (1) patients with late-occurring solitary pulmonary nodules should undergo initial surgery followed by chemotherapy; and (2) patients with rapidly progressive or multiple pulmonary metastases should receive initial chemotherapy, followed by surgery (if the metastatic disease regresses or remains stable for 2 to 6 months) and further postoperative chemotherapy.

C.P.

Benjamin RS, Baker LH, O'Bryan RM, et al: Chemotherapy for metastatic osteosarcoma—studies by the M.D. Anderson Hospital and the Southwest Oncology Group. Cancer Treat Rep 62:237–238, 1978.
Report provides a brief summary of Adriamycin combination chemotherapy.

Jeffree GM, Price CHG, Sissons HA: The metastatic patterns of osteosarcoma. Br J Cancer 32:87–107, 1975.
Article analyzes 91 patients with metastases from osteosarcoma.

Martini N, Huvos AG, Miké V, et al: Multiple pulmonary resections in the treatment of osteogenic sarcoma. Ann Thorac Surg 12:271–278, 1971.
In this report of 22 patients, 9 survived for two years after resection.

Ochs JJ, Freeman AI, Douglass HO Jr, et al: cis-Dichlorodiammineplatinum (II) in advanced osteogenic sarcoma. Cancer Treat Rep 62:239–245, 1978.
Objective regressions were observed in 5 of 8 patients with advanced disease.

Rosen G, Huvos AG, Mosende C, et al: Chemotherapy and thoracotomy for metastatic osteogenic sarcoma: A model for adjuvant chemotherapy and the rationale for the timing of thoracic surgery. Cancer 41:841–849, 1978.
In a retrospective analysis of 45 patients treated with chemotherapy and surgery, median survival was significantly prolonged (19 to 33+ months) when compared to historical data of untreated patients (6 months).

Rosen G, Suwansirikul S, Kwon C, et al: High-dose methotrexate with citrovorum factor rescue and adriamycin in childhood osteogenic sarcoma. Cancer 33:1151–1163, 1974.
Objective responses to these drugs were demonstrated in 7 of 13 children.

Rosenberg SA, Flye MW, Conkle D, et al: Treatment of osteogenic sarcoma: II. Aggressive resection of pulmonary metastases. Cancer Treat Rep 63:753–756, 1979.
Article gives results of thoracotomy in 18 patients with osteogenic sarcoma following adjuvant therapy relapse.

Simon R: Clinical prognostic factors in osteosarcoma. Cancer Treat Rep 62:193–197, 1978.
Discussion of such factors as histology, extent of disease, site of primary, duration of symptoms, and tumor size.

van Dongen JA, van Slooten EA: The surgical treatment of pulmonary
metastases. Cancer Treat Rev 5:29–48, 1978.
   *A comprehensive review including surgical selection criteria, treatment re-
   sults, and analysis of prognostic variables.*
Von Hoff DD, Rozencweig M, Louie AC, et al: "Single"-agent activity of
high-dose methotrexate with citrovorum factor rescue. Cancer Treat Rep
62:233–235, 1978.
   *Report emphasizes the limited experience in metastatic disease; objective re-
   sponses were documented in 11 of 26 patients.*

78. SOFT TISSUE SARCOMAS—RELAPSING OR METASTATIC

Local recurrence remains a difficult problem in the management of patients
with soft tissue sarcomas. Although these tumors may appear grossly encapsulated at presentation, they are poorly circumscribed microscopically, and simple
enucleation inevitably leaves behind unresected tumor. In most series such
excisions are associated with local recurrences in more than 80% of patients.
With more radical surgical procedures, the incidence of local recurrence is
dramatically reduced. Following soft part resection, fewer than 25% of patients
develop recurrence; and after amputation, fewer than 18%. For unresectable
lesions treated with high-dose radiation therapy, the recurrence rate is approximately 50% to 60%. Not only is the initial kind of therapy important in
influencing the rate of local recurrence, but histologic grade and tumor size are
also important determinants. Histologic type appears to be less important;
however, fibrosarcomas, neurofibrosarcomas, and synovial cell sarcomas are
associated with the highest rates of local recurrence.

Salvage rates of 30% to 50% are usually reported for recurrent soft tissue
sarcomas; and salvage therapies follow the principles outlined for primary
treatment. However, radical surgery may require amputation more frequently,
or may not be technically feasible at all. Radiation therapy may require larger
portals, leaving less normal tissue and thus increasing morbidity. Therefore
before initiating salvage therapy it is important to carefully assess the extent of
local disease as well as to rule out the presence of metastatic tumor.

Only 15% of patients with soft tissue sarcomas present initially with distant
metastases. Furthermore the majority of patients who ultimately do develop
distant disease do so only after, or at the same time as, they are found to
have locally recurrent tumor. Common sites of metastatic spread include lungs,
pleura, bones, liver, and retroperitoneum. In addition it has been emphasized
recently that central nervous system metastases may be detected in patients
receiving chemotherapy. More than 80% of local recurrences and/or distant
metastases will be detected within the first two years following primary treatment. The factors that influence the frequency of local recurrence are also those
that influence the incidence of distant metastases, namely, histologic type,
grade, and tumor size. Since metastatic lung involvement is so common at
relapse, it warrants particular attention. Full lung tomography and computed
tomography may detect small lesions not appreciated on routine examination.
Other possibly useful studies include bone scan, liver function tests, and liver
scan.

Once distant metastases are documented, fewer than 10% of patients survive
2 years. Chemotherapy is much less successful in adults than in children, and
experience with it is more limited. The single agents frequently used in child-

hood tumors include cyclophosphamide, vincristine, and actinomycin D. Their individual response rates in adults are poorly documented. Adriamycin is the most active single agent in adults, with reported objective response rates of 20% to 40%; however, the responses are transient, with a median duration of approximately 4 months. DTIC is another active agent, with a response rate of 15% to 20%. Several combination chemotherapy programs have been evaluated in adults, all utilizing Adriamycin and DTIC. The two drugs have been reported to achieve objective remissions in 40% to 50% of patients, with complete responses in 10%. In addition, responders survived significantly longer than nonresponders, with 70% of complete responders alive at 18 months. The objective response rate to a four-drug combination including cyclophosphamide, vincristine, Adriamycin, and DTIC has been reported to be 50% to 60%, with 15% complete remissions. Although the four-drug regimen appears superior, it has not been prospectively compared to Adriamycin plus DTIC alone. These chemotherapy programs appear to be effective for all histologic types, although the experience is limited.

Surgical resection of isolated pulmonary metastases has been reported to provide effective salvage in some selected patients. Factors considered prior to resection include the number of nodules and their technical resectability; whether there is evidence of metastatic disease outside the lung parenchyma; the initial disease-free interval prior to relapse; the tumor doubling time as assessed by sequential chest x-rays, tumor histology, and grade; and the patient's immune competence. Patients who are most likely to benefit from surgical resection are those with a solitary pulmonary metastasis, a disease-free interval of more than one year, a tumor doubling time of more than 40 days, and cutaneous delayed hypersensitivity.

C.P.

Band PR, Kocandrle C: Growth rate of pulmonary metastases in human sarcomas. Cancer 36:471–474, 1975.
The median tumor doubling time in 15 patients was 25 days.

Gercovich FG, Luna MA, Gottlieb JA: Increased incidence of cerebral metastases in sarcoma patients with prolonged survival from chemotherapy: Report of cases of leiomyosarcoma and chondrosarcoma. Cancer 36:1843–1851, 1975.
Of 14 patients with stable or responsive disease for at least 6 months, 5 developed cerebral metastases at relapse.

Gottlieb JA, Baker LH, O'Bryan RM, et al: Adriamycin (NSC-123127) used alone and in combination for soft tissue and bony sarcomas. Cancer Chemother Rep 6:271–282, 1975.
Article provides a complete summary of combination chemotherapy results.

Gottlieb JA, Baker LH, Quagliana JM, et al: Chemotherapy of sarcomas with a combination of adriamycin and dimethyl triazeno imidazole carboxamide. Cancer 30:1632–1638, 1972.
Of 100 patients who could be evaluated, objective responses were seen in 41%.

Holmes EC, Morton DL: Pulmonary resection for sarcoma metastases. Orthop Clin North Am 8:805–810, 1977.
Article discusses criteria and results of surgical resection for sarcoma metastases.

Pinedo HM, Kenis Y: Chemotherapy of advanced soft-tissue sarcomas in adults. Cancer Treat Rev 4:67–86, 1977.
A comprehensive review.

Russell WO, Cohen J, Enzinger F, et al: A clinical and pathological staging system for soft tissue sarcomas. Cancer 40:1562–1570, 1977.

A staging system based on tumor size and local extension, presence of lymph node or metastatic disease involvement, and tumor histopathologic grade is applied to 1215 cases of soft tissue sarcoma.

Shiu MH, Castro EB, Hajdu SI, Fortner JG: Surgical treatment of 297 soft tissue sarcomas of the lower extremity. Ann Surg 182:597–602, 1975.

A retrospective analysis of 297 patients. Histopathologic type and grade and tumor size were important prognostic variables.

PART V. LYMPHOMAS AND HEMATOLOGIC MALIGNANCIES

Hodgkin's disease is a malignancy that usually presents as painless lymph-adenopathy involving peripheral lymph nodes above the diaphragm. It may be associated with symptoms such as weight loss, fever, night sweats, pruritus, and/or alcohol-induced lymph node pain. Its diagnosis depends upon his-topathologic identification of characteristic giant cells (Reed-Sternberg cells) in an appropriate cellular and architectural background and can be further defined according to the Rye modification of the Lukes and Butler histologic classification (lymphocyte predominance, nodular sclerosis, mixed cellularity, and lymphocyte depletion), whose subtypes correlate well with anatomic sites of involvement, clinical stage at presentation, and survival.

The annual incidence of Hodgkin's disease is 35 per million for white males and 26 per million for white females in the United States. The incidence for nonwhites is slightly lower. There is a bimodal distribution of the age-specific incidence for Hodgkin's disease in the United States, with one peak at 15 to 34 years and the other at 50 and older. While the etiology of Hodgkin's disease is unknown, there is much speculation concerning the roles of immune compe-tence and immunologic mechanisms, exposure to infectious agents, and genetic and environmental factors.

Once the diagnosis has been established, it is necessary to document the extent of disease, so that appropriate therapy can be selected. The staging of Hodgkin's disease relies on both clinical (clinical stage—CS) and pathologic (pathologic stage—PS) data as defined by the Ann Arbor classification, and this staging system generally has a good correlation with histopathology and prog-nosis. For example, lymphocyte predominance and nodular sclerosis usually present with CS I or II, whereas lymphocyte depletion is usually CS III or IV.

In addition to a careful medical history (eliciting the "B" symptoms of weight loss greater than 10% of usual body weight in the prior 6 months, unexplained fever, and night sweats) and physical examination, several laboratory studies may be useful. Routine blood counts and liver and renal function tests are usually normal, whereas the serum alkaline phosphatase may be elevated nonspecifically or in association with liver, bone, or bone marrow disease. Likewise the sedimentation rate, serum copper, and ceruloplasmin are often high in active Hodgkin's disease. Delayed hypersensitivity may be assessed by testing with natural intradermal antigens and/or dinitrochlorobenzene. Al-though cutaneous anergy is associated with advanced clinical stage, it is by no means diagnostic. Mediastinal and hilar adenopathy may be demonstrated on routine chest x-ray, while full lung tomography is necessary to fully evaluate extent of anatomic disease. A bilateral lower extremity lymphogram opacifies iliac and para-aortic lymph node chains to the level of L-2. It does not opacify splenic hilar, celiac, porta hepatis, mesenteric, or presacral lymph nodes. It is a highly useful procedure, however, in identifying disease in 31% to 46% of patients. Follow-up films can be used subsequently in directing surgical sam-pling as well as in devising radiation therapy portals, demonstrating response to therapy, and detecting relapse. Less than 10% of lymphograms are false-negative studies, and 20% to 30% are false-positive when correlated with laparotomy findings. Other examinations used to evaluate the abdomen may be of lesser value, except in selected patients, including intravenous pyelogram, inferior vena cavagram, ultrasound or computerized tomography, gallium 67 abdominal scan, and liver-spleen scan.

Following the above noninvasive procedures, a clinical stage can be assigned to the patient's disease presentation. Unfortunately clinical stage is often in-adequate for determining therapy, since disease activity in the abdomen remains uncertain. Not only can the lymphogram be falsely positive or negative, but the spleen can be the only site of infradiaphragmatic disease in 8% to 14% of patients. The palpable size of the spleen and indirect methods of size assessment do not necessarily have a correlation with the presence or absence of pathologic involvement.

Invasive procedures that may document extranodal disease and preclude the need for staging laparotomy with splenectomy include percutaneous bone marrow biopsy and laparoscopy. Bone marrow disease may be identified in 5% to 14% of patients presenting with Hodgkin's disease and is most often associated with advanced clinical stage and systemic symptoms. Liver involvement alone without other extranodal disease is uncommon, and clinical assessment of liver disease is notoriously inaccurate (>70% false-positive). Percutaneous liver biopsy is not adequate for pathologic evaluation, whereas laparoscopy with multiple liver biopsies yields results comparable to open biopsy. Laparoscopy does not allow pathologic evaluation of abdominal lymph nodes or spleen, however.

Staging laparotomy includes biopsy of suspicious lymph nodes as well as selected nodes from the major lymph node chains, splenectomy, open liver and bone marrow biopsies, and oophoropexy in selected patients. It should be performed in all patients with CS I or II disease and those with CS IIIA. In those patients with unequivocal CS IIIB or IV, staging laparotomy does not usually add information that would change the therapeutic approach. Staging laparotomy's major advantage is accurate pathologic staging; however, it may also result in a smaller radiation portal to the left upper quadrant, an increased hematologic tolerance to therapy, and more accurate delineation of abdominal masses with metallic clips. In experienced hands the operative complication rate is less than 10% and the mortality less than 0.5%. Postsplenectomy sepsis with encapsulated bacteria (*Streptococcus pneumoniae* and *Haemophilus influenzae*) has been reported in 1% to 3% of patients, usually during or shortly following therapy. Vaccines prior to splenectomy and prophylactic antibiotics in children may be beneficial. In adults with febrile illness, antibiotic therapy should be promptly employed when indicated.

After complete pathologic staging the distribution of patients according to stage is approximately as follows: I = 13%, II = 38%, III = 35%, and IV = 14%. Systemic symptoms are correlated with disease extent, being present in fewer than 10% of patients with stage I disease and in more than 80% with stage IV.

C.P.

Beretta G, Spinelli P, Rilke F, et al: Sequential laparoscopy and laparotomy combined with bone marrow biopsy in staging Hodgkin's disease. Cancer Treat Rep 60:1231–1237, 1976.
Hepatic or bone marrow disease, or both, was documented in 9% of 121 previously untreated patients.
Desforges JF, Rutherford CJ, Piro A: Hodgkin's disease. N Engl J Med 301:1212–1222, 1979.
A good summary of pathology, pathogenesis, and clinical management, with extensive references.
Donaldson SS, Glatstein E, Vosti KL: Bacterial infections in pediatric Hodgkin's disease: Relationship to radiotherapy, chemotherapy, and splenectomy. Cancer 41:1949–1958, 1978.
Report analyzes the experience with bacterial infection in 181 children. Bacteremia-meningitis was found only postsplenectomy (2.5% incidence).
Kaplan HS: Hodgkin's disease: Unfolding concepts concerning its nature, management and prognosis. Cancer 45:2439–2474, 1980.
An excellent summary with extensive references.

Kaplan HS, Dorfman RF, Nelsen TS, Rosenberg SA: Staging laparotomy and splenectomy in Hodgkin's disease: Analysis of indications and patterns of involvement in 285 consecutive, unselected patients. Natl Cancer Inst Monogr 36:291–301, 1973.

A change of stage occurred in 18% of 272 patients who underwent laparotomy and the information obtained at laparotomy influenced treatment decisions in 97 of 272 cases (35%).

Siber GR, Weitzman SA, Aisenberg AC, et al: Impaired antibody response to pneumococcal vaccine after treatment for Hodgkin's disease. N Engl J Med 299:442–448, 1978.

Antibody concentrations were significantly reduced in 53 treated patients when compared to 10 normal controls.

Sweet DL Jr, Kinnealey A, Ultmann JE: Hodgkin's disease: Problems of staging. Cancer 42:957–970, 1978.

A comprehensive discussion.

Vianna NJ: The malignant lymphomas: Epidemiology and related aspects. Pathobiol Annu 7:231–255, 1977.

Article discusses environmental, genetic, and immune factors in Hodgkin's disease.

Young RC, Anderson T, De Vita VT: The treatment of Hodgkin's disease. Curr Probl Cancer 1:1–29, 1977.

Article discusses indications for staging laparotomy.

80. HODGKIN'S DISEASE—TREATMENT

Dramatic improvements have been made in the treatment of Hodgkin's disease during the last 20 years, so that it is now possible to cure as many as 70% of all patients. Radiation therapy offers curative potential in early stage disease, as does combination chemotherapy in advanced disease. Clearly the most critical factors affecting outcome are accurate initial staging combined with careful treatment planning and delivery appropriate to the patients' stage of disease. In addition, since cure is a realistic goal in the majority of patients, the choice of initial therapy must take into account not only its effectiveness in eradicating disease but its acute morbidity and long-term consequences for surviving patients.

Some of the features important to the radiation therapy of Hodgkin's disease include the use of megavoltage beam energies as obtained with linear accelerator or ^{60}Co teletherapy; the ability to encompass large shaped fields; and the ability to achieve tumoricidal doses of 3500 rads per 3.5 weeks to 4400 rads per 4 weeks. The typical radiotherapy fields include the mantle (mediastinal, hilar, cervical, axillary, supraclavicular, and infraclavicular lymph nodes); inverted Y (spleen or splenic pedicle; para-aortic, iliac, and femoral nodes); spade (an inverted Y without irradiation to pelvis or groin); and Waldeyer's ring (including preauricular nodes). Total nodal irradiation (TNI) refers to the mantle and inverted Y fields; subtotal nodal irradiation (STNI) refers to the mantle and spade fields; Waldeyer's ring is treated in addition if high cervical lymph nodes are involved.

The results of radiotherapy in nodal Hodgkin's disease are influenced by such factors as stage, histology, radiation portals, and technique. In general the relapse-free survival at 5 years (the "cure" rate) for radiation therapy alone according to stage is greater than 70% for stage I or IIA receiving STNI, 80% for I or IIB receiving TNI, and 50% to 70% for IIIA receiving TNI. Radiation therapy offers essentially no curative potential for stages IIIB and IV. Typical treatment-related complications may include radiation pneumonitis and/or carditis, hypothyroidism, myelosuppression, Lhermitte's syndrome (transient episodes of electric shock-like discomfort), infertility (if the gonads are not shielded), and arrest of bone growth in children. Recent treatment analyses in stage IIIA have suggested that there may be two prognostic subgroups: those with disease limited to the upper abdomen, involving the spleen, splenic hilum, and celiac and portal nodes (stage III_1A, 94% 5-year survival), and those with para-aortic, iliac, or mesenteric lymph node involvement in addition (stage III_2A, 65% 5-year survival). However, not all groups have confirmed these findings.

In contrast to radiation therapy, combination chemotherapy offers curative potential to patients with stage IIIB and IV disease. The drug program that has yielded the most consistent and reproducible results to date is MOPP: nitrogen mustard, 6 mg/M^2 IV days 1 and 8; vincristine, 1.4 mg/M^2 IV days 1 and 8 (total dose limited to 2 mg per injection); procarbazine 100 mg/M^2 po days 1 to 14; and prednisone 40 mg/M^2 po days 1 to 14 on cycles 1 and 4; 14-day treatment cycle repeated every 28 days for at least 6 cycles. Like radiotherapy, chemotherapy results are also influenced by the technique of treatment administration, and such considerations as optimal drug dose, scheduling, and documentation of pathologic complete remission are important factors in outcome. Approximately 80% of all patients with stage IIIB or IV disease will achieve a complete remission with MOPP chemotherapy. The complete remission rate is adversely affected by the presence of B symptoms or prior chemotherapy exposure, whereas prior irradiation has no adverse effect, and asymptomatic patients have an improved response rate and relapse-free survival. The disease-free survival for complete responders at 5 years is approximately 50% to 65%, and thus the "cure" rate is 40% to 50% overall. Some of the toxicities of MOPP therapy include nausea, vomiting, myelosuppression, neuropathy, effects of corticosteroids, and infertility.

At present there is little experience with MOPP alone in early stage Hodgkin's disease. However, MOPP has been added to radiation therapy in an attempt to improve the benefits of radiotherapy alone in nodal disease. Unfortunately the results to date remain inconclusive: radiation therapy plus MOPP yields significantly better relapse-free survival than radiotherapy alone but no significant survival benefit as yet. The reason for this discrepancy between relapse-free survival and survival appears to rest with the ability to "salvage" and "cure" patients who relapse following radiation therapy alone. Thus the survival results for both groups remain comparable. Similarly, radiation therapy to lymph nodes and areas of bulk disease has been added to combination chemotherapy in the treatment of advanced Hodgkin's disease. Again, the combined modality survival results do not yet appear significantly better than those achievable with chemotherapy alone. In addition, the toxicities of combined modality therapy include not only the additive side-effects of irradiation and chemotherapy but the apparent increased risk of second malignancies, particularly acute myelogenous leukemia.

C.P.

Canellos GP, Arseneau JC, De Vita VT, et al: Second malignancies complicating Hodgkin's disease in remission. Lancet 1:947–949, 1975.
  Of 452 patients with Hodgkin's disease 16 developed second tumors.
Coleman CN, Williams CJ, Flint A, et al: Hematologic neoplasia in patients treated for Hodgkin's disease. N Engl J Med 297:1249–1252, 1977.
  Of 680 patients, 9 developed acute nonlymphocytic leukemia—an actuarial

risk of 2.0% at 7 years; for those who received combined modality therapy (330 patients), the risk was 3.9% at 7 years.

Coltman CA Jr (Ed):   Hodgkin's disease. Semin Oncol 7:91, 1980.
An entire journal issue devoted to Hodgkin's disease. It includes reviews of epidemiology, pathology, immune deficits, all aspects of clinical management, and treatment complications.

De Vita VT Jr, Lewis BJ, Rozencweig M, Muggia FM: The chemotherapy of Hodgkin's disease: Past experiences and future directions. Cancer 42:979–990, 1978.
An excellent summary with complete references.

Hellman S, Mauch P, Goodman RL, et al: The place of radiation therapy in the treatment of Hodgkin's disease. Cancer 42:971–978, 1978.
A retrospective analysis of 216 patients with Hodgkin's disease.

Hoppe RT, Cox RS, Rosenberg SA, Kaplan HS: Prognostic factors in pathologic stage (PS) IIIA Hodgkin's disease (HD). Proc Am Soc Clin Oncol (Abstract) 20:429, 1979.
No differences in freedom from relapse according to anatomical substage were noted in 172 patients.

Krikorian JG, Burke JS, Rosenberg SA, Kaplan HS: Occurrence of non-Hodgkin's lymphoma after therapy for Hodgkin's disease. N Engl J Med 300:452–458, 1979.
Article gives a report of 6 cases of non-Hodgkin's lymphoma after therapy for Hodgkin's disease.

Portlock CS, Rosenberg SA, Glatstein E, Kaplan HS: Impact of salvage treatment on initial relapses in patients with Hodgkin's disease, stages I-III. Blood 51:825–833, 1978.
Article retrospectively analyzes 64 patients who had initial relapses.

Prosnitz LR, Farber LR, Fischer JJ, et al: Long term remissions with combined modality therapy for advanced Hodgkin's disease. Cancer 37:2826–2833, 1976.
Using combination chemotherapy plus low-dose irradiation, complete remissions were achieved in 60 of 80 patients; 5 have relapsed.

Rosenberg SA, Kaplan HS, Glatstein EJ, Portlock CS: Combined modality therapy of Hodgkin's disease: A report on the Stanford trials. Cancer 42:991–1000, 1978.
Prospective clinical trials in 244 patients compared radiotherapy alone with radiotherapy plus adjuvant MOPP for stages I, II, and III.

Stein RS, Golomb HM, Diggs CH, et al: Anatomic substages of stage III-A Hodgkin's disease: A collaborative study. Ann Intern Med 92:159–165, 1980.
A retrospective study of 130 patients: Relapse-free survival (74% vs. 46% at 5 years) and survival (94% vs. 65% at 5 years) were significantly better for stage III_1-A than for stage III_2-A.

Young RC, Canellos GP, Chabner BA, et al: Patterns of relapse in advanced Hodgkin's disease treated with combination chemotherapy. Cancer 42:1001–1007, 1978.
In an analysis of 52 patients relapse occurred at sites of prior disease, particularly lymph nodes (75%).

81. NON-HODGKIN'S LYMPHOMAS—"INDOLENT" HISTOLOGIES

The "indolent" non-Hodgkin's lymphomas are composed of four histopathologic subgroups—well-differentiated lymphocytic lymphomas of the nodular

(NLWD) or diffuse (DLWD) type, nodular poorly differentiated lymphocytic lymphoma (NLPD), and nodular mixed lymphocytic and histiocytic lymphoma (NML)—that compose approximately half of all non-Hodgkin's lymphomas. The median age at diagnosis is approximately 55 years; the sex ratio is 1:1. Slowly progressive lymphadenopathy is the typical presenting complaint. Other less common symptoms or signs may include lymphedema, hepatosplenomegaly, ascites, pleural effusions, peripheral nerve or epidural cord compression, and infiltration of skin or other extranodal sites. Systemic symptoms are present in 10% to 20% of patients and have a correlation with extent of disease.

The diagnosis is usually made by peripheral lymph node biopsy. Both tumor architecture and cytology must be adequately assessed. Immunofluorescence studies may document the B-cell origin of these indolent histologies. Laboratory evaluation includes blood counts, Coomb's test if anemia is present, serum protein electrophoresis, liver and renal function tests, chest x-ray, lymphogram, and intravenous pyelogram. Evidence of clinical stage III disease will be found in 50% to 75% of patients. Pathologic stage IV disease is most readily documented with percutaneous bone marrow biopsy: positive in 50% to 80% of cases of NLPD, 30% to 50% of NML, and more than 95% of DLWD. Liver involvement is also common; however, simultaneous bone marrow disease is often present, obviating the need for percutaneous or directed liver biopsy. Staging laparotomy with splenectomy is not an established procedure as it is in Hodgkin's disease. When it has been performed in clinical stage I and II patients with negative lymphograms and negative percutaneous bone marrow biopsies, mesenteric lymph node or splenic disease has been documented in up to 50% of cases.

Fewer than 10% of patients have stage I or II disease following complete pathologic staging. Radiation therapy (3000–4000 rads) to the involved regions is usually adequate treatment. There appears to be no significant improvement in relapse-free or survival results when extended field or total lymphoid irradiation is delivered. In one study relapse-free survival was 80% at 5 years following either involved field or total lymphoid treatment.

The incidence of pathologic stage III disease varies according to histology (NLPD, 10% to 30%; NML, 25% to 30%; DLWD, none). Total lymphoid irradiation has not been shown to be curative. Relapse-free survival was 43% at 5 years and 33% at 10 years in a retrospective study of 51 patients with nodular lymphoma. Consequently patients with stage III or IV disease most often receive similar systemic therapies. Commonly utilized approaches include single agent or combination chemotherapy, whole body irradiation, and combined chemotherapy and irradiation programs.

Objective response rates of at least 20% to 60% are reported for the alkylating agents, vinca alkaloids, corticosteroids, Adriamycin, bleomycin, nitrosoureas, procarbazine, and methotrexate. When tested prospectively in one study, single alkylating agent therapy was not significantly different from combination chemotherapy or a combined modality approach in terms of complete remission rate (65% to 83%), relapse-free survival (60% at 3 years), and survival (>80% at 5 years). On the other hand, results from the National Cancer Institute suggest that C-MOPP (cyclophosphamide, vincristine, procarbazine, and prednisone) may provide superior relapse-free survival in patients with NML (79% at 5 years).

Neither whole body irradiation nor combined chemotherapy and irradiation regimens have proved significantly better than chemotherapy alone. Complete response rates of 60% to 80% with a 2-year median relapse-free survival are reported with whole body irradiation.

Since most, if not all, treatment approaches are palliative rather than curative with stage III or IV disease, it is controversial whether initial therapy is required if patients are asymptomatic at presentation. A retrospective analysis of 44 such patients demonstrated that treatment could be deferred for a median of 3 years and that the overall median survival was 10 years in these selected patients.

Factors that may influence the choice of therapy for patients with stage III or IV disease include the anticipated benefits of treatment; whether the disease is symptomatic; sites and pace of disease; histopathology; potential acute and chronic morbidities of therapy; and the patient's age, general health, and psychological makeup. Whenever systemic treatment is initiated, the intent should be pathologically documented complete remission. Unnecessary continuous treatment should be avoided, if possible.

C.P.

Anderson T, Bender RA, Fisher RI, et al: Combination chemotherapy in non-Hodgkin's lymphoma: Results of long-term follow-up. Cancer Treat Rep 61:1057–1066, 1977.
The results of C-MOPP chemotherapy in nodular mixed lymphoma are discussed.

Carabell SC, Chaffey JT, Rosenthal DS, et al: Results of total body irradiation in the treatment of advanced non-Hodgkin's lymphomas. Cancer 43:994–1000, 1979.
In an analysis of 43 patients with nodular lymphoma and 15 with diffuse lymphoma the median relapse-free survival was 21 months.

Glatstein E, Donaldson SS, Rosenberg SA, Kaplan HS: The potential for combined modality therapy in malignant lymphomas. Cancer Treat Rep 61:1199–1207, 1977.
Article presents the Stanford clinical trials testing the benefits of combined modality therapy in non-Hodgkin's lymphomas.

Glatstein E, Fuks Z, Goffinet DR, Kaplan HS: Non-Hodgkin's lymphomas of Stage III extent: Is total lymphoid irradiation appropriate treatment? Cancer 37:2806–2812, 1976.
A retrospective analysis of total lymphoid irradiation in 51 patients with stage III non-Hodgkin's lymphoma.

Goffinet DR, Warnke R, Dunnick NR, et al: Clinical and surgical (laparotomy) evaluation of patients with non-Hodgkin's lymphomas. Cancer Treat Rep 61:981–992, 1977.
The pathological staging results in 423 patients are presented here.

Golomb H (Ed):   Non-Hodgkin lymphomas. Semin Oncol 7 (3): 1980.
An entire journal issue devoted to the non-Hodgkin's lymphomas with reviews of etiology, pathology, and all aspects of clinical management.

Jaffe ES, Braylan RC, Nanba K, et al: Functional markers: A new perspective on malignant lymphomas. Cancer Treat Rep 61:953–962, 1977.
B and T cell typing studies are discussed.

Portlock CS, Rosenberg SA: Chemotherapy of the non-Hodgkin's lymphomas: The Stanford experience. Cancer Treat Rep 61:1049–1055, 1977.
The results of a prospective trial comparing single alkylating agent therapy, combination chemotherapy, and combined modality therapy in patients with stage IV favorable histologies are presented.

Portlock CS, Rosenberg SA: No initial therapy for stage III and IV non-Hodgkin's lymphomas of favorable histologic types. Ann Intern Med 90:10–13, 1979.
Article provides a retrospective study of 44 patients with stage III or IV non-Hodgkin's lymphoma.

There are four "aggressive" histologic subtypes of non-Hodgkin's lymphomas—histiocytic lymphomas with nodular (NHL) or diffuse (DHL) architecture, diffuse poorly differentiated lymphocytic lymphoma (DLPD), and diffuse mixed lymphocytic and histiocytic lymphoma (DML). DHL is the most common subtype, representing almost 30% of all non-Hodgkin's lymphomas, whereas DLPD (15%), NHL (<5%), and DML (<5%) are infrequent. The median age at diagnosis is 50 to 60 years, and the sex distribution has a slight male preponderance. Patients usually present with rapidly progressive, occasionally tender, lymphadenopathy. The lymph nodes may be matted and fixed to the underlying tissues and skin. Retroperitoneal and/or mesenteric adenopathy may be so enlarged that an abdominal mass is appreciated. Lower extremity lymphedema is often present. Lymphatic obstruction of the upper extremities, superior vena cava syndrome, and/or tracheal compression may be seen occasionally. Extranodal disease is frequently symptomatic, involving such sites as liver, lung, skin, pleura, peritoneum, bone, and gastrointestinal tract. Sometimes there is peripheral nerve or epidural cord compression from large lymph node masses. Meningeal lymphoma may be documented infrequently at presentation, whereas it is an increasingly common finding at relapse or autopsy. Systemic symptoms are present in 10% to 20% at diagnosis and correlate with extent of disease.

Staging studies that may be useful include blood counts, Coomb's test if there is anemia, serum protein electrophoresis, liver and renal function tests, chest x-ray, lymphogram, and intravenous pyelogram. Radionuclide scans and x-ray studies of extranodal sites such as bone and gastrointestinal tract may be helpful in selected patients. Following clinical staging, approximately 15% of patients will be stage I, 30% stage II, 30% stage III, and 25% stage IV. Percutaneous bone marrow biopsy may be positive in up to 30% of patients, particularly those with DLPD or with clinical stage III or IV disease. With a normal lymphogram and negative bone marrow biopsy (clinical stage I or II), liver disease is documented in fewer than 5% and mesenteric lymph node or splenic involvement in fewer than 10%. Consequently percutaneous or directed liver biopsy as well as staging laparotomy with splenectomy add little additional information in this setting. Complete pathologic staging reveals that almost half of all patients with aggressive histologies have stage I or II disease.

Although DHL is considered an "unfavorable" histology, with aggressive radiation and chemotherapy programs cure may be a realistic goal. With pathologic stage (PS) I disease, radiation therapy is the treatment of choice. Relapse-free survival is reported to be more than 65% at 5 years. It remains unsettled, however, whether extended field or total lymphoid irradiation is superior to involved field treatment. Extranodal PS I_E presentations have a similar outcome with irradiation alone. Therefore it is important to rule out lymph node or other extranodal disease that would change both stage and therapy. Extended field or total lymphoid irradiation results for PS II DHL are less favorable and vary more widely (25% to 50% relapse-free at 5 years). Sites of disease, tumor bulk, and number of involved regions appear to be important prognostic variables. Adjuvant chemotherapy does not appear to improve significantly the results obtained with radiation therapy alone. On the other hand, Miller and Jones have recently reported excellent results with combination chemotherapy alone (100% complete response with only one relapse in 14 patients) in localized histiocytic lymphoma.

In stages III and IV DHL, the curative potential of combination chemotherapy has been dramatically demonstrated. Complete response (CR) rates of 40%

to 93% have been reported; and following pathologically documented CR, relapse is uncommon and usually occurs within the first 2 years after discontinuance of all treatment. The drug regimens with the most consistent CR rates (40% to 50%) and best relapse-free survivals (virtually 100%) are MOPP or C-MOPP (nitrogen mustard or cyclophosphamide, vincristine, procarbazine, and prednisone) and BACOP (bleomycin, Adriamycin, cyclophosphamide, vincristine, and prednisone). Variables that adversely affect rates of response include extranodal involvement, tumor bulk, and prior therapy. Histopathologically identifiable prognostic subgroups of DHL have recently been reported by Strauchen et al. [1978]. Combined modality approaches have not yielded superior results to chemotherapy alone. Lymphomatous meningitis has been reported in 25% to 30% of relapsing patients wth DHL or diffuse undifferentiated lymphoma following combination chemotherapy, and it is closely correlated with bone marrow involvement. Whether central nervous system prophylaxis can prevent this complication is yet to be tested prospectively.

There are few data available on the treatment of NHL and DML. In general their management is similar to DHL. Results in NHL appear comparable or perhaps superior to DHL, while those for DML are poor. Until recently, the histologic subtype DLPD has included lymphoblastic lymphoma (LL). Although often localized at diagnosis, LL should be treated systemically and in a like manner to acute lymphoblastic leukemia.

C.P.

Bitran JD, Kinzie J, Sweet DL, et al: Survival of patients with localized histiocytic lymphoma. Cancer 39:342–346, 1977.
Relapse-free survival at 5 years was 78% in 20 pathologically staged I and II patients receiving radiation therapy alone.

Bunn PA, Schein PS, Banks PM, DeVita VT: Central nervous system complications in patients with diffuse histiocytic and undifferentiated lymphoma: Leukemia revisited. Blood 47:3–10, 1976.
Occurrence of lymphomatous meningitis at relapse is described.

Fisher RI, DeVita VT, Johnson BL, et al: Prognostic factors for advanced diffuse histiocytic lymphoma following treatment with combination chemotherapy. Am J Med 63:177–182, 1977.
Article analyzes MOPP, C-MOPP, and BACOP chemotherapy programs.

Miller TP, Jones SE: Chemotherapy of localized histiocytic lymphoma. Lancet 1:358–360, 1979.
Reports the use of combination chemotherapy alone in patients with stage I and II diffuse histiocytic lymphoma.

Osborne CK, Merrill JM, Garvin AJ, et al: Nodular histiocytic lymphoma. An aggressive nodular lymphoma with potential for long-term survival. Proc Am Soc Clin Oncol (Abstract) 20:442, 1979.
Article provides a retrospective study of 16 patients with nodular histiocytic lymphoma.

Rosen PJ, Feinstein DI, Pattengale PK, et al: Convoluted lymphocytic lymphoma in adults: A clinicopathologic entity. Ann Intern Med 89:319–324, 1978.
Article gives a clinicopathologic description of 12 adults with lymphoblastic lymphoma.

Strauchen JA, Young RC, DeVita VT Jr, et al: Clinical relevance of the histopathological subclassification of diffuse "histiocytic" lymphoma. N Engl J Med 299:1382–1387, 1978.
The prognostic significance of DHL subtypes is analyzed.

Weinstein HJ, Vance ZB, Jaffe N, et al: Improved prognosis for patients with
mediastinal lymphoblastic lymphoma. Blood 53:687–694, 1979.
Treatment of 12 patients with this type of lymphoma is described.

Young RC, Howser DM, Anderson T, et al: Central nervous system complications of non-Hodgkin's lymphoma—the potential role for prophylactic therapy. Am J Med 66:435–442, 1979.
*In a retrospective study of 38 patients with lymphomatous meningitis aggres-
sive histologies and bone marrow or bone involvement correlated with its
development.*

83. ACUTE LYMPHOCYTIC LEUKEMIA

Acute lymphocytic leukemia (ALL) is the major neoplastic disease of childhood,
whereas it is an unusual form of leukemia in adults. Because of its infrequent
occurrence, the approach to diagnosis and management of adult ALL has been
taken almost exclusively from the successful experience in children.

The typical patient with ALL presents with symptoms of weakness, infection,
lymphadenopathy, bleeding, and/or anemia. On physical examination there
may be pallor and other signs of anemia, ecchymoses, lymphadenopathy and
hepatosplenomegaly. There is usually an elevated white blood cell count with
lymphocytosis, consisting of a uniform population of immature cells with scant,
pale blue, agranular cytoplasm and well-defined nuclei but indistinct chromatin and nucleoli. In addition, other laboratory abnormalities may include anemia,
thrombocytopenia, and hyperuricemia. Disorders that result in a lymphocytosis
and/or bone marrow failure should be considered in the differential diagnosis,
such as infectious mononucleosis, toxoplasmosis, cytomegalovirus or other
virus infection, tuberculosis, aplastic anemia, and tumor infiltration of the bone
marrow. The diagnosis is established by examination of the peripheral blood
and bone marrow cytology. At least 30% of the marrow cells should be leukemic, and in some instances the bone marrow is so replaced that biopsy rather
than aspirate is required to obtain adequate sampling.

Histochemically lymphoblasts are peroxidase-negative, periodic acid–
Schiff–positive, and Sudan red– or black–negative. By immunologic techniques
approximately 10% of adults will have T-cell leukemia, while the remainder
will be null-cell. B-cell disease is rarely seen and may indicate Burkitt's lymphoma or other forms of lymphosarcoma cell leukemia. Terminal deoxynucleotidyl transferase is present in both T-cell and null-cell ALL. The Philadelphia chromosome (Ph[1]) can be detected in up to 10% of patients with adult ALL,
and this chromosomal abnormality may represent the blastic phase of chronic
myelogenous leukemia rather than ALL.

Several prognostic factors have been identified in childhood ALL and most
are applicable to the adult disease, including kind of therapy, disease extent (a
white blood cell count of $>100,000/mm^3$; presence of lymphadenopathy and
hepatosplenomegaly), meningeal involvement, mediastinal enlargement, age
(patients <2 and >10 years), and race (black children). In addition, T-cell ALL
and Ph[1](+) ALL are associated with a poorer prognosis.

Chemotherapy is highly effective in the treatment of childhood ALL,
whereas the response rate, remission duration, and survival are substantially
lower in adults. The four most active single agents are prednisone, vincristine,
daunorubicin, and L-asparaginase, each achieving transient complete remissions in 25% to 50% of adult patients. When prednisone and vincristine are used

in combination with one or both of the other drugs, the complete response rate approaches 75% in adults and more than 90% in children. Remission induction usually occurs within 4 weeks, with normalization of the peripheral blood, bone marrow, and other evident systemic disease. Without the subsequent use of maintenance therapy, however, the bulk of patients will relapse. Standard continuation treatment consists of 6-mercaptopurine and methotrexate administered for at least 2.5 to 3 years following complete remission. The addition of other drugs to this maintenance regimen has not improved remission duration but has led to increased toxicity. Whether intermittent, intensive "consolidation" therapy adds to the benefits of standard maintenance is yet to be established.

In spite of effective systemic drug administration, the central nervous system (CNS) remains a "privileged" site for the proliferation of leukemic cells, presumably secondary to poor drug penetration. Therefore without prophylactic CNS treatment following remission induction, approximately 50% of children will develop meningeal disease, whereas this development is unusual with prophylaxis. CNS prophylaxis is equally important in the adult and is similarly administered: 2400 rads is given to the whole brain plus 5 doses of intrathecal methotrexate. At the time of the diagnosis, meningeal disease is documented in only 1% of children and up to 10% of adults. In addition to age, disease extent (WBC > 100,000/mm^3, hepatosplenomegaly, and lymphadenopathy) has a correlation with initial CNS involvement. All patients should receive careful cerebrospinal fluid examinations at presentation, comparing the CSF and bone marrow cytologies. Pleocytosis may be seen at diagnosis without demonstrable ALL. Unlike CNS prophylaxis, overt meningeal leukemia requires continued intrathecal therapy to prevent subsequent relapse.

Like the CNS, another privileged site is the testicle. It has recently been reported that testicular relapse may occur prior to or concurrent with initial bone marrow relapse. In one study, testicular relapse was documented in 5% of male patients. Since testicular relapse remains an unusual occurrence, prophylactic therapy is not yet recommended. However, testicular biopsy before maintenance therapy is discontinued is advocated by many.

Following successful induction therapy and CNS prophylaxis, approximately 50% of children will develop recurrent ALL during maintenance treatment, while another 10% will relapse after all drugs are discontinued. Therefore approximately 40% of all children with ALL appear to be cured by these treatment approaches. In contrast, among adults there are few long-term survivors, and the median disease-free interval is 11 to 25 months.

C.P.

Brouet JC, Seligmann M: The immunological classification of acute lymphoblastic leukemias. Cancer 42:817–827, 1978.
   Summarizes B and T cell marker studies and correlates immunologic markers with clinical features and prognosis.
Dow LW, Borella L, Sen L, et al: Initial prognostic factors and lymphoblast-erythrocyte rosette formation in 109 children with acute lymphoblastic leukemia. Blood 50:671–682, 1977.
   T-cell derived ALL was associated with a significantly higher frequency of relapse and central nervous system involvement at relapse.
Frei E III, Sallan SE: Acute lymphoblastic leukemia: Treatment. Cancer 42:828–838, 1978.
   A good review of current management strategy.
Gee TS, Haghbin M, Dowling MD Jr, et al: Acute lymphoblastic leukemia in

adults and children: Differences in response with similar therapeutic regimens. Cancer 37:1256–1264, 1976.

Response rate (78% in adults, 98% in children), median remission duration (25 months in adults, 54 months in children), and survival (at 3 years, 45% in adults, 75% in children) were found to be poorer in adults.

George SL, Aur RJA, Mauer AM, Simone JV: A reappraisal of the results of stopping therapy in childhood leukemia. N Engl J Med 300:269–273, 1979.

In this retrospective analysis of 639 patients approximately 20% had relapses after discontinuing maintenance; no relapses occurred after 4 years off all therapy.

Mauer AM, Simone JV: The current status of the treatment of childhood acute lymphoblastic leukemia. Cancer Treat Rev 3:17–41, 1976.

An excellent summary of the St. Jude's Hospital experience.

Nesbit ME Jr, Robison LL, Ortega JA, et al: Testicular relapse in childhood acute lymphoblastic leukemia: Association with pretreatment patient characteristics and treatment—A report for Children's Cancer Study Group. Cancer 45:2009–2016, 1980.

A retrospective analysis of 395 male patients. Testicular involvement was detected in 5% prior to or at time of bone marrow relapse.

Pinkel D: Treatment of acute lymphocytic leukemia. Cancer 43:1128–1137, 1979.

The ninth annual David Karnofsky Lecture summarizing the St. Jude Children's Research Hospital clinical trials.

Woodruff R: The management of adult acute lymphoblastic leukaemia. Cancer Treat Rev 5:95–113, 1978.

An excellent discussion.

84. CHRONIC LYMPHOCYTIC LEUKEMIA

Chronic lymphocytic leukemia (CLL) accounts for approximately one-quarter of all leukemias. The disorder is characterized by a persistent and progressive accumulation of monoclonal B-lymphocytes with defective immunoglobulin secretory function. It is a disease diagnosed in older adults (80% to 90% of patients are more than 50 years of age), with twice as many males as females affected. Examination of the peripheral blood reveals a lymphocytosis in excess of 5000 cells/mm³, and up to 25% of cases are incidentally diagnosed on routine blood count. Symptoms of the disease are usually minimal at presentation. However, fatigue, decreased exercise tolerance, complaints referable to bone marrow failure, sweating and weight loss, and symptomatic adenopathy and/or splenomegaly may be present. The physical examination may be entirely normal or reveal generalized lymphadenopathy with or without splenomegaly or hepatomegaly.

Laboratory studies that aid in diagnosis and evaluation of disease extent include: blood counts and examination of peripheral smear, to document a lymphocytosis with small, mature-appearing lymphocytes; bone marrow aspirate and biopsy to confirm the presence of an abnormal, diffuse lymphoid infiltrate and to identify its extent (usually >40% of marrow cells); Coomb's test, which may be positive and may be associated with an autoimmune hemolytic anemia; serum protein electrophoresis, which may reveal hypogammaglobulinemia; chest x-ray; intravenous pyelogram with or without lymphogram to assess ureteral compromise and extent of retroperitoneal adenopathy; and liver-spleen scan to document spleen size.

Diseases that may be confused with CLL include acute lymphoblastic leukemia, lymphosarcoma cell leukemia, hairy cell leukemia, and Waldenström's macroglobulinemia. In addition, lymphocytic leukemoid reactions may occur with tuberculosis and carcinomas of the breast or stomach.

The cells of CLL have membrane-bound immunoglobulin, which is restricted to one heavy chain class and a single light chain type in any given patient. This observation has led to the hypothesis that a single B-cell clone is responsible for the disease process. The kinetics of CLL demonstrate both increased production and delayed destruction of these abnormal cells, which leads to their exponential accumulation. The doubling time of CLL is estimated to be 4 to 19 months, with approximately 15 times the normal number of lymphocytes produced daily. The total daily production of lymphocytes in CLL is composed of short-lived cells with normal life span, increased 25-fold in number, and long-lived cells with abnormally long survival (5 times normal), increased 10-fold in number. In addition, there appears to be a disturbance in the normal exchange of lymphocytes between the intravascular and extravascular pools, resulting in tissue accumulation of these cells.

Although CLL cells are B-cell–derived, they have disturbed membrane dynamics and virtually absent immunoglobulin secretion. As a result, with compromise of the normal number of B- and T-cells, hypogammaglobulinemia becomes manifest and infection is the major cause of morbidity and mortality. Pneumococcal and staphylococcal infections are especially common, since they require antibody for clearance. Infections with gram-negative organisms, fungus, and herpes zoster are also frequently seen.

The prognosis for patients with CLL is good, with an overall median survival of more than 6 years. Using a clinical staging system such as that introduced by Rai et al. [1975], favorable and unfavorable prognostic groups can be identified according to disease extent. Patients with lymphocytosis with or without adenopathy have a median survival of more than 100 months, whereas those with hematologic compromise (anemia with hemoglobin <11 gm/100 ml and/or thrombocytopenia with platelets $<100,000$ cells/mm^3) have a median survival of only 19 months. Unfortunately few treatment results have been reported according to such a clinical staging system, making interpretation of data more difficult.

Although CLL is a highly responsive malignancy, there is no known curative treatment, and it is uncertain whether therapy prolongs survival. Therefore the goal of therapy is to palliate the signs and symptoms of the disease. Methods of systemic palliation include alkylating agent chemotherapy with chlorambucil or cyclophosphamide administered on a daily or intermittent schedule, whole body irradiation, thymic irradiation, the use of corticosteroids (usually daily or intermittent prednisone), leukapheresis, and extracorporeal irradiation of blood. The most effective therapies appear to be the first three, with similar objective response rates (approximately 50% clinical complete remissions), and remission durations (12 to 24 months). Radiation therapy may also be delivered to areas of bulky adenopathy or for splenomegaly. Splenectomy is reserved for those patients with hypersplenism and hematologic compromise, autoimmune hemolytic anemia, and/or painful splenomegaly.

C.P.

Binet JL, Leporrier M, Dighiero G, et al: A clinical staging system for chronic lymphocytic leukemia: Prognostic significance. Cancer 40:855–864, 1977.
   A retrospective analysis of 129 patients, suggesting a 5-stage clinical classification schema.
Brouet J-C, Seligmann M: Chronic lymphocytic leukaemia as an immunoproliferative disorder. Clin Haematol 6:169–184, 1977.
   This article discusses the monoclonal nature of CLL.

Huguley CM, Jr: Treatment of chronic lymphocytic leukemia. Cancer Treat
    Rev 4:261–273, 1977.
    A comprehensive review.
Johnson RE: Total body irradiation of chronic lymphocytic leukemia: Re-
    lationship between therapeutic response and prognosis. Cancer 37:2691–
    2696, 1976.
    *This article provides a retrospective analysis of 48 patients undergoing total
    body irradiation.*
Rai KR, Sawitsky A, Cronkite EP, et al: Clinical staging of chronic lympho-
    cytic leukemia. Blood 46:219–234, 1975.
    This article reports a staging system with prognostic utility.
Richards F II, Spurr CL, Ferree C, et al: The control of chronic lymphocytic
    leukemia with mediastinal irradiation. Am J Med 64:947–954, 1978.
    *In this report of 40 patients 15 of 27 previously untreated patients achieved
    clinical complete remissions.*
Rundles RW, Moore JO: Chronic lymphocytic leukemia. Cancer 42:941–945,
    1978.
    An excellent clinical discussion.
Sawitsky A, Rai KR, Glidewell O, Silver RT, participating members of CALGB:
    Comparison of daily versus intermittent chlorambucil and prednisone ther-
    apy in the treatment of patients with chronic lymphocytic leukemia. Blood
    50:1049–1059, 1977.
    *This article is a randomized study of 96 patients who could be evaluated with
    Rai stage III or IV disease.*
Theml H, Love R, Begemann H: Factors in the pathomechanism of chronic
    lymphocytic leukemia. Annu Rev Med 28:131–141, 1977.
    An excellent discussion.

85. ACUTE NONLYMPHOCYTIC LEUKEMIA

Acute nonlymphocytic leukemia (ANLL) is composed of several subtypes, including the myeloblastic, promyelocytic, myelocytic, myelomonocytic, monocy-
tic, and erythroleukemia variants. The most common form (>60% of cases) is
acute myelocytic leukemia. ANLL is not a common disease; it has an overall
incidence of approximately 2.5 per 100,000. There is no specific age peak, although it is less common in childhood; and there is a slight male preponderance. In most cases the etiology is unknown; however, radiation and/or chemical exposure as well as genetic or congenital factors are well-recognized causes.
A viral etiology has been hypothesized in humans but not yet established.

The clinical manifestations of ANLL are related to symptoms and signs of
bone marrow failure with anemia, thrombocytopenia, and granulocytopenia.
Besides bone marrow infiltration, there may be leukemic involvement of lymph
nodes, liver, spleen, skin, gingiva, and other organs. Bone and articular tenderness are also common. Meningeal or central nervous system mass lesions are
rare at diagnosis.

The diagnosis of ANLL rests upon the cytologic and histochemical characteristics of the leukemic marrow infiltrate. Generally the abnormal cells consti-
tute at least 50% of the nucleated cell population: they are large, with fine
nuclear chromatin and prominent nucleoli, grayish blue cytoplasm, a low
nuclear-cytoplasmic ratio, and Auer rods (in approximately 50% of cases). Histochemically, the myeloblasts are myeloperoxidase-positive, Sudan black B–
positive, and periodic acid–Schiff–negative. The peripheral white blood cell

count is usually elevated, although only one-fifth of patients have more than 100,000 cells/mm³ and one-quarter have fewer than 5000 cells/mm³. In most cases more than 75% of the circulating white cells are leukemic. A karyotype of the leukemic cells may reveal a chromosomal abnormality in 30% to 50% of patients and is constant for a given patient at diagnosis and relapse; however, unlike chronic myelogenous leukemia, the chromosomal abnormality is apparently random from patient to patient. An abnormal karyotype confers a poorer prognosis (a complete response rate of 25% and a median survival of 2.5 months) than a normal one (85% complete response, 18-month median survival). Bone marrow culture reveals a change from the normal growth pattern, with either excessive numbers of abnormal colonies or no colony formation at all. Following induction of complete remission, colony growth becomes normal; and with relapse, abnormal colony characteristics re-emerge.

Besides its use in following ANLL disease activity, bone marrow culture may aid in the diagnosis of preleukemia ("smouldering" leukemia). This disorder is found in older adults who are usually clinically well but have findings of mild bone marrow failure. Bone marrow examination reveals myeloblasts that make up fewer than 30% of the nucleated cells, and marrow culture most often yields normal colony formation. Unlike ANLL, it is unnecessary upon diagnosis to treat preleukemic patients aggressively, since their disease may remain stable for up to 2 years and sometimes longer before evolving into ANLL.

Other laboratory studies that may be useful in management of ANLL include coagulation parameters (particularly in promyelocytic leukemia, in which disseminated intravascular coagulation is a common complication); uric acid (allopurinol is routinely administered to prevent excess urate production); serum and/or urinary muramidase; liver and renal function tests; and routine x-rays and cultures to assess infection status.

The goal of treatment for ANLL is rapid induction of complete remission with return of normal blood and bone marrow function. Active single agents include the anthracyclines (daunomycin, Adriamycin), cytosine arabinoside, 6-thioguanine, hydroxyurea, methotrexate, and cyclophosphamide. Drug combinations that include both cytosine arabinoside and one of the anthracyclines have yielded complete response rates of 60% to 85% and median remission durations of at least 6 to more than 15 months. Moreover it has been reported recently that as many as one-third of complete responders may be long-term disease-free survivors. Factors that may influence prognosis include age, performance status, degree of bone marrow infiltration, abnormal cytogenetics, the presence of infection at onset of treatment, and prior therapy. Remission induction is often life-threatening, and the majority of patients who fail to achieve complete remission die of infectious and/or bleeding complications. Prophylactic antibiotics, the use of laminar airflow rooms, surveillance culture techniques, prompt and effective broad-spectrum antibiotic coverage, granulocyte transfusion, and awareness of fungal superinfection have served to reduce the infection hazard. Bleeding complications have been reduced with the use of donor-matched platelet transfusions and prompt treatment of central nervous system leukostasis. Although still controversial, prophylactic heparin during therapy of promyelocytic leukemia may decrease the risk of uncontrolled DIC.

Whether maintenance chemotherapy is of benefit following complete remission induction remains unsettled. Response to relapse therapy appears comparable to initial induction results; however, remission durations are brief. Another approach that has been used with some success is bone marrow transplantation in HLA-matched siblings. In identical twins such therapy is the initial treatment of choice.

C.P.

Arlin ZA, Fried J, Clarkson BD: Therapeutic role of cell kinetics in acute leukaemia. Clin Haematol 7:339 362, 1978.
This article provides a thorough discussion of cytokinetic principles.

Bodey GP, Rodriguez V: Approaches to the treatment of acute leukemia and lymphoma in adults. Semin Hematol 15:221–261, 1978.
An excellent summary.

Drapkin RL, Gee TS, Dowling MD, et al: Prophylactic heparin therapy in acute promyelocytic leukemia. Cancer 41:2484–2490, 1978.
This retrospective analysis suggests the benefit of prophylactic heparin in 9 patients.

Gale RP: Advances in the treatment of acute myelogenous leukemia. N Engl J Med 300:1189–1198, 1979.
This article gives a brief review of treatment advances.

Gallo RC, Meyskens FL Jr: Advances in the viral etiology of leukemia and lymphoma. Semin Hematol 15:379–398, 1978.
A comprehensive presentation of the field of RNA tumor viruses and human leukemia.

Gralnick HR, Galton DAG, Catovsky D, et al: Classification of acute leukemia. Ann Intern Med 87:740–753, 1977.
Morphology, cytochemistry, electron microscopy, surface markers, biochemistry, and cytogenetics of acute leukemia are discussed in this article.

Linman JW, Bagby GC Jr: The preleukemic syndrome (hemopoietic dysplasia). Cancer 42:854–864, 1978.
This article discusses clinical and laboratory features of the preleukemic syndrome as well as management.

Rodriguez V, Bodey GP, Freireich EJ, et al: Randomized trial of protected environment—prophylactic antibiotics in 145 adults with acute leukemia. Medicine 57:253–266, 1978.
Protected environment was associated with a significant reduction in fatal infections (13% vs. 28%) as compared to a conventional hospital room.

Rowley JD: The cytogenetics of acute leukemia. Clin Haematol 7:385–406, 1978.
An excellent summary, reviewing data for both nonlymphocytic and lymphocytic acute leukemias.

Sanders JE, Thomas ED: Bone marrow transplantation for acute leukaemia. Clin Haematol 7:295–311, 1978.
A complete review.

Spitzer G, Verma DS, Dicke KA, McCredie KB: Culture studies in vitro in human leukemia. Semin Hematol 15:352–378, 1978.
This article provides an excellent discussion of bone marrow culture characteristics and their clinical application to therapy.

86. CHRONIC MYELOGENOUS LEUKEMIA

Chronic myelogenous leukemia (CML) accounts for approximately 15% of all leukemias. It affects middle-aged adults (median age of 52 years), with a slight male predominance. Patients usually present with mild symptoms such as decreased energy, fatigue, anorexia, weight loss, dyspnea, pallor, low-grade fever, and night sweats. On physical examination there may be signs of anemia and tachycardia; however, the hallmark finding is splenomegaly, which is present in more than 90% of cases at diagnosis. The spleen may be tender to palpation, and a friction rub can sometimes be appreciated. In addition to splenomegaly, some patients may have hepatomegaly. Lymphadenopathy and bony percussion tenderness are usually limited to patients in blastic crisis. Typical blood findings include a mild anemia (mean hemoglobin of 10 gm/100 ml), thrombocytosis (mean of 500,000/mm³), and leukocytosis (mean of 225,000/mm³; range of 20–600,000/mm³). The peripheral smear demonstrates a complete spectrum of granulocytic forms as well as an absolute basophilia. Confirmatory laboratory studies include a low or absent leukocyte alkaline phosphatase, an elevated serum vitamin B_{12} and B_{12}-binding capacity, and the presence of the Philadelphia (Ph¹) chromosome.

The Philadelphia chromosome is documented in approximately 85% of patients with CML. It is due to a balanced, reciprocal translocation of the distal portion of the long arm of chromosome 22 to the long arm of 9, resulting in no detectable loss of total chromosomal DNA. This genetic abnormality is retained throughout the course of the disease; however, other karyotypic abnormalities may be superimposed, particularly at the onset of blastic crisis. Only 15% of patients will present with Ph¹(−) CML. These patients tend to be older (median age of 60 years as compared to 45 years for Ph¹(+) patients), have a poorer response to standard therapies during the chronic phase, have a more rapid evolution to blastic crisis, and have a shorter survival (a median of 18 months as compared to 40 months for those with Ph¹(+) CML).

CML can be divided into three phases: presentation and/or relapse, remission, and blastic crisis. The average survival of all patients is approximately 4 years, with a range of 1 to 11 years. After 2 to 5 years of waxing and waning disease, virtually all patients will develop blastic crisis characterized by a fever of unknown origin, musculoskeletal pain, malaise, hepatosplenomegaly, and the presence of more than 30% myeloblasts and promyeloblasts in the peripheral blood along with anemia and thrombocytopenia. Blastic crisis may be abrupt in onset or it may be preceded by an accelerated phase of CML lasting from 1 to 18 months. In general, blastic crisis is associated with a grave prognosis and a survival of less than 6 months.

During the chronic phase of CML the goals of therapy are palliative: to decrease symptomatic splenomegaly, improve normal peripheral blood counts, and reduce systemic symptoms. Some 20% of patients are asymptomatic at presentation and may require no specific therapy initially. For the remainder, busulfan is the usual drug of choice, achieving objective responses in 75% of patients. It is administered daily, 4 mg po, and over 3 to 4 months it obtains a gradual decrease in the white blood cell count (WBC) and splenomegaly. Because of the potential hazard of prolonged myelosuppression, busulfan is usually discontinued when the WBC reaches 10,000/mm³ and then reinstituted for maintenance when the count rises above 25,000/mm³. Busulfan's other chronic side effects include hyperpigmentation, pulmonary interstitial fibrosis, and infertility. Other drugs (such as chlorambucil, L-phenylalanine mustard, cyclophosphamide, dibromomannitol, and hydroxyurea) used as single agents or in aggressive combination chemotherapy programs have not yet been demonstrated to be superior to busulfan. Splenectomy during the chronic phase has not been shown to confer a survival advantage, although it may be a useful adjunct for the treatment of painful splenomegaly or thrombocytopenia. Another palliative therapy is leukapheresis, which can effectively decrease leukocytosis and hepatosplenomegaly; however, it has no apparent advantage over more standard approaches.

Approximately 20% of patients with blastic crisis will have immature cells whose morphologic, enzymic, and/or immunologic characteristics are compatible with lymphoblasts. It is this subset of patients who respond to vincristine and prednisone therapy (at least 50% objective response) and have improved survival (median of 6 months as compared to 3 months with no response). Studies that predict whether response will be favorable or unfavorable include lymphoblast morphology, presence of terminal deoxynucleotidyl transferase, and hypodiploid cytogenetics. Aggressive combination chemotherapy programs have also been used in blastic crisis, yielding remission rates of 30% to 40% and median survivals for responders of 8 to 10 months. During blastic crisis, disease complications may include leukostasis, meningeal leukemia, soft tissue and/or bony leukemic infiltrates, and hemorrhage and infection.

C.P.

Canellos GP: The treatment of chronic granulocytic leukaemia. Clin Haematol 6:113–139, 1977.
An excellent review of clinical management of both the chronic and blastic phases.

Cunningham I, Gee T, Dowling M, et al: Results of treatment of Ph¹ + chronic myelogenous leukemia with an intensive treatment regimen (L-5 protocol). Blood 53:375–395, 1979.
Intensive combination chemotherapy and prophylactic splenectomy yielded transient (1 to 43 months) reduction in or disappearance of Ph¹ positive marrow cells in 19 of 37 patients.

Fialkow PJ, Jacobson RJ, Papayannopoulou T: Chronic myelocytic leukemia: Clonal origin in a stem cell common to the granulocyte, erythrocyte, platelet and monocyte/macrophage. Am J Med 63:125–130, 1977.
CML granulocytes were found to have single-enzyme phenotypes in glucose-6-phosphate dehydrogenase heterozygotes.

Goldman JM: Modern approaches to the management of chronic granulocytic leukemia. Semin Hematol 15:420–430, 1978.
Preliminary experiences with combination chemotherapy, splenectomy, and autologous stem cell engraftment are summarized.

Marks SM, Baltimore D, McCaffrey R: Terminal transferase as a predictor of initial responsiveness to vincristine and prednisone in blastic chronic myelogenous leukemia: A co-operative study. N Engl J Med 298:812–814, 1978.
None of 9 patients whose terminal transferase was negative responded, whereas 8 of 13 with a positive study did.

Moore MAS: In vitro culture studies in chronic granulocytic leukaemia. Clin Haematol 6:97–112, 1977.
A clearly written summary of the in vitro findings in untreated and treated chronic myelogenous leukemia.

Rosenthal S, Canellos GP, DeVita VT Jr, Gralnick HR: Characteristics of blast crisis in chronic granulocytic leukemia. Blood 49:705–714, 1977.
Article provides a retrospective analysis of 73 patients with this type of leukemia.

Rosenthal S, Canellos GP, Whang-Peng J, Gralnick HR: Blast crisis of chronic granulocytic leukemia: Morphologic variants and therapeutic implications. Am J Med 63:542–547, 1977.
Lymphoblastic morphology and hypodiploid cytogenetics were favorable prognostic variables.

Rowley JD: Ph¹-positive leukaemia, including chronic myelogenous leukaemia. Clin Haematol 9:55–86, 1980.
An excellent review of Ph¹ and other chromosomal abnormalities in chronic myelogenous leukemia.

Spiers ASD: The clinical features of chronic granulocytic leukaemia. Clin Haematol 6:77–95, 1977.
Excellent, practical review.

Wolf DJ, Silver RT, Coleman M: Splenectomy in chronic myeloid leukemia. Ann Intern Med 89:684–689, 1978.
Article provides a review of clinical trials.

87. MULTIPLE MYELOMA

Multiple myeloma (MM) is a disease characterized by the malignant, monoclonal proliferation of plasma cells that synthesize and secrete immunoglobulin. The M-proteins produced are homogeneous and contain a single type of heavy and/or light chain. The most common form of myeloma is IgG-secreting (52%), followed by IgA (21%), light-chain disease (11%), IgD (2%), and IgE (<0.01%) myeloma. IgM disease, or Waldenström's macroglobulinemia, constitutes 12% of cases of MM and is a distinct clinicopathologic entity. Fewer than 1% of patients may be found to have nonsecretory myeloma.

The median age for all types of MM is 55 to 65, and the disease is rare before age 30. The disease is equally common in males and females except for IgD myeloma, which predominates in men, 3:1. Making the diagnosis of MM is often challenging, since the hallmark of the disease is secretion of monoclonal protein—a "benign" laboratory abnormality that may be present in more than 3% of adults over age 70. Features that may help to distinguish a "benign" monoclonal gammopathy from MM include the amount of serum M-protein (if >2 gm/100 ml, it is more likely to be MM), the presence of Bence Jones proteinuria (usually indicates MM), the absence of a plasma cell bone marrow infiltrate (however, bone marrow involvement with MM may be spotty), and the presence of lytic bone disease (compatible with MM, although it may be seen with metastatic carcinoma). Nevertheless, it may be impossible to differentiate these two entities at first discovery, requiring that such patients be followed indefinitely.

The majority of patients with MM are symptomatic at presentation, however, complaining of bone pain and symptoms of anemia, hypercalcemia, renal insufficiency, and/or infection. Diagnostic studies should include serum protein electrophoresis and quantitative immunoelectrophoresis, urine protein studies (grams of protein per 24 hours, Bence Jones assay, electrophoresis, immunoelectrophoresis), skeletal bone survey to assess lytic lesions, and bone marrow aspirate to document a malignant plasma cell infiltrate. In addition to benign monoclonal gammopathy, other diseases that may be associated with M-proteins include the hematologic malignancies, carcinoma, collagen diseases, chronic infections, and hepatic cirrhosis. Once the diagnosis has been established, other laboratory studies that are helpful include serum calcium, BUN, creatinine, creatinine clearance, uric acid, and complete blood count. Assessment of hyperviscosity and the presence of cryoglobulins or pyroglobulins should also be considered. An intravenous pyelogram, if necessary, should be done only with extreme caution, since dehydration and contrast material may result in renal failure.

Although the diagnostic triad of serum and/or urine M-protein, marrow plasmacytosis, and osteolytic bone disease is present in most patients with MM, some may have only the first two plus findings of diffuse osteopenia or even normal bones. And occasionally, patients may have only a soft tissue or bony mass lesion (a localized plasmacytoma) without other associated findings. By taking into account the level of M-proteins in serum and/or urine, the extent of osteolytic bone disease, and the levels of serum hemoglobin and calcium, one can assess disease extent and calculate the probable tumor cell mass. Such a clinical staging system has a good correlation with response to therapy (stage I, $<0.6 \times 10^{12}$ cells/M² = 78%; stage III, $>1.2 \times 10^{12}$ cells/M² = 30%) and median survival (stage I = 5+ years, stage III = 2 years). Another prognostic factor is the type of M-protein secreted: patients with λ-chain myeloma have a shorter survival overall than those with κ-chain disease. Median survivals according to immunoglobulin class are IgG (κ = 35 months, λ = 25 months), IgA (κ = 22, λ = 19), light-chain disease (κ = 28, λ = 11), and IgD = 9 months.

The treatment of MM requires attention to all sites of disease activity as well as to the management of disease complications. In general, chemotherapeutic effect is most easily assessed by following the level of M-protein. Although osteolytic lesions may heal, they do not do so commonly. An objective response is usually defined as a greater than 75% decrease in M-protein and the absence of Bence Jones proteinuria. A standard chemotherapy program is intermittent melphalan 10 mg/M²/day for 4 days and prednisone 60 mg/M²/day for 4 days repeated every 4 to 6 weeks for approximately 1 year. On this regimen about 30% to 50% of patients achieve an objective response. Continuing therapy in responders beyond 1 year does not appear to improve median unmaintained remission duration (11 months) or survival (24 months). Since the development of acute myelogenous leukemia has been associated with long-term alkylating agent therapy, it would seem wise to discontinue all unnecessary maintenance therapy. Other drugs that have activity in MM include cyclophosphamide, Adriamycin, vincristine, and BCNU. A drug combination using all these drugs other than Adriamycin has been reported recently to yield improved response and survival results but has not yet been tested prospectively.

Complications of MM that must be managed expectantly include bone pain (which may require analgesics, local radiation therapy, and/or surgical fixation); hypercalcemia (exacerbated by bed rest, dehydration); renal failure; hyperuricemia; pancytopenia; hyperviscosity; and infection.

C.P.

Alexanian R, Gehan E, Haut A, et al: Unmaintained remissions in multiple myeloma. Blood 51:1005–1011, 1978.
Maintenance chemotherapy was of no significant benefit in terms of remission duration and survival in 28 responders after 1 year of induction therapy.

Alexanian R, Salmon S, Bonnet J, et al: Combination therapy for multiple myeloma. Cancer 40:2765–2771, 1977.
This article provides a retrospective analysis of 6 treatment protocols in 462 previously untreated patients.

Case DC Jr, Lee BJ III, Clarkson BD: Improved survival times in multiple myeloma treated with melphalan, prednisone, cyclophosphamide, vincristine and BCNU: M-2 protocol. Am J Med 63:897–903, 1977.
Response (87% in previously untreated patients), median remission duration (20+ months), and median survival (22+ months) in patients given this treatment were significantly better than in historical controls treated with melphalan and prednisone.

Cohen HJ, Rundles RW: Managing the complications of plasma cell myeloma. Arch Intern Med 135:177–184, 1975.
A retrospective analysis of 102 patients with a discussion of illustrative cases.

DeFronzo RA, Cooke CR, Wright JR, Humphrey RL: Renal function in patients with multiple myeloma. Medicine 57:151–166, 1978.
This study of 35 patients correlated renal histopathology and myeloma protein patterns.

Durie BGM, Salmon SE: A clinical staging system for multiple myeloma: Correlation of measured myeloma cell mass with presenting clinical features, response to treatment, and survival. Cancer 36:842–854, 1975.

A retrospective analysis of 71 patients correlating clinical characteristics and prognosis with calculated tumor cell mass.

Durie BGM, Salmon SE, Moon TE: Pretreatment tumor mass, cell kinetics, and prognosis in multiple myeloma. Blood 55:364–372, 1980.

Pretreatment labeling index of bone marrow plasma cells was measured in 79 patients. With LI% < 1, median survival was approximately 34 months; with LI% ≥ 1, median survival was 24 months.

Gonzalez F, Trujillo JM, Alexanian R: Acute leukemia in multiple myeloma. Ann Intern Med 86:440–443, 1977.

Of 476 patients with myeloma, 6 developed acute myelogenous leukemia while on continuous melphalan-prednisone therapy for a median duration of 3 years.

Kyle RA: Monoclonal gammopathy of undetermined significance: Natural history in 241 cases. Am J Med 64:814–826, 1978.

Myeloma developed in 18 patients; the median interval to diagnosis was 64 months.

Shustik C, Bergsagel DE, Pruzanski W: κ and λ light chain disease: Survival rates and clinical manifestations. Blood 48:41–51, 1976.

In a retrospective study of 97 patients median survival was 30 months for patients with κ-LCD and 10 months for those with λ-LCD.

Wiltshaw E: The natural history of extramedullary plasmacytoma and its relation to solitary myeloma of bone and myelomatosis. Medicine 55:217–238, 1976.

A comprehensive retrospective review.

PART VI. TREATMENT

Postoperative problems common to all types of surgery may affect patients undergoing surgery for malignant diseases.

Respiratory Problems

Postoperative atelectasis and pneumonitis are the most common postoperative complications. Fevers 24 to 48 hours after surgery are usually due to atelectasis. This complication may be minimized by discontinuation of smoking, preoperative breathing exercises, and the use of blow bottles or nebulizers, with encouragement of cough and early mobilization in the postoperative period. Respiratory insufficiency may ensue when patients with poor pulmonary reserve or function develop atelectasis or pneumonitis postoperatively. A chest radiograph may reveal atelectasis or pulmonary infiltrates. Serial evaluations of the degree of respiratory insufficiency are best made by arterial blood gas determinations. Patients with poor respiratory reserve who need prolonged tracheal intubation and assisted ventilation postoperatively may also require a tracheostomy.

Shock

Postoperative shock may have several causes. Myocardial infarction or cardiac failure may result in decreased cardiac output. In this case it may be necessary to obtain left atrial (pulmonary wedge) pressures, measured by a Swann Ganz catheter, to guide fluid replacement. If cardiac failure is present, fluid restrictions, diuretics, digitalis, and positive end-expiratory pressure ventilation may all be needed. Hypovolemic shock may be due to an unrecognized low preoperative blood volume but may also result from intraoperative blood or fluid loss and postoperative hemorrhage. Extracirculatory fluid losses into the GI tract, peritoneal cavity, or soft tissues after trauma may also reduce the effective blood volume and produce shock. Once hypovolemia is diagnosed, the central venous pressure (CVP) should be used as a guide for fluid replacement, while urinary output is kept at between 25 and 50+ cc/hour. If shock occurs and a bleeding source is not apparent, the possibility of coagulation abnormalities due to disseminated intravascular coagulation, platelet abnormalities, or liver dysfunction should be considered.

Cardiac Arrest

Cardiac arrest is a potential anesthetic complication. Its risk is greatly increased in hypoxic patients and in those with arrhythmias or electrolyte imbalances. Electrolyte imbalances may result from sodium and/or fluid excess or depletion or acid-base imbalances. Electrolyte abnormalities in surgical patients are most commonly due to uncorrected, unreplaced vomiting losses. Hypoventilation most commonly produces respiratory acidosis, while metabolic acidosis is noted with renal failure. Hyperventilation induces respiratory alkalosis, while metabolic alkalosis follows prolonged vomiting and loss of gastric hydrochloric acid; potassium deficiency ultimately results, with further hydrogen ion loss and hence greater degrees of alkalosis.

Oliguria

Postoperative oliguria (urinary volumes <400 m/day) may have prerenal, renal, or postrenal causes. Such prerenal causes of oliguria as reduced blood volume, myocardial infarction, and heart failure should be recognized and treated. A concentrated urine with low urine sodium concentration is noted in prerenal oliguria. Mannitol, 25 gm, or furosemide, 40 mg IV, will usually produce a diuresis if the diagnosis of prerenal oliguria is in doubt. Intrarenal oliguria usually follows kidney injury or acute tubular necrosis (ATN) secondary to diminished renal perfusion. In ATN the urine specific gravity is usually 1.014 or less, BUN and creatinine are elevated, and there is increased urinary sodium loss. ATN is treated by restricting fluid intake to 400 cc daily (plus replacement of insensible losses); ion exchange enemas or dialysis is used if hyperkalemia occurs. Postrenal oliguria or anuria from ureteral or bladder outlet obstruction should be treated appropriately.

Jaundice
Postoperative jaundice occurs in 20% of patients but is severe in only 4%. Postoperative jaundice and/or hepatic failure may be caused by hemolysis, fluothane anesthesia, prolonged shock with liver hypoxia, chlorpromazine ingestion, viral hepatitis, sepsis, or extrahepatic biliary tract obstruction.

Mental Changes
Mental changes may also occur postoperatively. In restless, confused postoperative patients, hypoxia should be ruled out by performing arterial blood gas determinations. Prolonged unresponsiveness may follow lengthy anesthesia and resolves spontaneously with time. However, cerebrovascular accidents, clot or fat emboli, or electrolyte imbalance may produce permanent changes in mentation.

Gastrointestinal Problems
Gastrointestinal complications, such as prolonged ileus, may be due to electrolyte abnormalities, technical surgical complications, or intraperitoneal infections. Tube decompression, parenteral nutrition, and reoperation may all be indicated.

Vascular Complications
Such vascular complications as phlebitis and pulmonary emboli also occur. A pulmonary embolus (20% or more of which are unrecognized) should be suspected in patients who develop chest pain, dyspnea, tachycardia, and unexplained hypoxia 5 to 10 days postoperatively. A chest radiograph may show a peripheral infiltrate or cardiac enlargement. An electrocardiogram may reveal right ventricular strain. The diagnosis of pulmonary emboli may be confirmed by a ventilation-perfusion lung scan, since the involved pulmonary segment is ventilated but not perfused after embolization has occurred. Anticoagulation is the treatment of choice, but for selected patients with massive emboli, pulmonary angiography and surgical removal of the clot may also be indicated. Wound, catheter tip, or systemic infections usually occur more than 48 hours postoperatively, with leukocytosis, local symptoms, and fever. Wound infections are usually treated by opening the incision, draining it, obtaining a culture, and administering appropriate antibiotics.

Structural Deformities
Structural deformities may be minimized by carefully planning operations, obtaining maxillofacial prosthedontic consultation prior to major head and neck surgical procedures, fitting of prostheses immediately after amputations, carefully preparing ostomies, and carefully planning surgery to maintain the postoperative integrity of normal tissues.

Complications of Head and Neck Surgery
Following head and neck surgery (especially for thyroid neoplasms), hemorrhage into tightly closed tissue spaces may cause respiratory distress. Post-

operative hypertension may also increase the risk of hemorrhage into the wound. If respiratory obstruction occurs, the wound must be reopened and the clot evacuated; insertion of an endotracheal tube for 24 to 48 hours maintains an adequate airway. Hypoparathyroidism and recurrent laryngeal nerve injury may also occur during thyroid resections. A thoracic duct fistula may follow a left-sided radical neck dissection. Neck dissections are performed with thin skin flaps, which may necrose and produce partial loss of the flap and exposure of the carotid artery. If orocutaneous or pharyngocutaneous fistulae occur, the carotid artery may rupture, unless tissue coverage is reestablished. Head and neck surgery may also result in injury to the hypoglossal nerve, with articulation and swallowing difficulties; the recurrent laryngeal nerve, resulting in vocal cord paralysis and hoarseness; or the superior laryngeal nerves, causing both loss of pharyngeal sensation and severe difficulty in swallowing. There may be dysphagia and aspiration after supraglottic laryngectomy, and impaired speech and dysphagia following tongue or oropharyngeal surgery.

Post-tracheostomy Complications
Post-tracheostomy complications have been minimized by the recent introduction of large volume, low pressure cuffs and by planned operations (with prior endotracheal intubation). If the tracheostomy site is too high, cricoid cartilage stenosis may be produced; if the incision is placed too low in the neck, late vascular injury and hemorrhage may result. Hemorrhage, arrythmias, cardiac arrest, mediastinal emphysema, pneumothorax, and aspiration may all occur after tracheostomy. In the early postoperative period a tracheostomy tube may be inadvertently removed or may become obstructed, the patient may aspirate, or local infection or atelectasis may develop. Such late complications as tracheal stenosis and tracheoesophageal or tracheoarterial fistulae, although rare, also do arise. A tracheoesophageal fistula is best confirmed by bronchoscopy, although radiographs or the ingestion of methylene blue may also document the presence of a fistula. Tracheal stenosis is best demonstrated by tracheal tomograms. Granulomas at the tracheostomy site or tracheomalacia may also narrow the airway after a tracheostomy. After decannulation, the tracheal stoma rarely fails to heal spontaneously, requiring surgical closure.

Complications of Thoracic Surgery
Special complications can occur after thoracic surgery. Postoperative bleeding from chest tubes of more than 250 m/hour for 4 to 6 hours is an indication for reexploration, if clotting factors and platelet function are normal. Hypotension and shock from hypovolemia may occur after thoracic surgery, but other causes of shock, such as cardiac tamponade, myocardial infarction, and heart failure, should also be considered. If fluid administration raises the CVP, but cardiac output does not improve, left atrial pressure (LAP) should be measured by a Swann Ganz catheter; if the LAP is low, additional fluid replacement is indicated. Digitalis is administered in acute heart failure, but for a slow heart rate isoproterenol or dopamine by drip infusion is an effective inotropic agent. The use of pressor drugs that produce only peripheral vasoconstriction should be avoided. Atrial fibrillation or flutter may be managed by digitalis, quinidine, or cardioversion. Intravenous lidocaine (1500 mg bolus), procainamide, or dilantin are all useful drugs for ventricular tachycardias. Atropine, 0.5 to 1.5 mg IV, isoproterenol, and a pacemaker may all be necessary if bradycardia ensues. For second- or third-degree heart block not due to digitalis intoxication, the administration of atropine or Isuprel is indicated. A pacemaker may also be required.

For a patient with pulmonary edema, diuretics, rotating tourniquets, digitalis, oxygen, and positive end-expiratory pressure may all be required. Vigorous postoperative pulmonary care, including IPPB and frequent endotracheal suction, are all important in minimizing postoperative atelectasis and pneumonitis. Arterial blood gases, intubation, and mechanical ventilation may be indicated for patients with respiratory insufficiency. Respiratory insufficiency may be avoided by meticulous surgical technique and careful preoperative estimation of pulmonary reserve. The recognition and treatment of oliguria has already been described. Pneumothorax, empyema, and bronchopleural fistulae may all be seen after thoracic operations. A tube thoracostomy may be necessary with a pneumothorax, but closure of a bronchopleural fistula may require additional surgery. With empyema, prolonged tube drainage followed by thoracotomy may be required.

Fistulae

Fistulae following head and neck operations are usually managed with antibiotic treatment, tube feedings, and ultimately resection and flap closure to restore continuity and close the fistula if it does not close spontaneously. Abdominal fistulae extend either from one viscus to another, from viscus to surrounding soft tissues, or from viscus to skin. Most occur after operative trauma to the bowel, but they may also result from abdominal trauma, inflammatory conditions such as Crohn's disease or ulcerative colitis, following radiotherapy to the abdomen, or with intra-abdominal neoplastic diseases, with or without surgery. High-output fistulae (over 500 ml/24 hours) carry the worst prognosis for spontaneous fistula closure. Abdominal pain and tenderness usually occur 24 to 48 hours postoperatively, the white count becomes elevated and a fistula develops.

Oral indigo carmine or charcoal may appear at the cutaneous opening of a fistula; but barium studies, including fistulograms, UGI series, or barium enemas, may also be necessary to demonstrate the extent and origin of a fistula. The prognosis and treatment plan depend on the age of the patient, the segment of bowel involved by the fistula, the magnitude of the fluid losses, the presence of associated infection, the underlying cause of the fistula, and the presence or absence of distal obstruction. Complications such as electrolyte and fluid depletion, peritonitis and sepsis, nutritional deficits, skin injury, gastrointestinal obstruction, and pneumonitis may all occur. The most important items in successful management of fistulae are nutritional support and careful monitoring of fluid losses; replacement of fluid, electrolytes, albumin, and calories; control of infection; proper skin care; and surgical correction of the fistula if necessary. Fistulae involving distal bowel segments may be managed by oral feedings; a feeding tube may be placed distal to a fistula involving the duodenum or proximal jejunum. Antibiotic administration and drainage of infections or abscesses are also indicated. If a fistula does not close spontaneously after optimal local measures and nutritional support, distal obstruction, neoplasm, abscess, foreign body, or tract epithelization should all be ruled out.

Ostomies

When an ileostomy is performed, a perfect fit of the drainage bag should be obtained, so that irritating small bowel secretions do not macerate the skin. Karaya gum rings, bag, and foreplate should be applied and changed at least two times a week. Colostomies are also managed by bag drainage, either with spontaneous evacuation and bag collection or by "training" the colostomy through irrigation at 2-day intervals with 1 to 2 pints of solution and the dietary avoidance of fruit and highly spiced foods. A karaya gum washer seal and appliance bag are necessary. Colostomy complications such as necrosis (impaired blood supply or too tight an orifice), retraction, stricture (avoided by primary suture techniques), prolapse or herniation, hemorrhage, infection, and perforation may all occur. An ileal loop ureteral diversion should be made to function optimally by choosing flat skin for the stoma, so that a cemented bag can be used. If a protruding stoma is made, either a cemented or strap-on bag may be used. The bowel should be everted and sewn to the skin, the bag should be cemented into place during the recovery period, the stoma should be dilated to prevent strictures, and scrupulous cleanliness must be maintained. Inflammatory skin reactions may be treated by removing the bag, using heat lamps, catheter stomal drainage, and antibiotics if necessary. A belt appliance may be used if the cement is irritating to the skin. Complications may be prevented by avoiding tight clothing over the bag and not allowing the bag to become overfilled with urine.

D.G.

Bartlett R: Studies on the pathogenesis and prevention of postoperative pulmonary complications. Surg Gynecol Obstet 137:925–933, 1973.
Maximal inspiration maneuvers prevented postoperative alveolar collapse and shunting.

Chew J, Cantrell R: Tracheostomy: Complications and their management. Arch Otolaryngol 96:538–545, 1972.
The complication rate of tracheostomy in this study, 15.8%, was due mostly to hemorrhage, infection, obstruction, and a displaced tube. Mortality was 1.6%.

Evans C, Evans M, Pollock A: The incidence and causes of postoperative jaundice. A prospective study. Br J Anaesth 46:520–525, 1974.
180 patients had 218 operations; severe jaundice occurred in 3.7%, mild jaundice in 16.5%. The most common cause of the jaundice was bilirubin overload (from transfusions) inadequately excreted by liver due to impaired postoperative function.

Roback S, Nicoloff D: High output enterocutaneous fistulas of the small bowel. An analysis of 55 cases. Am J Surg 123:317–322, 1972.
The most frequent cause of fistulas was bowel injury at surgery. The most common associated diseases were colorectal cancer, chronic cholecystitis, hernia, and regional enteritis.

Sheldon G, Gardner B, Dunphy J: Progress in the management of intestinal fistulae. Rev Surg 27:452, 1970.
This is a short review of the treatment of 51 fistulas.

89. PROBLEMS AND TOXICITIES OF RADIATION THERAPY

Skin

The severity of postirradiation skin reactions depends upon radiation dose, fraction size, length of treatment course, beam quality, volume of tissue irradiated, and anatomic location of the treated skin. Megavoltage radiation, in contrast to orthovoltage, delivers maximum doses beneath the skin surface, thus sparing the skin and causing it less radiation injury than did the superficial x-rays formerly used.

Acute skin reactions occur after 2 to 3 weeks of treatment at 1000 rads per week (orthovoltage) or when the skin dose is increased by bolus with megavoltage beams. The first noticeable skin changes (after 10 to 14 days) are skin erythema (due to capillary dilatation) and epilation. Next, dry desquamation occurs due to decreased basal cell activity, thinning of the epidermis, decreased sebaceous and sweat gland function, and shedding of superficial cells. After the fourth week of radiation therapy, epidermal bullae, superficial slough, and a moist desquamative reaction may appear, followed by necrosis of the epidermis and destruction of the epithelium if the skin receives excessive radiation doses. In most instances the epidermis will regenerate through epithelial cell migration from the periphery. Six to twelve months after high-dose irradiation, the skin may become atrophic and ulcerated. After one year or more, cutaneous atrophy and marked subcutaneous fibrosis also occur. These late radiation changes may be differentiated from recurrent carcinoma, since no neoplasm is evident, the skin changes conform closely to the prior radiation fields, and the underlying bone may also be involved in the irradiated area. There is also an increased risk of late carcinogenesis in heavily irradiated skin, with a latent period of 5 to 25 years.

Acute radiation skin reactions may be reduced by minimizing the following: excessive sun exposure, skin trauma, the use of topical agents containing heavy metals, excessive washing, hyperthermia, administration of cutaneous sensitizing drugs such as erythromycin, and the use of adhesive tape. Drug allergies must be differentiated from radiation skin reactions, but the former are usually not confined to the irradiated area.

Erythematous skin should be kept clean, while topical corticosteroids promote healing. When dry desquamation occurs, topical steroids should be used initially, followed by daily applications of lanolin ointment after the skin has healed. More severe moist desquamative or ulcerative reactions should be treated by frequent soaks in Burrow's solution and dressing changes. Any co-existing infections should also be treated, while severely damaged skin may require excision, grafting, or skin flap coverage of necrotic areas.

Skin grafts appear to have an increased radiosensitivity during the first 3 months, but become similar to skin in their radiation tolerance between 3 months and 1 year, and less radiosensitive after 12 months. The relatively hypoxic split-thickness skin grafts appear to be less sensitive to the effects of radiation than full-thickness grafts. If grafts must be included in radiation fields, at least 1 month should elapse from the time of surgery to allow capillaries to enter the graft, begin its vascularization, and provide organic union.

Cardiopulmonary

Lung

Acute radiation pneumonitis usually occurs 1 to 6 months after the completion of a radiotherapy course. This early, exudative pneumonitis may subside spontaneously but may also be followed by severe pulmonary fibrosis. Interstitial fibrosis also occurs without acute symptoms and may be noted months to years after irradiation. Acute, symptomatic radiation pneumonitis is noted in 11% of patients undergoing postmastectomy irradiation and in 5% to 15% of those who have radiotherapy for lung cancer. Radiographic changes are present in 40% of the former and occur in 33% of the latter by 6 months, in 66% by 12 months, and in 100% 30 months after irradiation. The risk of radiation pneumonitis increases when large lung volumes are irradiated; 6% of patients become symptomatic when only the mediastinum is irradiated, but 33% have pulmonary symptoms following treatment of both lung and mediastinum. Swelling of the alveolar lining cells, septal edema, and capillary engorgement, followed by fibrosis and alveolar obliteration, are common histologic findings in radiation lung injury.

Clinically a nonproductive cough, dyspnea on exertion, fever, elevated white blood count and erythrocyte sedimentation rate, and no pathogens in sputum cultures are the usual findings in acute radiation pneumonitis. Radiographs reveal infiltrates or areas of fibrosis generally confined to the radiation ports; late in the course they may demonstrate decreased lung volume and pulmonary fibrosis. The presence of infection, lymphangitic tumor spread, or recurrence of an irradiated carcinoma should also be considered before the diagnosis of radiation pneumonitis is made. Radiation pneumonitis is best prevented by limiting the radiation dose to a lung to less than 1800–2000 rads in 2 to 3 weeks. These maximum doses should be decreased when chemotherapeutic agents are used concurrently. The lung volume irradiated should always be kept to a minimum when possible, since the risk of radiation pneumonitis increases sharply when large volumes are treated. Superimposed infections should be treated, if present. If the pneumonitis is mild, the patient may need only observation, but if severe symptoms occur, the use of prednisone (60 to 100 mg daily in divided doses) is recommended, with a prolonged taper to minimize flaring the pneumonitis as the drug is withdrawn.

Esophagus

When radiation doses of 3000 rads in 2 weeks or more are delivered to the esophagus, dysphagia and/or localized pain is often noted. This mucosal reaction is self-limited; it may be minimized by either decreasing the daily radiation dose or temporarily discontinuing treatment, or by the use of antacids, a bland diet, and topical anesthetics such as Oxaine M or Viscous Xylocaine. Acute esophagitis usually heals rapidly after completion of the radiation therapy course.

Heart

Radiation-induced pericarditis, pancarditis, or coronary artery disease may all occur, especially in patients who are irradiated for neoplasms of the lung, esophagus, or breast, or for lymphomas that involve the mediastinum. A 6.6% incidence of radiation pericarditis was noted when patients who were treated for Hodgkin's disease received radiation doses of 4000 rads to more than 50% of the heart. There was a very high risk of developing this complication after retreatments with radiation. At present, the risk of developing radiation pericarditis after mantle irradiation is 2.5% or less.

Postirradiation pericarditis may present with dyspnea, cough, or precordial pain. If a pericardial effusion is present, cardiac tamponade may occur, producing edema, hepatomegaly, and increasing dyspnea on exertion. Acute pericarditis may be noted 6 to 48 months after irradiation; pericardial effusions usually occur 6 to 12 months after irradiation; constrictive pericarditis, if it occurs, is usually noted after 6 to 36 months. The diagnosis of pericarditis may be suspected when a postirradiation chest radiograph demonstrates widening of the cardiac configuration. The presence of a pericardial effusion may be confirmed by an echo cardiogram. Pericardiocentesis and cardiac catheterization should be performed on symptomatic patients: an elevated pre-tap and post-tap right atrial pressure (RAP) is evidence for constrictive pericarditis. A decreased RAP following pericardiocentesis allows an estimate of the degree of tamponade. A pericardial fluid cytologic examination should be performed, although the fluid is usually sanguineous, with elevated protein but cytologically benign. Therapy consists of salicylate administration or observation in mild cases and pericardiocentesis if symptomatic amounts of fluid are present. Two-thirds of patients with pericardial effusions improve without surgical intervention. Systemic corticosteroids may also be indicated in the acute phase. For increasingly symptomatic patients, or in those with severe constrictive pericarditis, pericardiectomy may be necessary. The entire pericardium should be resected for optimum results. Radiation pericarditis may be almost completely prevented by limiting the left ventricular radiation dose to 1500 rads in 1.5 weeks, by using carefully shaped mediastinal radiotherapy fields, and by inserting a subcarinal block at 3000–3500 rads to further protect the base of the heart.

A few deaths from coronary artery disease in young patients who received mediastinal and cardiac irradiation have been reported. It has been postulated that radiotherapy in certain rare instances may result in both increased coronary artery fibrosis and accelerated athrogenesis, but the mechanism of this process is unknown, and such events are extremely rare.

Gastrointestinal

Stomach

Fractionated total radiotherapy doses of 2000 rads to the stomach may decrease gastric acid production. Higher doses, over 4500–5000 rads, may produce gastric ulcers and should be avoided if possible. Antacids and bland diets usually control the symptoms of radiation gastritis.

Gastrointestinal Tract

The incidence of gastrointestinal injury varies from 8% to 11% in patients receiving pelvic irradiation for bladder cancers to 30% in those receiving larger radiation portals for ovarian carcinomas. Nausea, vomiting, diarrhea, crampy abdominal pain, and occasional gastrointestinal bleeding may all be noted during an abdominal irradiation course. Acute rectal bleeding may be followed by chronic radiation enteritis. The severity of the symptoms are partially due to the radiation fractionation, volume of bowel irradiated, total radiation dose, and prior surgery, which increases the risk of intra-abdominal adhesions. Chronic radiation enteritis or colitis may produce crampy abdominal pain, nausea and vomiting, chronic diarrhea, partial or complete bowel obstruction, and, rarely, bowel perforation or fistula formation.

A history of the foregoing symptoms and recent abdominal irradiation will confirm the diagnosis of suspected radiation enteritis or colitis. Physical examination may elicit signs of an acute abdomen if perforation has occurred but usually reveals hyperactive bowel sounds without rebound tenderness. A fecal occult blood test may be positive. During irradiation acute GI reactions may be managed by antiemetics, antidiarrheal drugs (Lomotil, paregoric, Kaopectate), antispasmodics, or anticholinergics. Patients should avoid dairy or spiced foods; and low residue, elemental, or gluten-free diets may be necessary. Severe acute radiation enteritis may require systemic corticosteroid therapy, whereas cortisone enemas may be necessary for acute radiation colitis. These symptoms may be minimized by reducing the daily radiation doses, interrupting therapy, decreasing the irradiated volume, and dietary manipulation, and possibly by hyperalimentation in severe cases.

Late radiation-induced GI tract injury must be differentiated from neoplastic involvement. Usually, long involved bowel segments, "saw-tooth" mucosal pattern, and no sharp demarcation between normal and damaged bowel are characteristic GI series findings in radiation enteritis. Intestinal stricture and obstruction may both be noted. Malabsorption may be documented. Parenteral hyperalimentation is occasionally necessary in severe radiation enteritis. If surgery is required, the simplest procedure that will obtain the best results is recommended. Depending on the condition of the patient, the affected bowel may be either resected or bypassed. A colostomy may be necessary with severe radiation colitis. There are increased risks of postoperative intraperitoneal infections, fistula formation, and bowel infarction in these patients.

Genitourinary

Kidney

When the entire kidney is irradiated, the radiation dose should be less than 1500–2000 rads in 2 weeks. However, one-third to one-half of a kidney may receive radiation doses of 4000 rads or more without development of radiation nephritis. If both kidneys receive high-dose irradiation (>3000 rads), however, radiation nephritis may occur 6 to 12 months later. Edema, shortness of breath, headache, hypertension, and pleuroperitoneal effusions may all be present in severe radiation nephritis. If high-dose irradiation is delivered to only one kidney, hypertension may result. Radiation nephritis may produce debilitation similar to that seen with carcinomatosis, while the severe headache, vomiting, and papilledema of malignant hypertension secondary to radiation renal injury may be mistaken for symptoms due to cerebral metastases. Malignant hypertension may also be attributed to other causes, delaying the diagnosis of radiation nephritis.

A history of the above symptoms, with prior abdominal irradiation that included the kidneys, when there is no evidence of intra-abdominal involvement by carcinoma, allows the presumptive diagnosis of radiation nephritis to be made. Albuminuria, serum BUN and creatinine elevation, and hypertension all occur in radiation nephritis, but hematuria is absent. The characteristic lesion is arteriolonephrosclerosis, with secondary degeneration of glomeruli and renal tubules. The acute phase of radiation nephritis may be managed in the same way as acute renal failure from other causes: by decreased dietary protein and fluid and salt restriction; peritoneal or hemodialysis may also be necessary pending restoration of renal function. Corticosteroids may worsen radiation nephritis and are contraindicated. Twenty-five percent of patients with severe renal radiation injury may die, especially when the BUN is greater than 100 mg/100 ml and massive edema is present.

Bladder

The bladder may be injured when neoplasms of the bladder, cervix, prostate, colorectum, ovary, or endometrium are irradiated. During a pelvic radiation therapy course for bladder cancer, acute cystitis develops during the third and fourth week in 50% to 60% of patients. Urgency, frequency, dysuria, and hematuria all occur. There may also be an associated urinary tract infection. Mucosal hyperemia is found in acute radiation cystitis; the vesical epithelium may desquamate, and in rare instances, bladder perforation or fistulae have occurred. The acute reaction subsides after irradiation. Acute cystitis may be minimized by reducing the daily radiation dose; temporarily discontinuing therapy; or administering Urispas, 100 mg po qid, or pyridium, 100 to 200 mg po qid. The urine should also be cultured, and appropriate antibiotics begun if an infection is present.

Subacute and chronic radiation cystitis occurs from 6 months to more than 2 years after a pelvic treatment course. Painless hematuria is the most common symptom. When patients have had intracavitary radium treatments for carcinoma of the cervix, cystoscopy may reveal an ulcer on the posterior bladder wall or a bleeding point without the induration characteristic of malignant tumors. Conservative therapy is indicated. If there is a contracted bladder (usually 6 to 24 months after irradiation), urinary frequency, urgency, and nocturia may all be severe problems. Cystoscopy and a cystogram may establish the diagnosis; since the contracted bladder has been caused by perivesicular ischemia, ileal loop diversion may be necessary, since the vesical fibrosis is unlikely to improve. A postirradiation contracted bladder is uncommon (found in only 2% to 7% of patients undergoing pelvic irradiation) but is noted more frequently in patients with chronic cystitis or in those with large, invasive carcinomas. The risk of bladder injury may be minimized by waiting 4 to 6 weeks after a transurethral resection before starting irradiation, eliminating urinary obstruction if possible, avoiding prolonged catheterization during the treatment course, eradicating infections, and controlling bulky tumor masses that predispose to bladder infections.

Ureter
Ipsilateral ureteral obstruction is rarely a complication of radiation. Ureteral obstruction at the ureterovesical junction is usually due to a malignancy, whereas postirradiation strictures arise 4 to 6 cm superior to the ureterovesical junction, at the site of high-dose intracavitary irradiation. A ureter may also be blocked by recurrent carcinoma, by fibrosis secondary to eradication of an invasive carcinoma, or by an ascending infection. Ureteral dilatation may be necessary for obstruction due to fibrosis or, in rare instances, ureteral diversion may be necessary.

Prostate
The prostate is a very radioresistant organ. Postirradiation prostatic urethral strictures may occur but can be minimized by irradiating without an indwelling urethral catheter and by starting a radiotherapy course at least 4 to 6 weeks post-transurethral resection.

Uterus
The uterus is very resistant to radiation. Cervical or vaginal necrosis, atrophy, and fibrosis may all occur, however, following radiotherapy of cervical carcinomas. Vaginal fibrosis and shortening may be minimized by the resumption of intercourse or by regular dilations with an obturator after irradiation.

Ovary and Testis
The ovaries and the testis are both very sensitive to radiation. Radiation doses as low as 150–500 rads may produce amenorrhea or infertility.

Thyroid
Low-dose head and neck irradiation in childhood may result in thyroid carcinoma after a long latent period (see Part II, Chapter 17). When the thyroid was incidentally included in external beam radiotherapy ports, a high incidence of postirradiation thyroid dysfunction was noted in previously untreated patients with Hodgkin's disease who received high-dose mantle irradiation; 36% were euthyroid, whereas 44% had compensated hypothyroidism, and 20% became hypothyroid. In patients with untreated head and neck cancers, 62% were euthyroid; another 25% had compensated hyperthyroidism, and 13% were hypothyroid following high-dose irradiation that included the thyroid gland. Graves' ophthalmopathy, occurring 18 to 84 months after neck radiotherapy for non-thyroid-related neoplasms, has been reported in 7 patients, while thyroid carcinomas have also been noted in a very limited number of adults following mantle irradiation for Hodgkin's disease.

Pituitary
The pituitary gland may be irradiated for the treatment of eosinophilic, basophilic, or chromophobe adenomas or may be incidentally included in the radiation fields for brain tumors, nasopharyngeal or sinus malignancies, or other head and neck neoplasms. Hypothalamic-pituitary endocrine deficiencies were detected in 14 of 15 adult patients who underwent high-dose nasopharyngeal irradiation. In these patients, both serum growth hormone and plasma cortisol levels were determined before and during insulin-induced hypoglycemia. Prolactin was measured before and after the intramuscular administration of chlorpromazine by the intravenous injection of thyrotrophin-releasing hormone (TRH). TSH levels were also measured before and after TRH injections, and luteinizing hormone (LH) before the administration of LH-releasing hormone. Other authors have confirmed the presence of pituitary dysfunction after radiation doses of 4500 rads or more to the gland.

Musculoskeletal

The most common osseous complication from therapeutic irradiation is osteoradionecrosis of the mandible (ORN). One-third of cases occur less than 6 months after the completion of irradiation. This complication is noted when high-dose radiation fields include the mandible, and it is especially common in patients with mucosal trauma, advanced periodontal disease or periapical infections, or neglected dental caries, or after postirradiation extractions performed without antibiotic coverage or meticulous alveolar closure. It occurs in 10% to 20% of patients receiving high-dose external beam irradiation for oral, oropharyngeal, or pharyngeal carcinomas.

A patient with mandibular ORN may have painful exposed bone, with associated cellulitis and edema of the surrounding tissues. A mandibular radiograph may show lucent areas, bony sequestra, and pathologic fractures. Physical examination may reveal exposed mandible and adjacent soft tissue edema, induration and inflammation, and carious teeth. This complication may be prevented or minimized by carefully planned radiotherapy courses and possibly by the combined use of interstitial irradiation and lower external beam doses, by dental evaluation and prophylaxis prior to radiation therapy, by extraction of nonrestorable teeth, and by prophylactic fluoride treatments. Extractions performed after irradiation require antibiotic coverage, with meticulous closure of the mucosa over the alveolar ridge to protect the underlying bone. When osteoradionecrosis is present, antibiotics, conservative debridement as necessary, and resection and closure only in selected cases are the usual methods of treatment.

When cartilage (especially of the larynx, nose, and ear) is infected, exposed, or invaded by carcinomas, high-dose radiation may result in further cartilaginous exposure and painful chondritis. This risk may be minimized by the use of appropriate antibiotics, carefully planned radiation treatments, and protracted radiation courses.

Pathologic fractures, especially of the pelvis and femur, usually occur 1 to 5 years after irradiation in patients over the age of 50. These fractures are caused by decreased blood supply to the bone secondary to the irradiation. No osteocyte activity is noted, while osteoporosis and reactive sclerosis are both present. Rest and supported ambulation are important factors in management. Recurrent or metastatic carcinoma should also be ruled out. Femoral fractures may require fixation, while in selected patients joint replacement may be necessary. Postmastectomy chest wall radiation doses exceeding 5000 rads in 5 weeks may produce rib fractures. Most of these fractures heal spontaneously, but they may be prevented in large part by decreasing the total radiation dose and by the use of careful radiotherapy techniques.

Radiation doses greater than 2000–2500 rads to bones of children may produce skeletal growth arrest, scoliosis, or structural deformities, depending on the site irradiated, the total radiation dose, and whether or not the entire bone was included in the radiation field. A dose below 2000 rads in a fractionated course probably does not cause significant height retardation, even though the axial skeleton is irradiated at the most vulnerable ages (6 to 9 and 12 to 15 years).

Skeletal muscle is not radiosensitive and is rarely injured by therapeutic doses of radiation.

Neurologic

Brain

Brain necrosis may occur not only after the primary irradiation of brain tumors, but also when the brain is incidentally included in radiotherapy fields used in the treatment of nasopharyngeal, scalp, pituitary, or sinus neoplasms.

It is uncertain whether vascular changes or neuronal injury are the underlying mechanism in radiation-induced brain necrosis. Early in a course of brain irradiation, acute cerebral edema may occur and may require corticosteroid therapy, reduction of daily radiation doses, therapy "splits" or a shunt procedure.

Brain necrosis may develop 6 to 12 months or more after radiotherapy, mimicking the original symptoms of the brain tumor. Factors important in brain necrosis are the total radiation dose, the size of the fractions, the volume of brain irradiated, the location of the tumor, and concomitant use of antitumor drugs. The brain stem appears to be more radiosensitive than the cerebral hemispheres or cerebellum. A history and careful neurologic examination should be performed to reveal recurrent neoplasm or a brain abscess, if possible. A history should elicit symptoms referable to the anatomic location of the area of radionecrosis. With radionecrosis of the brain, there is usually none of the papilledema that characterizes recurrent brain tumors, which produce increased intracranial pressure. A cerebral angiogram or pneumoencephalogram may reveal only an avascular mass lesion, without characteristic findings of a brain tumor. A CT scan may demonstrate a low density area with irregular contrast enhancement, suggestive of radiation necrosis (a glioma may produce a similar appearance, however). No repeat radiotherapy course should be given without biopsy proof of recurrent neoplasm, if at all possible, due to the extreme risks run in re-irradiating an area of brain necrosis.

Rarely, late secondary neoplasms (primary brain tumors or fibrosarcomas) have occurred after radiotherapy to the brain or pituitary regions, but these have usually been noted in patients who were re-treated with orthovoltage irradiation.

Spinal Cord

Following spinal cord irradiation, Lhermitte's syndrome may occur 1 to 6 months after the completion of radiation therapy. This self-limited syndrome, characterized by lightning-like sensations along the spine with head flexion, appears to have no relationship to severe late postirradiation spinal cord sequelae. The rare but extremely serious complication of radiation myelitis usually occurs 6 to 15 months or more after the completion of radiation therapy and may be associated with progressive paresis, paralysis, and, if severe, ultimately loss of bowel and/or bladder function. There is usually a sensory level at the site of prior irradiation. A careful neurologic examination is mandatory. In radiation myelitis the process is localized to an area that received prior high-dose irradiation, there is no evidence of metastatic carcinoma, appropriate radiographs do not demonstrate metastases, a lumbar puncture is usually normal, CSF cytology is negative, and a *myelogram is normal*. Radiation myelitis is rarely seen unless doses of 5000 rads in 5 weeks or its equivalent are given to the spinal cord. There is no known effective therapy. Spinal cord injury due to trauma, a primary spinal cord neoplasm, vascular accident, or metastatic carcinoma must be ruled out when myelitis is suspected.

D.G.

Brisman J, Roberson G, Davis K: Radiation necrosis of the brain. Neuroradiological considerations with computed tomography. Neuroradiol 12:109–113, 1976.
In the 3 patients studied CT revealed a low density area with irregular contrast enhancement.

Carmel R, Kaplan H: Mantle Irradiation in Hodgkin's disease. Cancer 37:2813-2825, 1976.
Pericarditis (asymptomatic cardiac enlargement) occurred in only 2.5% of patients treated with a subcarinal block.

Cram A, Pearlman N, Jochimsen P: Surgical management of complications of radiation-injured gut. Am J Surg 133:551-553, 1977.
In 1824 patients who had abdominal XRT gut radiation injury occurred in 89 (5.1%). Surgery was needed in 31 of the 89 (35%).

Donaldson S: Nutritional consequences of radiotherapy. Cancer Res 37:2407-2413, 1977.
All aspects of radiation injury and nutrition are reviewed.

Fajardo L: Radiation induced coronary artery disease. Chest 71:563-564, 1977.
This is a rare complication, only 16 reported cases. It is difficult to produce experimentally with radiation alone.

Fuks Z, Glatstein E, Marsa G, et al: Long-term effects of external radiation on the pituitary and thyroid glands. Cancer 37:1152-1161, 1976.
In previously untreated Hodgkin's disease thyroid dysfunction occurred in 64% of patients. In previously untreated head and neck cancers 48% of patients had thyroid dysfunction.

Goffinet D, Schneider M, Glatstein E, et al: Bladder cancer—results of radiation therapy in 384 patients. Radiology 117:149-153, 1975.
Report analyzes acute bladder and chronic bowel complications secondary to XRT.

Green N, Iba G, Smith W: Measures to minimize small intestine injury in the radiated pelvis. Cancer 35:1633-1640, 1975.
Prone treatment position (to minimize amount of small bowel in pelvis) and careful attention to total XRT dose and volume of irradiation are recommended.

Grise J, Rubin P, Ryplansky A, et al: Factors influencing response to recovery of grafted skin to ionizing radiation: Experimental observations. Am J Roentgenol 83:1087-1096, 1960.
Article goes into effects of XRT on skin grafts.

Gross N: Pulmonary effects of radiotherapy. Ann Intern Med 86:81-92, 1977.
Pulmonary effects of radiation are related to the volume irradiated and radiation dose. Exacerbating factors are concomitant chemotherapy, steroid withdrawal, and repeat radiation courses.

Kopelson G, Herwig K: The etiologies of coronary artery disease in cancer patients. Int J Radiat Oncol Biol Phys 4:895-906, 1978.
In this literature review 10 young patients with CAD after XRT are studied.

Levene M, Harris J, Hellman S: Treatment of carcinoma of the breast by radiation therapy. Cancer 39:2840-2845, 1977.
Sixteen of 150 patients who underwent radiation therapy had complications (10.7%): rib or clavicle fractures, radiation pneumonitis, or skin desquamation.

Libshitz H, Southard M: Complications of radiotherapy: The thorax. Semin Roentgenol 9:41-49, 1974.
This is a review article in an issue devoted to radiation effects and complications.

Luxton R, Kunkler P: Radiation nephritis. Acta Radiol 2:169-178, 1962.
This is a classic description of radiation nephritis.

Regezzi J, Courtney R, Kerr D: Dental management of patients irradiated for oral cancer. Cancer 38:994-1000, 1976.
In this study of 130 patients all aspects of management are reviewed.

Samann N, Bakdash M, Caderao J, et al: Hypopituitarism after external irradiation. Ann Intern Med 83:771–777, 1975.
*Fourteen of 15 patients irradiated for nasopharyngeal neoplasms had evidence
of endocrine deficiency.*

Stewart J, Fajardo L: Dose response in human and experimental radiation-
induced heart disease. Radiology 99:403–408, 1971.
This is a clinical and laboratory study of radiation-induced heart disease.

VonEssen C: A spatial model of time-dose area relationships in radiation
therapy. Radiology 81:881–883, 1963.
*This article discusses XRT dose-time volume relationships re tumor cures and
effects on skin.*

Wara W, Phillips T, Margolis L, Smith V: Radiation pneumonitis: A new
approach to the derivation of time-dose factors. Cancer 32:547–552, 1973.
*The recommendations of this report are that 1500 rads in 10 fractions to whole
lung (with a drug such as actinomycin D) and 2500 rads in 20 fractions
without drugs are the maximum radiation doses.*

Wolf E, Berdon W, Cassady J, et al: Slipped femoral capital epiphysis as a
sequela to childhood irradiation for malignant tumors. Radiology 125:781–
784, 1977.
*Five patients whose XRT ports included the femoral head and neck developed
this complication.*

90. CHEMOTHERAPY—PRINCIPLES

The success of cancer chemotherapy depends upon several factors: the relative
antitumor activity of a given agent; its mechanism of action; its dose, schedule,
and route of administration; its interaction with other drugs or other treatment
modalities; its acute and chronic toxicities for the host; and the biology of the
tumor itself. The clinical factors that are used to judge antitumor activity
include the response rate, freedom-from-relapse or remission duration, and
survival. The response rate may be composed of pathologically documented
complete responders (CRs), in which case biopsy proof of remission is required;
clinical CRs, for which clinical assessment is all that is required; and partial
responders (PRs), in which case tumor diameters are monitored (usually a reduction in size of >50% in the product of the two largest perpendicular dimensions). In some series, patients with stable disease or symptomatic improvement may even be considered responders. Furthermore, response rates may be
affected by a multitude of variables, such as prior therapy, tumor histopathology, disease extent or site, and age. To date in vitro methods of evaluating
antitumor activity are rudimentary but promising. The remission duration and
survival curves may demonstrate cure or prolongation of survival. Even if there
is no significant improvement in survival, however, there may be palliative
benefit (for example, reduction in pain or shortness of breath).

Depending upon their mechanisms of action, antitumor agents may affect
both proliferating and resting tumor cells (nonspecific agents), proliferating
cells only (cycle-specific), or only a portion of the proliferative pool (phase-
specific). Animal studies have shown that the effectiveness of phase-specific
drugs depends upon a repeating schedule or infusion, whereas cycle-specific
drugs are most effective in large single doses. In order to maximize cell kill,
these drug regimens must be repeated for a number of cycles, and the interval
between cycles must be long enough to allow recovery of normal elements.

Drugs used in combination should be individually active and ideally should have different mechanisms of action. If two drugs have the same mechanism of action, their antitumor activity is usually greatest when they are administered at separate times. When combinations are employed, full single-agent drug doses should be given whenever possible, and overlapping drug toxicities avoided. Drug scheduling can often minimize overlapping toxicity (e.g., myelo-suppression).

The toxicities of chemotherapy may be enhanced or ameliorated by the administration of other drugs. For example, the nephrotoxicity of methotrexate may be exacerbated by the aminoglycoside antibiotics or cis-Diamminedichloroplatinum but is diminished by alkalinization and hydration. In addition, combined modality approaches may produce enhanced or unexpected toxicities (for example, the increased risk of congestive cardiomyopathy following Adriamycin and mediastinal irradiation, and the increased risk of acute nonlymphocytic leukemia following combined chemotherapy and irradiation for Hodgkin's disease).

Whenever cancer chemotherapy is considered, one must ask whether the benefits of treatment outweigh the potential acute and chronic toxicities. When cure or improved survival is the goal, then more acute toxicity may be acceptable than if the goal is only palliation. With prolonged survival or the potential for cure, however, chronic or delayed toxicities become important, particularly if there are two equally effective drug regimens. These considerations are even more important when drugs are administered in the adjuvant setting. Here there is no clinically apparent tumor, just the probability of persistent disease. Therefore some patients will receive chemotherapy who have already been cured by surgery or irradiation and are subject only to its toxicities and not its benefits.

Besides tumor histology, tumor burden is an important prognostic variable in animal studies. Small tumors have a higher proportion of proliferating cells and are more sensitive to chemotherapy than large tumors, and often large tumors have diminished blood flow and poor drug distribution as well. Adjuvant chemotherapy attempts to maximize this biologic difference by treating microscopic disease only. Factors that reduce the effectiveness of chemotherapy in experimental animals include increasing primary tumor stage, prolonging interval from primary treatment to chemotherapy initiation, and decreasing effective drug dosage.

Drug resistance may develop for several reasons: inherent resistance of the tumor cell population at initiation of treatment, spontaneous mutation (occurring in $1/10^6$ cells), alteration of the cellular membrane to decrease permeability, enhanced drug metabolism, and other intracellular mechanisms of resistance. Animal data suggest that a major cause of chemotherapy failure after initial tumor response is the selection of drug-resistant tumor cells and their rapid regrowth. This has led to the conclusion that combinations of drugs are superior to single agents and that drug scheduling as well as dose is a critical factor.

C.P.

Capizzi RL, Keiser LW, Sartorelli AC: Combination chemotherapy—theory and practice. Semin Oncol 4:227–253, 1977.
   An excellent review of pharmacologic principles.
Carter SK: The analysis of adjuvant trials. Cancer Treat Rev 5:1–5, 1978.
   A critique of clinical studies.
Mihich E, Grindey GB: Multiple basis of combination chemotherapy. Cancer 40:534–543, 1977.
   A clear discussion.

Norton L, Simon R: Tumor size, sensitivity to therapy, and design of treatment schedules. Canccr Treat Rep 61:1307–1317, 1977.
Given here is a mathematical hypothesis, based on cell kinetics, that suggests that microscopic disease is more resistant to chemotherapy than macroscopic disease.

Salmon SE, Hamburger AW, Soehnlen B, et al: Quantitation of differential sensitivity of human-tumor stem cells to anticancer drugs. N Engl J Med 298:1321–1327, 1978.
Article describes laboratory methods and preliminary clinical correlations in 18 patients.

Schabel FM Jr: Rationale for adjuvant chemotherapy. Cancer 39:2875–2882, 1977.
Experience with adjuvant chemotherapy in animal model systems is given.

Skipper HE, Schabel FM Jr, Lloyd HH: Experimental therapeutics and kinetics: Selection and overgrowth of specifically and permanently drug-resistant tumor cells. Semin Hematol 15:207–219, 1978.
This article discusses animal studies and the strategy of intensification chemotherapy.

Tannock I: Cell kinetics and chemotherapy: A critical review. Cancer Treat Rep 62:1117–1133, 1978.
This report emphasizes the difficulty of applying animal studies directly to man.

Valeriote FA, Edelstein MB: The role of cell kinetics in cancer chemotherapy. Semin Oncol 4:217–226, 1977.
A general introduction to the subject of cell kinetics in cancer chemotherapy is provided here.

Warren RD, Bender RA: Drug interactions with antineoplastic agents. Cancer Treat Rep 61:1231–1241, 1977.
Laboratory and clinical data on drugs and antineoplastic agents are summarized.

Weiss RB, DeVita VT: Multimodal primary cancer treatment (adjuvant chemotherapy)—current results and future prospects. Ann Intern Med 91:251–260, 1979.
This article is a review of laboratory and clinical data on multimodal cancer treatment.

91. ALKYLATING AGENTS—CYCLOPHOSPHAMIDE

The alkylating agents are a diverse group of drugs that share a common ability to undergo strongly electrophilic chemical reactions to form covalent linkages with nucleophilic substances. Their clinical cytotoxicity results from their effects on nucleic acids (DNA and RNA) and, in particular, alkylation at the 7-position of guanine. The molecular events may include miscoding of DNA, since alkylated guanine codes for thymine rather than cytosine; imidazole ring cleavage or depurination with DNA scission; and cross-linkage of two adjacent nucleic acid chains by bifunctional agents. Although the alkylating agents are not cell cycle–specific and may act on cells at any stage in the cell cycle, they are proliferation-dependent and express their toxicity when the cell enters S-phase. Drugs that are members of this class include: mechlorethamine (nitrogen mustard), cyclophosphamide, chlorambucil, melphalan, busulfan, thiotepa, the nitrosoureas, DTIC, and *cis*-Diamminedichloroplatinum. Even though they are all alkylating agents, resistance to one drug does not necessarily predict resistance to another. The mechanisms of resistance are unknown but may be due to increased DNA repair and/or increased production of nucleophilic substances by the cell, which act as a "sink" to protect DNA.

Cyclophosphamide is the most commonly used alkylating agent. It has a broad spectrum of antitumor activity, against carcinomas of the breast, lung, ovary, and cervix as well as against sarcomas and lymphomas. The drug may be administered orally or intravenously but must be hepatically metabolized for activation. The active principles are phosphoramide mustard and acrolein. Both the active metabolites and the unchanged parent compound are excreted in the urine. Like most alkylating agents, the major dose-limiting toxicity of cyclophosphamide is bone marrow depression. The myeloid series is more often affected than the other elements. Nadir leukopenia occurs at 10 to 14 days after bolus administration, with recovery within 3 to 4 weeks. Other frequently found toxicities include alopecia, mucositis, nausea, and vomiting. Sterile, hemorrhagic cystitis may occur in up to 10% of patients receiving cyclophosphamide and is thought to be secondary to the renal excretion of active alkylating metabolites. The bladder may develop chronic inflammatory changes, with fibrosis and telangiectasia. If the drug is not discontinued after the development of hemorrhagic cystitis, the bladder changes may be progressive, and life-threatening hemorrhage may arise. Fluids and frequent emptying of the bladder are recommended during drug therapy. Some other reported toxicities of cyclophosphamide include the syndrome of inappropriate antidiuretic hormone secretion with water intoxication during vigorous hydration and diuresis; the development of cardiomyopathy at high dosage; and pulmonary fibrosis.

In addition to myelosuppression, other side-effects that are often seen with alkylating agents are infertility (particularly in males) and immunodepression. Recently it has been emphasized that acute nonlymphocytic leukemia may occur following alkylating agent therapy.

C.P.

Carter SK, Livingston RB: Cyclophosphamide in solid tumors. Cancer Treat Rev 2:295–322, 1975.
   A comprehensive review of the single agent activity of cyclophosphamide and its role in combination chemotherapy programs.
Reimer RR, Hoover R, Fraumeni JF, Young RC: Acute leukemia after alkylating-agent therapy of ovarian cancer. N Engl J Med 297:177–181, 1977.
   The relative risk of developing leukemia was significantly increased with this therapy, particularly in those women surviving for 2 years.
Schabel FM Jr, Trader MW, Laster WR Jr, Wheeler GP, Witt MH: Patterns of resistance and therapeutic synergism among alkylating agents. Antibiot Chemother 23:200–215, 1978.
   This report discusses the animal data that support the lack of cross-resistance among alkylating agents.
Sherins RJ, DeVita VT Jr: Effect of drug treatment for lymphoma on male reproductive capacity: Studies of men in remission after therapy. Ann Intern Med 79:216–220, 1973.
   Of 16 men studied, 12 had azospermia or oligospermia after therapy.
Wall RL, Clausen KP: Carcinoma of the urinary bladder in patients receiving cyclophosphamide. N Engl J Med 293:271–273, 1975.
   Article reports on 5 patients receiving cyclophosphamide and suggests an etiologic relationship.

5-Fluorouracil (5-FU) is a fluorinated pyrimidine with single agent activity against carcinomas of the colon, stomach, pancreas, breast, and ovary. Its mechanism of action is the inhibition of thymidylate synthetase with subsequent inhibition of DNA synthesis. Following administration of 5-FU, the drug is rapidly converted to a series of metabolites, including 5-fluorouridine, 5-fluorodeoxyuridine, 5-fluorouridine monophosphate (FUMP), and 5-fluorodeoxyuridine monophosphate (FdUMP). It is FdUMP that binds covalently to the active center of thymidylate synthetase and produces 5-FU's lethal action. Although FUMP is incorporated into RNA as well, it does not appear to contribute significantly to the lethal mechanism of 5-FU. Neither FUMP nor FdUMP crosses cell membranes, therefore their formation must occur within the target cell in order for 5-FU to have tumoricidal activity. If there is rapid catabolism of 5-FU or deletion of the enzymes capable of converting 5-FU to FdUMP, then apparent tumor resistance will develop. Other proposed mechanisms of 5-FU resistance include altered affinity of thymidylate synthetase for FdUMP; a rapid accumulation of deoxyuridine monophosphate, which leads to the protection of newly synthesized thymidylate synthetase from FdUMP inhibition; and an increased velocity of thymidylate synthetase production, serving to overcome FdUMP inhibition.

5-FU diffuses rapidly into all tissue compartments and has a volume of distribution equivalent to the total body water. The drug also enters the central nervous system and is detectable in cerebrospinal fluid after intravenous administration. Peak plasma levels of 10^{-3} to 10^{-4} Molar are obtained after a single intravenous dose of 15 mg/kg with a plasma half-life of only 10 to 20 minutes. 5-FU is primarily eliminated by hepatic metabolic degradation, with the remainder excreted by the kidneys. Since there is a dual route of elimination, modification of drug dose for hepatic or renal dysfunction is unnecessary.

Objective response rates to single agent 5-FU therapy hover around 20% for susceptible neoplasms. Because response rates and remission durations are low and brief, assessment of optimal drug dose and schedule is difficult. It appears that the most effective dose is 10 to 15 mg/kg IV, administered daily as an intensive 5-day course, repeated every 4 to 6 weeks. Other schedules include a (5-day or more) loading course followed by weekly therapy, weekly therapy without an initial loading course, and continuous intravenous infusion. Oral 5-FU is erratically absorbed and produces widely variable plasma levels; clinical trials have demonstrated its inferiority to intravenous therapy. Direct hepatic artery 5-FU infusion has also been used for the treatment of hepatic metastases (discussed in Part VII, Chapter 110), but has not been clearly shown superior to intravenous 5-FU.

The toxicities of 5-FU include nausea, vomiting, diarrhea, stomatitis, alopecia, leukopenia, thrombocytopenia, and neurotoxicity. All these side-effects are rapidly reversible and should be closely monitored with loading course therapy. Neurotoxicity occurs in approximately 2% of patients and is characterized by somnolence, cerebellar ataxia, and pyramidal tract signs. There is chromatolysis of neurons in the olivary and dentate nuclei as well as diffuse loss of neurons in the granular layer of the cerebellum. These changes are attributed to the formation of fluorocitrate, a neurotoxic metabolite.

C.P.

Ansfield G, Klotz J, Nealon T, et al: A phase III study comparing the clinical utility of four regimens of 5-fluorouracil: A preliminary report. Cancer 39:34–40, 1977.

An intravenous loading course of 5-FU achieved a significantly better objective response rate (33%) and remission duration (median of 20 weeks) as compared to weekly intravenous or oral schedules (<15%, median of 10-15 weeks) in 198 patients with metastatic colorectal cancer.

Hahn RG, Moertel CG, Schutt AJ, Bruckner HW: A double-blind comparison of intensive course 5-fluorouracil by oral vs. intravenous route in the treatment of colorectal carcinoma. Cancer 35:1031–1035, 1975.

In this 100-patient study the objective response (19.1% vs. 26%) and response duration (11.1 weeks vs 20 weeks) were superior for the intravenous route of drug administration.

Moertel CG: Chemotherapy of gastrointestinal cancer. Clin Gastroenterol 5:777–793, 1976.

This broad overview discusses 5-FU therapy.

Myers CE, Diasio R, Eliot HM, Chabner BA: Pharmacokinetics of the fluoropyrimidines: Implications for their clinical use. Cancer Treat Rev 3:175–183, 1976.

An excellent review of 5-fluorouracil.

93. METHOTREXATE

Methotrexate is a folate antagonist that inhibits dihydrofolate reductase, thus stopping the conversion of folic acid to reduced folate cofactors. These reduced folates are necessary for the biosynthesis of both DNA and RNA precursors; and it is the inhibition of thymidylate synthesis with its subsequent inhibition of DNA synthesis that appears to be methotrexate's primary mechanism of action. Since the drug acts by inhibiting DNA synthesis, methotrexate is highly cell cycle–dependent and primarily affects those cells that are in S-phase. Consequently tumor insensitivity is most often related to a low number of cells in S-phase. However, other possible mechanisms of drug resistance include an inability to transport methotrexate across the cell membrane, an increase in the production of dihydrofolate reductase, and the formation of a "resistant" form of dihydrofolate reductase.

Methotrexate was one of the first antineoplastic agents used in clinical practice. Currently it is employed in the treatment of choriocarcinoma, breast cancer, squamous carcinomas of the head and neck, osteogenic sarcoma, lymphomas, leukemias, and meningeal tumor. In addition it is sometimes prescribed for psoriasis, rheumatoid arthritis, dermatomyositis, and Wegener's granulomatosis. A number of treatment regimens have been developed, including low-dose methotrexate (intermittent or continuous), high-dose methotrexate (bolus or infusion) with citrovorum factor rescue, and intrathecal methotrexate. Whether high-dose schedules with citrovorum factor rescue are superior (in terms of single agent tumor response and remission duration) to those that use low-dose methotrexate without rescue remains an unsettled question. The standard low-dose schedule is 2.5 to 10 mg/day or 40 to 80 mg/M^2/week, titrated to tumor response and host toxicity.

High-dose methotrexate schedules with citrovorum factor (CF) rescue were developed to take advantage of possible increased intracellular drug concentration, selective rescue of normal cells, and the potential amelioration of host toxicity. Citrovorum factor (i.e., leucovorin or folinic acid) is converted to tetrahydrofolate and enters the reduced folate cycle distal to the enzymatic block caused by methotrexate, thus allowing the repletion of reduced folate stores. It is not known, however, whether CF can selectively rescue normal cells without also rescuing tumor cells at the same time.

Host toxicity of methotrexate is correlated with drug exposure of those tissues with rapid cell proliferation (large numbers of cells in S-phase), such as the bone marrow, gastrointestinal tract, and skin. The severity of these toxic effects is dependent upon the duration of drug exposure (thus affecting more cells entering S-phase) at plasma concentrations greater than 8×10^{-8} Molar and not just the peak plasma levels achieved. Citrovorum factor is effective in ameliorating methotrexate's toxicity if initiated within 42 hours of drug administration and continued until the plasma levels of methotrexate fall below 8×10^{-8} Molar. If CF is not begun promptly or is discontinued prematurely, then irreversible host toxicities may develop.

High-dose methotrexate is fraught with additional hazard because the drug is excreted unchanged in the urine; and at high concentrations it has limited solubility, which may lead to tubular precipitation of methotrexate and renal dysfunction. With reduced excretion, there is prolonged drug exposure at elevated plasma levels, as well as a potential for increased drug toxicity. Therefore high-dose programs require close monitoring of renal function, methotrexate plasma levels, state of hydration, and urinary output. Alkalinization of the urine also helps to prevent renal drug precipitation. When reduced renal function is demonstrated, excess toxicity may possibly be avoided by increasing the dose of CF administered. Hemodialysis is an inefficient means of removing methotrexate and is limited to the anuric patient; peritoneal dialysis is of no value. In addition to renal dysfunction, other toxicities associated with high-dose methotrexate include vomiting, acute desquamative dermatitis, seizures, vasculitis of the hands and feet, and reactivation of solar dermatitis or of prior radiation injury. Chronic low-dose methotrexate has been associated with hepatic cirrhosis, interstitial pneumonitis, osteoporosis, and immunosuppression.

The use of methotrexate for intrathecal therapy is discussed in Part I, Chapter 6. After intrathecal administration methotrexate is slowly released into the plasma and may result in systemic toxicity if the plasma levels exceed 8×10^{-8} Molar. "Third space" reservoirs such as pleural effusions or ascites may also result in slow release of methotrexate, prolonged drug exposure, and increased host toxicity.

C.P.

Bertino JR: "Rescue" techniques in cancer chemotherapy: Use of leucovorin and other rescue agents after methotrexate treatment. Semin Oncol 4:203–216, 1977.
  This report discusses the use of citrovorum factor (leucovorin), thymidine, L-asparaginase, and carboxypeptidase G-1 as rescue agents.
Bleyer WA: The clinical pharmacology of methotrexate: New applications of an old drug. Cancer 41:36–51, 1978.
  An excellent review of all aspects.
Jaffe N, Frei E III, Traggis D, Watts H: Weekly high-dose methotrexate-citrovorum factor in osteogenic sarcoma: Pre-surgical treatment of primary tumor and of overt pulmonary metastases. Cancer 39:45–50, 1977.
  Of 9 patients with pulmonary disease, 5 obtained objective responses.
Pitman SW, Frei E III: Weekly methotrexate-calcium leukovorin rescue: Effect of alkalinization on nephrotoxicity; pharmacokinetics in the CNS; and use in CNS non-Hodgkin's lymphoma. Cancer Treat Rep 61:695–701, 1977.
  Describes the beneficial use of urinary alkalinization in 18 patients and the role of monitoring serum methotrexate levels.

Von Hoff DD, Rozencweig M, Louie AC, Bender RA, Muggia FM: "Single"-agent activity of high-dose methotrexate with citrovorum factor rescue. Cancer Treat Rep 62:233–235, 1978.
A brief synopsis of the reported activity of high-dose methotrexate.

94. CYTOSINE ARABINOSIDE

Cytosine arabinoside is a synthetic nucleoside that substitutes the sugar moiety arabinose for the ribose or deoxyribose of the naturally occurring nucleosides cytidine or deoxycytidine. The drug is used primarily in the treatment of acute nonlymphocytic leukemia (see Part V, Chapter 85), in which it has a single agent complete remission rate of approximately 25%. When it is used in combination chemotherapy programs with daunomycin, 6-thioguanine, and/or alkylating agents, the complete remission rate is in excess of 50%. In addition cytosine arabinoside may be administered intrathecally and has been used effectively for the treatment of meningeal leukemia (see Part I, Chapter 6).

Cytosine arabinoside is an S-phase specific–drug, inhibiting DNA synthesis only, without directly affecting RNA or protein synthesis. Its mechanism of action is the competitive inhibition of DNA polymerase by cytosine arabinoside triphosphate (Ara-CTP). The ara-nucleotides are also incorporated into DNA, but this is of lesser cytocidal importance. The mechanisms of drug resistance that have been demonstrated in vitro include a decreased affinity of DNA polymerase for Ara-CTP; increased intracellular pools of the competitive substrate for DNA polymerase (deoxycytidine triphosphate); and alterations in the levels of activating or degrading enzymes for cytosine arabinoside.

Cytosine arabinoside is inactive when orally administered because of rapid deamination in the gastrointestinal tract and liver. When given intravenously, it is inactivated rapidly, with an initial distribution half-time of 7 to 17 minutes followed by an elimination phase half-time of 30 to 200 minutes. The drug is deaminated in the liver by cytidine deaminase, and almost all the metabolic product, arabinosyl uracil, is recovered in the urine within 24 hours. Although cytosine arabinoside crosses the blood-brain barrier, the drug concentrations achieved are only 40% of plasma levels Therefore it is necessary to administer the drug intrathecally for treatment of meningeal disease.

Because cytosine arabinoside is an S-phase–specific drug and is rapidly deactivated after intravenous administration, its tumoricidal activity and host toxicities are dose- and duration-dependent. In order to affect rapidly proliferating cells, the drug must be administered in multiple repeated doses or as a continuous infusion. For example, following a single intravenous dose of 2 gm/M^2 there is no myelosuppression, whereas after a continuous infusion of 1 gm/M^2 for 48 to 96 hours there is severe myelosuppression. When it is given in doses of 1 to 3 mg/kg/day for 5 days, the nadir white blood cell count is found on day 8, with recovery by day 15.

In addition to myelosuppression, other toxicities of cytosine arabinoside include nausea, vomiting, and diarrhea; alopecia; mucositis; and transient elevations in liver transaminases. Hepatic dysfunction is documented in 10% to 20% of patients, with transaminase levels of 2 to 4 times normal. This abnormality is dose-related and is not a reason for discontinuing therapy. With intrathecal administration, cytosine arabinoside may cause arachnoiditis.

Investigative approaches to improving the therapeutic index of cytosine arabinoside include the concurrent use of tetrahydrouridine, a drug that inhibits cytidine deaminase and thereby prevents the deactivation of cytosine arabinoside; and the development of cyclocytidine, a "sustained-release" depot form of cytosine arabinoside.

C.P.

Cohen SS: The mechanisms of lethal action of arabinosyl cytosine (ara C) and arabinosyl adenine (ara A). Cancer 40:509–518, 1977.
A thorough discussion of these mechanisms is given.
Ho DHW: Potential advances in the clinical use of arabinosyl cytosine. Cancer Treat Rep 61:717–722, 1977.
A brief discussion of continuous infusion therapy is presented.

95. THE ANTHRACYCLINE ANTIBIOTICS—DAUNOMYCIN AND ADRIAMYCIN

The anthracycline antibiotics, daunomycin (daunorubicin) and Adriamycin (doxorubicin), are derived from the fermentation products of *Streptomyces peucetius* var. *caesius*. Structurally, Adriamycin is an analogue of daunomycin, differing from it only by the addition of a hydroxyl group attached to the alkyl side chain. Both drugs bind specifically to DNA by intercalation between adjacent base pairs, and inhibition of DNA synthesis appears to be their primary mechanism of action. In addition there is inhibition of DNA polymerase activity as well as disruption of RNA synthesis by template disordering and steric changes, with subsequent inhibition of protein synthesis. Following intravenous administration there is rapid tissue distribution without drug penetration of the central nervous system. Both drugs are primarily metabolized by the liver, then excreted in the bile. Approximately one-half of administered Adriamycin is excreted unchanged and another 30% excreted as conjugates. Due to Adriamycin's hepatic metabolism and excretion, preexistent hepatic dysfunction can lead to significant prolongation of the plasma levels of Adriamycin and its metabolites. As a result, clinical drug toxicity is exaggerated and may be severe. Therefore dose reduction is indicated when there is elevation of the plasma bilirubin (with a total bilirubin of 1.2 to 3 mg/100 ml, there should be a 50% reduction; and with >3 mg/100 ml, a 75% reduction). The anthracyclines are also excreted in the urine; however, this represents only 10% of the total drug administered and is of little consequence when there is abnormal renal function.

Although daunomycin and Adriamycin are similar in their chemical structure and pharmacology, they are very different in their clinical activity and usefulness. Daunomycin has a narrow therapeutic index due to severe myelosuppression and is limited to the treatment of acute leukemia. On the other hand Adriamycin has acceptable clinical toxicity and is active against a broad range of malignancies. Single agent objective response rates of 20% to 40% have been reported for such diverse diseases as sarcomas, breast cancer, lung cancer, lymphoma, neuroblastoma, acute leukemia, testicular cancer, ovarian cancer, and bladder cancer. The usual dose of Adriamycin is 60 mg/M^2 intravenously once every 3 or 4 weeks. There appears to be a dose-response relationship for this intermittent schedule, with single doses in excess of 60 mg/M^2 conferring no increased response benefit.

The clinical toxicities of the anthracycline antibiotics include dose-limiting myelosuppression (particularly leukopenia and thrombopenia); gastrointestinal distress with nausea, vomiting, and diarrhea; mucositis; universal alopecia; reactivation of radiation injury (such as dermatitis, esophagitis); intravenous extravasation tissue damage; and cardiac toxicity. Because of Adriamycin's clinical usefulness, cardiotoxicity has been extensively investigated. There are both early toxicities and late effects. The acute cardiac changes that may be seen include pericarditis-myocarditis (which is fatal in 25% of affected patients); acute reversible congestive heart failure; rhythm disturbances, most commonly sinus tachycardia; and possible drug-induced vasospasm (myocardial infarction has been reported). The late cardiac toxicity is subclinical or overt left ventricular dysfunction, which may be irreversible. This abnormality is related to cumulative drug dose administered, and below a total dose of 500 mg/M² the incidence of clinical cardiotoxicity is low. In addition there is some evidence suggesting that a low-dose weekly schedule rather than a high-dose intermittent one may reduce the risk of cardiotoxicity above a cumulative dose of 500 mg/M². Factors that may contribute to the development of congestive cardiomyopathy include prior mediastinal irradiation (particularly above 4000 rads), age greater than 70 years, concurrent cyclophosphamide, and other underlying heart disease.

Serial endomyocardial biopsy studies have demonstrated progressive, dose-related myocyte damage with repetitive drug administration. Myocyte changes include myofibrillar loss and vacuolar degeneration followed by focal cell death with no inflammatory cell infiltrate. The amount of myocyte damage has also been correlated with the development of congestive heart failure; however, the myocardial degenerative process begins prior to any functional abnormality of left ventricular function. Noninvasive methods such as electrocardiogram (decreased voltage), echocardiography, systolic time interval determination, and radionuclide angiocardiography are relatively insensitive indicators of Adriamycin myocardial damage. Left ventricular dysfunction may occur late, and often precipitously, without early clinical warning. Invasive studies such as right-heart catheterization and endomyocardial biopsy are better early predictors of cardiotoxicity, but in most settings they are impractical. Limiting the total cumulative dose to 450 mg/M², following the noninvasive parameters of left ventricular function (as listed above), and paying special attention to those at high risk will reduce the risk of congestive heart failure in most patients.

C.P.

Alexander J, Dainiak N, Berger HJ, et al: Serial assessment of doxorubicin cardiotoxicity with quantitative radionuclide angiocardiography. N Engl J Med 300:278–283, 1979.
  Of 55 patients studied, 5 had severe cardiotoxicity preceded by a decline in left ventricular ejection fraction to ≤45%.
Billingham ME, Mason JW, Bristow MR, Daniels JR: Anthracycline cardiomyopathy monitored by morphologic changes. Cancer Treat Rep 62:865–872, 1978.
  Article describes histopathological endomyocardial changes and presents a pathology grading scale.
Blum RH, Carter SK: Adriamycin: A new anticancer drug with significant clinical activity. Ann Intern Med 80:249–259, 1974.
  A complete review of Adriamycin.
Bristow MR, Billingham ME, Mason JW, Daniels JR: Clinical spectrum of anthracycline antibiotic cardiotoxicity. Cancer Treat Rep 62:873–879, 1978.
  A good summary with guidelines for cumulative drug administration is provided.

Bristow MR, Mason JW, Billingham ME, Daniels JR: Doxorubicin car-
  diomyopathy: Evaluation by phonocardiography, endomyocardial biopsy,
  and cardiac catheterization. Ann Intern Med 88:168–175, 1978.
  Studies performed in 33 adults to assess Adriamycin cardiac toxicity.
Bristow MR, Thompson PD, Martin RP, Mason JW, Billingham ME, Harrison
  DC: Early anthracycline cardiotoxicity. Am J Med 65:823–832, 1978.
  Eight patients with anthracycline cardiotoxicity are described.
O'Bryan RM, Baker LH, Gottlieb JE, et al: Dose response evaluation of ad-
  riamycin in human neoplasia. Cancer 39:1940–1948, 1977.
  In a study of 870 patients those given 60 mg/M² of Adriamycin every 3 weeks
  appeared to achieve the highest remission rate.
Reilly JJ, Neifeld JP, Rosenberg SA: Clinical course and management of
  accidental adriamycin extravasation. Cancer 40:2053–2056, 1977.
  Extravasation causes an intense inflammatory response, which may progress
  to full thickness skin loss and irreversible damage to underlying tendons and
  neurovascular structures.
Von Hoff DD, Rozencweig M, Slavik M: Daunomycin: An anthracycline antibiotic effective in acute leukemia. Adv Pharmacol Chemother 15:1–50, 1978.
  A comprehensive review of daunomycin is given.
Weiss AJ, Manthel RW: Experience with the use of adriamycin in combination with other anticancer agents using a weekly schedule, with particular
  reference to lack of cardiac toxicity. Cancer 40:2046–2052, 1977.
  63 patients receiving more than 600 mg/M² cumulative total dose of Adria-
  mycin are reported.

96. BLEOMYCIN

Bleomycin is an antitumor antibiotic isolated from *Streptomyces verticillus* and
consisting of a mixture of low molecular weight glycopeptides. The drug is
active in the treatment of testis cancer, squamous cell carcinomas (of the head
and neck, esophagus, uterine cervix, and penis), Hodgkin's disease, and non-
Hodgkin's lymphomas. Objective response rates range from 20% to 60%; however, remission durations are usually brief (<8 weeks).

The drug's mechanism of action is to inhibit DNA synthesis selectively by
inducing single-strand breaks in DNA. Thus, rapidly proliferating cells are
most sensitive to bleomycin, particularly during mitosis; and in vitro studies
have demonstrated progression delay during G_2, with subsequent cell syn-
chronization. Following intravenous infusion approximately 60% of the administered bleomycin is excreted unchanged in the urine. The remainder is
degraded by aminopeptidases present in the liver, kidneys, and malignant
tumor. Because the majority of drug is excreted unchanged, increased host
toxicity may be seen with renal dysfunction. Even with renal failure, however,
bleomycin cannot be detected in the blood 48 to 72 hours after bolus therapy
and is probably not dialyzable.

Bleomycin does not cause myelosuppression. Its host toxicities include transient fever, chills, nausea, and vomiting following drug administration. Rarely,
patients develop acute fulminant reactions characterized by profound fever,
hypotension, and sustained cardiorespiratory collapse. However, the most important clinical toxicities are pulmonary and mucocutaneous. It is of interest
that neither lung nor skin contain aminopeptidases necessary for bleomycin
degradation.

The pulmonary toxicity is characterized by the insidious onset of nonproductive cough, dyspnea, pleurisy, and sometimes fever. On physical examination

there may be bibasilar fine dry rales and, rarely, cyanosis. The chest x-ray may demonstrate a diffuse bibasilar interstitial pattern; and pulmonary function tests may reveal decreased diffusion capacity, vital capacity, and arterial oxygen saturation. Lung biopsy shows findings of diffuse alveolar damage progressing to interstitial pneumonitis. Electron microscopy reveals interstitial edema, collagen deposition, and the accumulation of fibroblasts. Type I alveolar epithelial cells disappear and type II cells proliferate. Tne alveoli contain proteinaceous material and a mixture of macrophages and type II cells. There is no known therapy for bleomycin pulmonary toxicity other than discontinuation of the drug. Lung function may improve after the drug is stopped; however, irreversible pulmonary toxicity and fatal acute respiratory failure have been reported. Patients at high risk for developing pulmonary toxicity include those over 70 years of age, with preexistent lung disease and prior or concurrent irradiation to the thorax. Single doses in excess of 25 mg/M^2 and total cumulative doses of more than 400 mg or 200 mg/M^2 have been associated with increased lung toxicity. Patients have developed lung damage after much smaller drug doses, however.

The cutaneous toxicity of bleomycin is manifested by reversible induration, erythema, and hyperpigmentation of the skin at points of stress and in scars. There may be exacerbation of prior radiation injury to the skin and/or mucous membranes resulting in erythema, desquamation, and ulceration. This is a particular problem in the treatment of head and neck neoplasms with resultant mucositis and/or esophagitis.

C.P.

Blum RH, Carter SK, Agre K: A clinical review of bleomycin—A new antineoplastic agent. Cancer 31:903–914, 1973.
Drug response and toxicity data in 1,174 patients are reviewed.
Broughton A, Strong JE, Holoye PY, Bedrossian CWM: Clinical pharmacology of bleomycin following intravenous infusion as determined by radioimmunoassay. Cancer 40:2772–2778, 1977.
Continuous infusion of bleomycin in 9 patients is studied.
DeLena M, Guzzon A, Monfardini S, Bonadonna G: Clinical, radiologic, and histopathologic studies on pulmonary toxicity induced by treatment with bleomycin (NSC-125066). Cancer Chemother Rep 56:343–356, 1972.
An excellent review of the experience in 168 patients.
Holoye PY, Luna MA, MacKay B, Bedrossian CWM: Bleomycin hypersensitivity pneumonitis. Ann Intern Med 88:47–49, 1978.
Article provides a report of 3 cases of this syndrome.
Krakoff IH, Cvitkovic E, Currie V, et al: Clinical pharmacologic and therapeutic studies of bleomycin given by continuous infusion. Cancer 40:2027–2037, 1977.
Toxicity and response results are compared to historical data of daily injection therapy.
Muller WEG, Zahn RK: Bleomycin, an antibiotic that removes thymine from double-stranded DNA. Prog Nucleic Acid Res Mol Biol 20:21–57, 1977.
A comprehensive review of the biochemistry of bleomycin.

97. THE VINCA ALKALOIDS—VINCRISTINE AND VINBLASTINE

The vinca alkaloids, vincristine and vinblastine, are dimeric indole-indoline–containing alkaloids derived from the periwinkle plant, *Vinca rosea*. They differ from one another by a single carbon, and both are related to colchicine, a tropolone alkaloid. Their mechanism of action is related to their ability to enter cells rapidly and quantitatively and bind to tubulin. Consequently those cellular processes that require intact microtubular systems are disrupted, including mitosis, maintenance of cell shape, and cell surface mobility. The most important event is mitotic arrest, which results in actual dissolution of the spindle structure rather than simple fixation of the mitotic apparatus in metaphase. Mitotic arrest is probably not the sole basis for cytotoxicity, however. Both drugs have been shown to inhibit RNA and protein synthesis in vitro, and vincristine inhibits DNA synthesis in vivo as well. Mechanisms of drug resistance have not been elucidated. It is of interest that there is no cross-resistance between vinblastine and vincristine.

Both drugs are available only as intravenous preparations, although vinblastine may be orally absorbed (albeit erratically). After intravenous administration, there is rapid clearing from the blood followed by biliary excretion (whether hepatic metabolism is clinically significant is not known). The biphasic half-lives in humans are approximately 5 minutes and 160 minutes, respectively. There is extensive binding of drug to leukocytes and platelets, with microtubular crystallization, forming cellular inclusions. Although both drugs are excreted in the bile, there are no established guidelines for dose modification. It is the usual practice, however, to reduce the dose with hepatic dysfunction.

The spectrum of single agent activity is different for the two agents; vincristine is used in the treatment of acute lymphoblastic leukemia, Wilms' tumor, Hodgkin's disease, non-Hodgkin's lymphomas, brain tumors, and choriocarcinoma; and vinblastine in neuroblastoma, histiocytosis X, carcinomas of the testis and breast, and Hodgkin's disease. Unlike vincristine (which causes no myelosuppression), the dose-limiting toxicity of vinblastine is myelosuppression. The granulocytes are affected primarily, with sparing of the platelets and erythrocytes. Nadir leukopenia is documented 4 to 7 days after therapy, with rapid recovery. The usual dose is 6 mg/M² intravenously every 1 to 3 weeks. Recently, high-dose vinblastine regimens have been developed for the treatment of testis cancer. At these doses myelosuppression may be severe, and the neurotoxicities commonly associated with vincristine may become evident.

These neurotoxicities include peripheral neuropathy with depressed deep tendon reflexes, paresthesias, motor weakness, sensory impairment, and muscle pain; autonomic neuropathy with constipation, abdominal pain, paralytic ileus, bladder atony, impotence, and orthostatic hypotension; cranial nerve dysfunction with ptosis, ophthalmoplegia, facial weakness, hoarseness, and loss of corneal reflex; mental changes such as depression, agitation, insomnia, and hallucinations; seizures (rarely); and the syndrome of inappropriate antidiuretic hormone production. There is no known treatment for these neurotoxicities other than modification or discontinuance of the drug. If these neurologic abnormalities are permitted to progress, they may become severe and, in some cases, irreversible. The neuropathy appears to be due to alterations in the neurotubular system with subsequent disruption of axon function. Because of the potential severity of neurotoxicity with vincristine the dose (1.4 mg/M²) is usually limited to 2 mg per injection and modified in the presence of preexisting neurologic impairment. Other toxicities of the vinca alkaloids include phlebitis, severe extravasation skin injury, and alopecia (with vincristine only).

C.P.

Bender RA, Castle MC, Margileth DA, Oliverio VT: The pharmacokinetics of {³H}-vincristine in man. Clin Pharmacol Ther 22:430–438, 1977.
A study in 4 patients of pharmacokinetics metabolism and excretion of labelled vincristine.

Holland JF, Scharlau C, Gailani S, et al: Vincristine treatment of advanced cancer: A cooperative study of 392 cases. Cancer Res 33:1258–1264, 1973.
Article describes single agent activity and host toxicities.

Krikorian JG, Daniels JR, Brown BW, Hu MSJ: Variables for predicting serious toxicity (vinblastine dose, performance status, and prior therapeutic experience):   Chemotherapy for metastatic testicular cancer with *cis*-dichlorodiammineplatinum (II), vinblastine, and bleomycin. Cancer Treat Rep 62:1455–1463, 1978.
Toxicity of the drug combination correlated best with the dose of vinblastine administered.

Rosenthal S, Kaufman S: Vincristine neurotoxicity. Ann Intern Med 80:733–737, 1974.
A good review.

98. NITROSOUREAS

The nitrosoureas are highly lipid soluble drugs, rapidly transported into cells and across the blood-brain barrier. Of the synthetic chloroethyl nitrosoureas, methyl-CCNU is the most lipid-soluble, CCNU is intermediate, and BCNU is the least lipid-soluble. After bolus administration all three drugs are rapidly distributed and metabolized by hepatic microsomal enzymes. The metabolites generated by the liver have both alkylating and carbamoylating activities; however, their cytotoxicity is probably related primarily to alkylation. They kill both cycling and noncycling cells, causing DNA strand breakage and altering RNA structure and function. The parent compounds, their active metabolites, and their degradation products are excreted primarily by the kidneys. Drug levels in the cerebrospinal fluid are approximately 15% to 30% of those found in the peripheral blood.

The antitumor activities are slightly different among the chloroethyl nitrosoureas. BCNU has activity in brain tumors, myeloma, lymphomas, melanoma, and carcinomas of the breast and stomach; CCNU has activity in brain tumors, lymphomas, and carcinomas of the lung and breast; and methyl-CCNU has activity in brain tumors, melanoma, and carcinomas of the colon and breast. The treatment-limiting toxicity of all three drugs is delayed, cumulative, bone marrow suppression. Following bolus administration, nadir platelet counts are encountered at 4 weeks and nadir granulocyte counts at 5 to 6 weeks. Recovery of all elements may require an additional 1 to 2 weeks. With subsequent drug administrations there is cumulative myelotoxicity, so that at a given dose there are lower and earlier nadirs as well as longer periods of myelosuppression. As a result the drug dosage must be attenuated with continued treatment as well as modified for prior radiation or chemotherapy. In addition to nausea and vomiting these drugs may cause stomatitis, alopecia, anemia, anorexia, abnormal liver function tests, and neuro-ophthalmologic toxicity. BCNU may also cause severe local phlebitis and rarely, pulmonary interstitial fibrosis. As single agents, these drugs are usually administered as follows: BCNU, 225 mg/M^2 IV every 6 weeks; CCNU, 130 mg/M^2 po every 6 weeks; and methyl-CCNU, 225 mg/M^2 po every 6 weeks.

Streptozotocin is a naturally occurring methyl nitrosourea isolated from the fermentation of *Streptomyces achromogenes*. Unlike the synthetic chloroethyl nitrosoureas, streptozotocin does not produce dose-limiting myelosuppression, and its major clinical usefulness is in the treatment of islet cell tumors, carcinoid, and Hodgkin's disease. Its treatment-limiting toxicity is renal dysfunction, first manifested by proteinuria, diminished creatinine clearance, and hypophosphatemia; and, if not discontinued, by progressive azotemia, renal glycosuria, and tubular acidosis. Although streptozotocin is toxic to pancreatic islet beta cells in rodents, there is no diabetogenic effect in man. The usual single agent dose is 1 gm/M^2 IV once per week.

C.P.

Aronin PA, Mahaley MS Jr, Rudnick SA, et al: Prediction of BCNU pulmonary toxicity in patients with malignant gliomas: An assessment of risk factors. N Engl J Med 303:183–188, 1980.
  Of 93 patients treated with BCNU, 20% developed symptomatic lung disease.
Schein PS, Heal J, Green D, Woolley PV: Pharmacology of nitrosourea antitumor agents. Antibiot Chemother 23:64–75, 1978.
  Article discusses mechanisms of action and the synthesis of new compounds.
Schein PS, O'Connell MJ, Blom J, et al: Clinical antitumor activity and toxicity of streptozotocin (NSC-85998). Cancer 34:993–1000, 1974.
  Retrospective evaluation of use of streptozotocin in 106 patients is provided.
Wasserman TH: The nitrosoureas: An outline of clinical schedules and toxic effects. Cancer Treat Rep 60:709–711, 1976.
  Summarizes effective dose schedules and drug toxicities.
Wasserman TH, Slavik M, Carter SK: Clinical comparison of the nitrosoureas. Cancer 36:1258–1268, 1975.
  A review of the comparative pharmacology and clinical efficacy of BCNU, CCNU and methyl-CCNU.

99. *CIS*-DIAMMINEDICHLOROPLATINUM (CDDP)

Cis-Diamminedichloroplatinum (CDDP) is an inorganic drug composed of a central atom of platinum surrounded by chlorine and ammonia atoms in the *cis* position. As a single agent CDDP produces objective responses in approximately two-thirds of patients with carcinoma of the testis or ovary and in one-third of those with bladder cancer or squamous carcinomas of the head and neck. It also has activity in pediatric neoplasms, prostate cancer, and osteogenic sarcoma. The drug's mechanism of action is not fully established. Although it is known that CDDP cross-links complementary strands of DNA and inhibits DNA synthesis in vitro, the drug does not demonstrate cell-cycle phase specificity. CDDP is handled biologically like other heavy metals. There is biphasic disappearance of the drug in humans, with an initial half-life of 40 minutes and a second phase half-life of 65 hours. CDDP is excreted in the urine, albeit slowly, with only 45% eliminated within the first 5 days following drug administration.

The dose-limiting toxicity of CDDP is nephrotoxicity manifested by a reduction in creatinine clearance without proteinuria or abnormalities in the urinary sediment. Renal biopsy demonstrates acute tubular necrosis with tubular degeneration and interstitial edema. The glomeruli appear normal. The mechanism of CDDP renal failure is unknown, and there is some data to suggest that the resultant renal damage may not be completely reversible. Nephrotoxicity appears to be at least partially ameliorated by hydration and forced diuresis (with furosemide or mannitol) and exacerbated by the concomitant use of other nephrotoxic drugs (such as aminoglycosides or methotrexate). With the usual drug dose of 50 to 75 mg/M^2 intravenously every 3 weeks, approximately 25% of patients may develop mild to moderate renal dysfunction, which is clinically reversible.

Other toxicities of CDDP include dose-related myelosuppression, nausea and vomiting (which may be severe), ototoxicity with tinnitus and high frequency hearing loss, occasional elevations in hepatic transaminases, peripheral neuropathy, and, rarely, anaphylaxis, seizures, and hemolysis.

C.P.

Dentino M, Luft FC, Yum MN, et al: Long term effect of cis-diammine-dichloride platinum (CDDP) on renal function and structure in man. Cancer 41:1274–1281, 1978.
   Subclinical renal dysfunction persisted in 7 patients for 2 years after therapy.
Getaz EP, Beckley S, Fitzpatrick J, Dozier A: Cisplatin-induced hemoly-sis. N Engl J Med 302:334–335, 1980.
   Report of two cases: cis-diamminedichloroplatinum was found to cause a positive direct-antiglobulin test and one patient developed overt hemolysis.
Madias NE, Harrington JT: Platinum nephrotoxicity. Am J Med 65:307–314, 1978.
   A complete review.
Prestayko AW, D'Aoust JCD, Issell BF, Crooke ST: Cisplatin (cis-diammine-dichloroplatinum II). Cancer Treat Rev 6:17–39, 1979.
   A review of the drug's therapeutic efficacy and pharmacology.
Rozencweig M, Von Hoff DD, Slavik M, Muggia FM: Cis-diammine-dichloroplatinum (II): A new anticancer drug. Ann Intern Med 86:803–812, 1977.
   Describes pharmacology, clinical use, and drug toxicities.

100. OTHER ANTINEOPLASTIC AGENTS AND MODALITIES

The following references discuss some of the other commonly used antineoplas-tic agents and modalities. An excellent summary of laetrile is included, since it is also administered, legally or illegally, to many cancer patients.

Bender RA, Zwelling LA, Doroshow JH, Locker GY, Hande KR, Murinson DS, Cohen M, Myers CE, Chabner BA: Antineoplastic drugs: Clinical phar-macology and therapeutic use. Drugs 16:46–87, 1978.
   Article provides an excellent discussion of alkylating agents, antibiotics, an-timetabolites, plant alkaloids, and epipodophyllotoxins.
Dorr RT, Paxinos J: The current status of laetrile. Ann Intern Med 89:389–397, 1978.
   This complete summary of laetrile includes a discussion of potential cyanide poisoning and its treatment.
Field SB, Bleehen NM: Hyperthermia in the treatment of cancer. Cancer Treat Rev 6:63–94, 1979.
   An excellent and complete review.
Goodnight JD, Morton DL: Immunotherapy for malignant disease. Annu Rev Med 29:231–283, 1978.
   An excellent review with exhaustive references.
Issell BF, Crooke ST: Etoposide (VP-16-213). Cancer Treat Rev 6:107–124, 1979.
   A review of therapeutic activity and pharmacology is given.
Kreis W: Hydrazines and triazenes. *In* FF Becker (Ed), Cancer: A comprehen-sive treatise. New York, Plenum Press, 1977. Vol. 5, pp. 489–519.
   The pharmacology of DTIC is presented in this chapter.

Mouridsen H, Pashof T, Patterson J, Battersby L: Tamoxifen in advanced breast cancer. Cancer Treat Rev 5:131–141, 1978
A comprehensive summary of clinical pharmacology and clinical trials.
Rozencweig M, Von Hoff DD, Henney JE, Muggia FM: VM 26 and VP 16-213: A comparative analysis. Cancer 40:334–342, 1977.
Reviews pharmacology, clinical efficacy and toxicity.
Spivack SD: Procarbazine. Ann Intern Med 81:795–800, 1974.
Discusses therapeutic efficacy and clinical pharmacology.

101. ORGAN-SPECIFIC CHEMOTHERAPY TOXICITIES

Toxicities of commonly used chemotherapeutic agents are discussed according to the specific drug utilized in Part VI, Chapters 91–99. The following references discuss potential acute and chronic toxicities according to the organ affected.

Cadman E: Toxicity of chemotherapeutic agents. *In* FF Becker (Ed), Cancer: A comprehensive treatise. New York, Plenum Press, 1977. Vol. 5, pp. 59–111.
A comprehensive summary.
Chapman RM, Rees LH, Sutcliffe SB, Edwards CRW, Malpas JS: Cyclical combination chemotherapy and gonadal function: Retrospective study in males. Lancet 1:285–289, 1979.
Only 4 of 74 males regained spermatogenesis following therapy for Hodgkin's disease.
Chapman RM, Sutcliffe SB, Malpas JS: Cytotoxic-induced ovarian failure in women with Hodgkin's disease: I. Hormone function. JAMA 242:1877–1881, 1979.
Complete or partial ovarian failure was documented in 34 of 41 women following combination chemotherapy.
Chapman RM, Sutcliffe SB, Malpas JS: Cytotoxic-induced ovarian failure in Hodgkin's disease: II. Effects on sexual function. JAMA 242:1882–1884, 1979.
41 patients with cytotoxic-induced ovarian failure are analyzed.
Friedman MA, Carter SB: Serious toxicities associated with chemotherapy. Semin Oncol 5:193–202, 1978.
Excellent compilation of drug toxicities according to antineoplastic agent.
Green MR: Pulmonary toxicity of antineoplastic agents. West J Med 127:292–298, 1977.
Article reviews clinical data on toxicity of these agents.
Levine N, Greenwald ES: Mucocutaneous side effects of cancer chemotherapy. Cancer Treat Rev 5:67–84, 1978.
A complete review of the clinical characteristics of mucocutaneous toxicities seen with antineoplastic agents.
Weiss HD, Walker MD, Wiernik PH: Neurotoxicity of commonly used antineoplastic agents. N Engl J Med 291:75–81; 127–133, 1974.
An excellent review.

In the treatment of malignant diseases, surgery may be used to debulk the primary cancer, and radiation therapy to eradicate tumor cells not only at and beyond the surgical margins, but also in the regional lymph nodes. Combined surgery and radiation therapy are often used in treating patients with certain head and neck, breast, bladder, colorectal and lung cancers, and soft tissue sarcomas, and in such pediatric tumors as Ewing's sarcoma and rhabdomyosarcomas. Radiation therapy may be given either preoperatively or postoperatively; in addition, the primary cancer may be irradiated, while the lymph nodes are treated surgically, or the primary cancer may be treated by surgery and the regional lymph nodes irradiated. Surgery may also be used to salvage recurrent cancers after full-dose irradiation, or radiotherapy may be used after surgical failure. Finally, surgery may increase the effectiveness of a planned course of radiation by relieving obstructions or by draining abscesses prior to radiotherapy. Each of these methods will be discussed.

Preoperative Irradiation
Preoperative irradiation is used to decrease the size of the tumor preoperatively, to destroy tumor cells in lymphatic transit, and (possibly) to decrease the incidence of distant metastases, tumor cell seeding, or shedding at the time of surgery. Radiotherapy may also decrease the capacity of the "tumor bed" to support postoperative tumor cell growth. With preoperative irradiation, the exact extent and size of the cancer is often not known. Wound healing may be decreased by high-dose preoperative irradiation (>4500–5000 rads), resulting in such increased complications as suture line disruptions, soft tissue necroses, and increased intraoperative hemorrhagic tendencies if the procedure is carried out too soon after high-dose irradiation. The hyperemia after high-dose preoperative irradiation usually resolves 1 to 2 weeks after the course is completed.

Postoperative Irradiation
With postoperative irradiation, the margins and extent of the cancer are known. Postoperative radiation therapy may also eradicate residual neoplasm at the surgical margins, destroy tumor cells seeded locally at the time of surgery, and sterilize unresectable lymph node or soft tissue disease. Postoperatively cancer cells may be hypoxic due to a diminished blood supply, with resultant decreased radiosensitivity. Surgical complications may be decreased by postoperative irradiation, but there appears to be a slightly increased risk of distant metastases when radiation treatments follow surgery. Wound breakdowns and fistula formation are rare if postoperative irradiation is begun after complete wound healing has occurred. When 49 patients with hypopharyngeal head and neck cancers randomly received either preoperative irradiation (5500 rads in 5½ weeks) or similar radiation doses postoperatively, significantly decreased survival and a greater incidence of postoperative complications were noted in the group that received preoperative irradiation. There were 6 carotid ruptures, a 38% incidence of soft tissue necroses and wound breakdowns, and an average hospitalization of 98 days in the group with preoperative irradiation; whereas no carotid ruptures occurred, necroses and wound breakdowns were less frequent, and an average hospitalization of only 23 days was necessary in the group which received postoperative radiotherapy.

In combined treatment, the total radiation therapy dose is an important variable. Two thousand to 3000 rads usually do not increase postoperative complications but also may not effectively eradicate cancer cells, whereas 4000 to 5000 rads (at 1000 rads per week) may be more effective in destroying neoplastic cells but may also increase the risk of complications. The anatomic location of the cancer is also important, since fewer postoperative complications arise in patients after buccopharyngeal surgery and irradiation than after laryngopharyngeal surgery and radiotherapy.

The extent and magnitude of the surgical procedure is also important; in a retrospective review, patients with laryngopharyngeal carcinomas who underwent *both* laryngectomy and radical neck dissection had a threefold increase in carotid ruptures compared to other patients who had laryngectomies but no radical neck dissections. Meticulous, careful surgical technique is also required: incisions must be placed properly, meticulous hemostasis and operative technique, careful wound closure to avoid carotid exposure, and placement of ostomies away from anticipated radiation fields are all mandatory.

Surgical Salvage
After a full-dose curative radiation attempt has failed, salvage operations are usually performed through tissues that have developed postirradiation fibrosis and a reduced blood supply. In a retrospective review of 155 patients with laryngopharyngeal cancers, however, major complication rates were similar in patients who received surgery alone, combined preoperative irradiation (5000 rads), or salvage surgery after radiotherapy failure. No increased incidence of complications was detected after postirradiation salvage surgery. Other authors believe, however, that surgery performed months to years after a radiation therapy course is associated with an increased risk of complications.

Radiotherapy Salvage
For many years, prior to the concept of combined modality cancer treatment, the primary use of radiotherapy was to treat surgical failures. This method is often less successful than planned combined treatment, especially for patients with advanced head and neck cancers.

Breast Irradiation
In the postoperative irradiation of breast carcinomas there is a 6% risk of such local complications as subcutaneous fibrosis, pathologic rib fractures, and radiation pneumonitis. These sequelae may be minimized by such careful setup and treatment techniques as minimizing the volume of lung irradiated in both the internal mammary and tangential chest wall radiation portals, treating all fields each day, limiting the weekly radiation dose to 900–1000 rads, and carefully positioning patients to avoid areas of overdosage or underdosage.

Abdominal Irradiation
Abdominal irradiation following resection of gastrointestinal malignancies may result in injury to the liver, genitourinary tract, gastrointestinal tract, or soft tissues. When anterior colorectal resections were performed and preoperative pelvic radiation doses of 5000 rads in 5 weeks were used, a retrospective review revealed a reduced local recurrence rate, fewer tumor-related deaths, and fewer fatal complications, but an increased incidence of postoperative adhesions, small bowel obstructions, and anastomotic leaks as compared to patients who underwent surgery alone. There were no differences in wound dehiscences or postoperative infection rates when the patients who received combined treatment were compared to those who had resection and not irradiation. When preoperative irradiation was used prior to abdominoperineal resections, there was no increase in postoperative complications in the irradiated group. When 62 patients received postoperative radiotherapy after resections of

colorectal cancers, complications were increased when an extended radiation field, from the pelvis to the L2 level, was irradiated (4 of 12 patients). Overall, 7 of the 62 patients (11%) developed radiation enteritis. Small bowel obstructions also occurred, from either adhesions, strictures, or radiation enteritis. Self-limited cystitis and proctitis were also noted. Postirradiation complications may be decreased by using careful setup techniques, avoiding extended field irradiation if possible in patients with pelvic carcinomas, and limiting large volume radiation doses to 5000 rads or less. Treatment techniques that minimize bowel irradiation by placing patients in the prone position, which tends to force the small bowel out of the pelvis during radiation treatments, are under investigation.

Irradiation of Extremities

When irradiating extremities, late radiation-induced morbidity may be minimized by sparing the medial-situated lymphatics and soft tissues to prevent girdling of the limb by radiation; treating multiple fields daily; using shrinking field techniques; and carefully immobilizing the limb during each radiation treatment. At least 75% of irradiated limbs may remain functional and pain-free (without excessive edema, fibrosis, joint immobility, or neurologic vascular injury) if these refinements of technique are adhered to.

Benefits of Combined Surgery and Irradiation

Patients who have undergone resections for lung cancer appear to have no greater risk of developing radiation pneumonitis, esophagitis, or pericarditis than patients who did not receive radiotherapy; and since the tumor was debulked, more lung may be spared, reducing the risks from radiation.

Surgery may also be necessary to increase the effectiveness of a curative course of radiation, for example, in transurethral resection of bladder or prostate cancers to relieve urinary obstruction prior to a radiation course. For certain patients with head and neck cancers, a preradiotherapy tracheostomy may be necessary, or dental extractions may be indicated to avoid osteoradionecrosis of the mandible. Patients with esophageal neoplasms may need feeding tubes or a gastrostomy, while fixation of impending pathologic fractures may be necessary prior to beginning radiotherapy.

D.G.

Cachin Y, Eschevage F: Combination of radiotherapy and surgery in the treatment of head and neck cancers. Cancer Treat Rev 2:177–191, 1975.
A complete review of preoperative and postoperative radiation therapy is provided.
Cady B: Pre-operative radiation. Surg Gynecol Obstet 126:851–868, 1968.
Older but comprehensive review.
Chung CT, Sagerman RH, King GA, et al: Complications of high dose preoperative irradiation for advanced laryngeal-hypopharyngeal cancer. Radiology 128:467–470, 1978.
In this retrospective analysis of 155 patients no significant differences in either major or minor postoperative complications were found in those receiving: (1) surgery alone, (2) planned 5000 rad preoperative radiation therapy, or (3) surgical salvage after failure of high-dose radiation therapy.
Kligerman MM: Radiotherapy and rectal cancer. Cancer 39:896–900, 1977.
Complications after abdominoperineal resections are similar in those having surgery alone or those having surgery and radiation therapy.
Potter JF: Preoperative irradiation and surgery for certain cancers. Cancer 35:84–90, 1975.

Article reviews experimental data and clinical trials in breast, lung, bladder, and colorectal cancer.

Romsdahl MM, Withers HR: Radiotherapy combined with curative surgery. Arch Surg 113:446–453, 1978.

There was an 11% complication rate (primarily radiation enteritis and/or bowel obstruction) with this therapeutic approach. Excessive complications (4/12) occurred in patients who received extended field radiation therapy to L2 levels. Authors recommend pelvic irradiation only.

Stevens KR, Fletcher WS, Allen CV: Anterior resection and primary anastomosis following high dose preoperative irradiation for adenocarcinoma of the rectosigmoid. Cancer 41:2065–2071, 1978.

There was no change in incidence of abdominal wound or dehiscence rates, but there was a higher frequency of anastomotic leaks, postoperative adhesions, and bowel obstructions in preoperatively irradiated patients compared to those having only surgery. But, there were fewer fatal complications, cancer deaths, and recurrences in the group undergoing preoperative irradiation.

Suit HD, Russell WO, Martin RG: Sarcoma of soft tissue: Clinical and histopathologic parameters and response to treatment. Cancer 35:1478–1483, 1975.

A retrospective analysis of 100 patients treated with radical irradiation or limited surgery plus irradiation; 75% of the patients retained a functional pain-free limb without edema.

Vandenbrouck C, Sancho H, LeFur R, et al: Results of a randomized clinical trial of preoperative irradiation versus postoperative in treatment of tumors of the hypopharynx. Cancer 37:1445–1449, 1977.

There was a statistically significant improvement in survival with fewer complications and shorter hospitalizations for the group randomly assigned to receive postoperative radiation therapy.

Weichselbaum RR, Marck A, Hellman S: The role of postoperative radiation in carcinoma of the breast. Cancer 37:2682–2690, 1976.

In 352 patients studied there was a 6.2% complication rate, including fibrosis, radiation pneumonitis, and rib fractures.

103. COMBINED MODALITY PROBLEMS—RADIATION THERAPY AND CHEMOTHERAPY

Increased normal tissue reactions may occur when chemotherapy and radiation therapy are combined. In some instances adjustments in radiation dose must be made to protect sensitive normal tissues from the combined side-effects of the two modalities. Radiation therapy is often used to treat both the primary cancer and the regional lymph nodes, while concomitant or sequential chemotherapy may improve the chances of local control but may also be used as an adjuvant to eradicate micrometastases. Untoward interactions of chemotherapy and radiation therapy have been reported for most anatomic sites. Combined modality interactions may produce hematologic toxicity, enhanced immunosuppression, increased local complications, and possibly an increased risk of developing late second neoplasms in certain situations. Further experience will be necessary to determine the ideal sequence of drug administration and radiotherapy to minimize normal tissue injury while still obtaining the desired antitumor effects. Untoward normal tissue effects may be decreased by administering drugs either before or after irradiation, but "recall" phenomena (heightened skin reactions), such as those reported with Adriamycin, may be noted when the drug is given after irradiation. Unfortunately, severe side-effects may occur long after the treatments have been completed; examples are cerebral leukoencephalopathy and the appearance of second neoplasms.

Some of the sites where heightened effects have been noted are as follows.

Breast

When 26 patients received postoperative irradiation to the regional lymph nodes and chest wall (5000 rads) and adjuvant CMF chemotherapy, marked skin reactions were seen in 81%; however, of 43 control patients who did not receive chemotherapy, only 33% developed similar skin reactions. There were no differences in tracheal or esophageal symptoms. These skin reactions, which peaked 1 to 2 weeks after irradiation and subsided in 4 to 6 weeks, were definitely worse when the two treatment modalities were combined.

Skin

Skin sensitization from the concomitant use of radiation therapy and actinomycin D was first described in 1959. More recently, Adriamycin, 6 mercaptopurine, 5-FU, bleomycin, hydroxyurea, and methotrexate have all been reported to accentuate radiation skin reactions. When both intrathecal and intravenous methotrexate were combined with a radiation dose to the scalp of 3000 rads, severe skin injury in the radiation field was reported. In addition to radiation skin reactions, alopecia, hyperpigmentation (after administration of many anticancer drugs), hemorrhage (from thrombocytopenia or disseminated intravascular coagulation), and infections in immunosuppressed patients, most commonly with gram-negative bacteria or fungi, may all occur.

Head and Neck

Increased radiation mucositis, local pain, and dysphagia may occur when 5-FU or methotrexate are administered during radiation therapy. Increased normal tissue reactions also occurred when radiosensitizing drugs were infused during a radiation therapy course. No definite increased local reactions with combined cis-Diamminedichloroplatinum (CDDP) chemotherapy and radiation have been reported, but the modalities in combination may increase the ototoxicity of CDDP.

Heart

Many studies have documented the cardiotoxicity potential of Adriamycin. Myocardial degeneration occurs prior to clinical evidence of heart failure, which is usually noted only after total Adriamycin doses of 330 to 545 mg/M^2. The risk of Adriamycin cardiomyopathy is increased in patients older than 70 and in those who have received mediastinal radiation doses greater than 600 rads. Clinical studies, including a phonocardiogram with systolic time intervals, and invasive tests (endomyocardial biopsy and right heart catheterization) may be necessary to establish the maximum tolerated dose of Adriamycin prior to the appearance of overt heart failure.

Lung

In irradiated patients, the abrupt withdrawal of corticosteroids may flare latent radiation pneumonitis or pericarditis. Therefore patients who have received mantle irradiation for Hodgkin's disease and are undergoing MOPP chemotherapy should have prednisone omitted. Heightened radiation lung reactions have been noted with many chemotherapeutic agents. Those that have apparently produced severe radiation pneumonitis are hydroxyurea, actinomycin D, vincristine, Adriamycin, bleomycin, and procarbazine. When the BACO regimen (consisting of bleomycin, Adriamycin, vincristine, and cyclophosphamide) was used in 29 patients with small cell carcinomas without radiotherapy, no significant pulmonary fibrosis was seen. However, when 13 other patients received combined BACO and mediastinal-lung irradiation, 3 fatal and 2 severe cases of radiation pneumonitis subsequently occurred, including widespread pulmonary fibrosis beyond the radiation portals. These reactions developed 6 weeks after a 90-unit bleomycin course, but did not appear in 20 patients who received "ACO" therapy (bleomycin omitted).

Esophagus
Drugs that may increase radiation esophagitis include bleomycin, actinomycin D, procarbazine, and vinblastine. When the COMA regimen (cyclophosphamide, vincristine, methotrexate, and Adriamycin) and irradiation were used for small cell pulmonary carcinomas, severe radiation esophagitis developed in 6 of 8 patients when the two were used concomitantly. When COMA was begun 1 week after radiation, 2 of 5 patients developed esophagitis, but when the drug combination was started 2 weeks or more after radiation therapy, no esophagitis occurred in 9 patients.

Gastrointestinal Tract
Increased gastrointestinal symptoms may occur during a radiotherapy course with concomitant use of actinomycin D, Adriamycin, 5-FU, or bleomycin. When these agents are used in patients receiving gastrointestinal irradiation, consideration should be given to reducing the total radiation dose, fraction size, and volume of gut irradiated. Special techniques of setting up may also be needed to minimize the amount of bowel in the radiation therapy portals.

Kidney
The original observation on the interaction of actinomycin D and radiation in producing radiation nephritis was made many years ago. Bleomycin and vinblastine in combination have also been reported to increase the risk of radiation nephritis.

Liver
Actinomycin D and Adriamycin either alone or in combination have both been suspected of producing low-dose radiation hepatitis. The hepatic volume irradiated, the total radiation dose and fractionation, and prior hepatic surgery all place a patient at greater risk of developing radiation hepatitis.

Bladder
Severe cyclophosphamide cystitis has occurred when the pelvis and bladder were irradiated simultaneously with the administration of cyclophosphamide. The combined chemotherapy regimen VAC (vincristine, actinomycin D, and cyclophosphamide) plus Adriamycin has also produced severe radiation cystitis.

Central Nervous System
When systemic methotrexate (>40 to 80 mg/M^2/week) is combined with a total intrathecal methotrexate dose greater than 750 mg and cranial irradiation (more than 2000 rads) in patients with acute leukemia, a 45% risk of leukoencephalopathy has been noted. This syndrome, consisting of varying degrees of blindness, dementia, or mental retardation, occurs months to years after therapy and may also be associated with cortical atrophy. Attempts are now being made to reduce both the radiation and methotrexate doses in patients with more favorable leukemic presentations.

Neoplasia

Two recent reports have documented an increased frequency of late second malignancies in cured Hodgkin's disease patients treated with combined radiation and drugs. The risk at 6 years for developing acute leukemia in relapse-free patients with Hodgkin's disease who were treated by combined chemotherapy and radiotherapy was 3.9% in one study. A similar risk of 4.4% (after 10 years) of developing abdominal involvement by a second lymphoma (non-Hodgkin's lymphoma) was noted in the same group of patients with Hodgkin's disease who received both radiation and chemotherapy. Therefore the risk of developing late second neoplasms is at least 8% after combined modality treatment of Hodgkin's disease. Another report revealed a 29-fold greater risk of developing a second tumor in patients with Hodgkin's disease after combined treatment. Combined modality treatment is one of the most important ways of treating malignancies; but drug-radiotherapy interactions on normal tissues, organs, and in the genesis of late neoplasms should also be considered when making therapeutic decisions.

Arseneau J, Canellos G, DeVita V, Sherins R: Recently recognized complications of cancer chemotherapy. Ann NY Acad Sci 230:481–488, 1974.
There was an increased risk of secondary malignancies in patients with Hodgkin's disease who received both XRT and MOPP chemotherapy.
Bleyer W: Methotrexate: Clinical pharmacology, current status and therapeutic guidelines. Cancer Treat Rev 4:87–101, 1977.
Article reviews effects of methotrexate on all critical organs.
Bristow M, Mason J, Billingham M, Daniels J: Doxorubicin cardiomyopathy: Evaluation by phonocardiography, endomyocardial biopsy and cardiac catheterization. Ann Intern Med 88:168–175, 1978.
Radiation of the heart and advanced age were two important risk factors in Adriamycin-induced cardiac failure.
Castellino R, Glatstein E, Turbow M, et al: Latent radiation injury of lungs or heart activated by steroid withdrawal. Ann Intern Med 80:593–599, 1974.
Abrupt steroid withdrawal in 7 patients "flared" latent radiation pneumonitis.
Chabora B, Hopfan S, Wittes R: Esophageal complications in the treatment of oat cell carcinoma with combined irradiation and chemotherapy. Radiology 123:185–187, 1977.
COMA therapy (CTX, VCR, MTX, and adriamycin) plus XRT resulted in esophagitis in 6 of 8 patients; when chemotherapy was begun within 1 week of XRT 2 of 5 developed esophagitis; when chemotherapy was begun 2 weeks after XRT 0 of 9 developed esophagitis.
Churchill D, Honf K, Gault M: Radiation nephritis following combined abdominal radiation and chemotherapy (bleomycin-vinblastine). Cancer 41:2162–2164, 1978.
Radiation nephritis was reported after use of bleomycin-velban and radiation.
Coleman C, Williams C, Flint A, et al: Hematologic neoplasia in patients treated for Hodgkin's disease. N Engl J Med 297:1249–1252, 1977.
There were no cases of hematologic neoplasia when XRT or chemotherapy alone was given; the 7-year risk of developing leukemia with combined therapy is 3.9%.
D'Angio G, Farber S, Maddock C: Potentiation of skin effects by actinomycin D. Radiology 73:175–177, 1959.
This is a classic description of increased skin reactions with the combined use of the two modalities.
Einhorn L, Krause M, Hornback N, Furnas B: Enhanced pulmonary toxicity with bleomycin and radiotherapy in oat cell lung cancer. Cancer 37:2414–2416, 1976.

When BACO alone was given to 29 patients there was no pulmonary fibrosis. When BACO plus XRT was used in 13 patients 3 developed fatal and 2 significant, generalized pulmonary fibrosis. There was no fibrosis in 20 subsequent patients treated with ACO and XRT (omitting bleomycin).

Foucar K, McKenna RW, Bloomfield CD, et al: Therapy-related leukemia: A panmyelosis. Cancer 43:1285–1296, 1979.
This article reports on 15 patients who developed leukemia following chemotherapy and/or radiotherapy.

Greco F, Brereton H, Kent H, et al: Adriamycin and enhanced radiation reaction in normal esophagus and skin. Ann Intern Med 85:294–298, 1976.
Eight of 10 patients treated for oat cell carcinoma had severe esophagitis and 5 also developed moist cutaneous desquamation at low radiation doses (1200–2800 rads).

Hahn P, Hallberg O, Vikterlof K: Acute skin reactions in post-operative breast cancer patients receiving radiotherapy plus adjuvant chemotherapy. Am J Roentgenol 130:137–139, 1978.
When XRT plus CMF was used there were 81% chest wall reactions, compared to only 33% in patients treated by XRT alone to similar total doses (~5000 rads).

Krikorian J, Burke J, Rosenberg S, Kaplan H: Occurrence of non-Hodgkin's lymphoma after therapy for Hodgkin's disease. N Engl J Med 300:452–458, 1979.
Seven patients who developed non-Hodgkin's lymphoma all received both XRT and chemotherapy. The 10-year risk of developing this complication is 4.4%.

Kun L, Camitta B: Hepatopathy following irradiation and adriamycin. Cancer 42:81–84, 1978.
When 2300–2500 rads were given to the liver, liver injury resulted.

Littman P, Davis LW, Nash J, et al: The hazard of acute radiation pneumonitis in children receiving mediastinal irradiation. Cancer 33:1520–1525, 1974.
Two deaths occurred after whole lung and mediastinal boost XRT in children who were also receiving drug chemotherapy.

Muggia F, Cortes-Funes H, Wasserman T: Radiotherapy and chemotherapy in combined clinical trials: Problems and promise. Int J Radiat Oncol Biol Phys 4:166–171, 1978.
Review of combined modality clinical trials (and complications).

Phillips T, Fu K: Quantification of combined radiation therapy and chemotherapy effects on normal tissues. Cancer 37:1186–1200, 1976.
Detailed review.

PART VII. MANAGEMENT PROBLEMS

Few diagnoses convey so dramatically and unambiguously the specter of death as does cancer. From the moment of detection and diagnosis, the certainty of mortality influences the behavior of both the patient and the medical care team. Consequently it is important that those involved in patient treatment and support examine their own attitudes toward cancer and death before attempting to care for others. To most, life with cancer implies social unacceptability—fear of painful suffering, disability, disfigurement, impaired body function, loss of sexual attractiveness, and loss of self-esteem. In addition, death from cancer may imply failure of the patient's battle against his disease and of the medical team in providing effective treatment.

The relationship of patient and caregiver should be open, honest, and based on trust. Goals of treatment should be realistic, recognizing that both quality and quantity of survival are important. Whatever therapy is chosen, the patient must be informed not only of its potential benefits but of its potential hazards and disabilities as well. Although the patient may be anxious to begin treatment, he will also be reluctant to suffer its side-effects. Communication, accessibility, and consistent support assist in lessening this ambivalence. This applies not only to the patient but also to his family. Open, honest communication among patient, family, and caregivers should be encouraged.

For those patients who are "cured," stress and anxiety do not end with the completion of treatment but may be present, continuously or intermittently, for many years to come. For those whose disease recurs or who cannot be cured, there is a persistent confrontation with mortality. However, "incurable" cancer does not mean that death is imminent. Physicians cannot predict with certainty the course of a given patient with cancer. Although definitive antitumor therapy may not be available, supportive measures may alleviate symptoms and promote survival.

Caregivers should bear in mind such fundamental features of human worth as respect for the individual, inclusion in a community, concern for the physical body, and personal meaning beyond the self. Competent and compassionate care requires that neither the patient nor his family be abandoned; that the patient not be isolated from his family or caregivers by a conspiracy of silence; that the patient be allowed to live and die with dignity; and that the family be aided in accepting the patient's death without guilt.

C.P.

Cassileth BR, Zupkis RV, Sutton-Smith K, March V: Information and participation preferences among cancer patients. Ann Intern Med 92:832–836, 1980.
A study of 256 patients with metastatic cancer, revealing that the majority desired maximum information and participation in medical decisions.

Creech RH: The psychologic support of the cancer patient: A medical oncologist's viewpoint. Semin Oncol 2:285–292, 1975.
A useful guide.

Holland J: Psychological aspects of oncology. Med Clin North Am 61:737–748, 1977.
An essay on the psychological aspects of oncology.

Kennedy BJ, Tellegen A, Kennedy S, Havernick N: Psychological response of patients cured of advanced cancer. Cancer 38:2184–2191, 1976.
Questionnaires and interviews of 22 patients are analyzed. Patients had increased appreciation of time, life, people, and interpersonal relationships.

Kübler-Ross E: On Death and Dying. New York: Macmillan, 1969.
  *This book presents five stages of response to incurable illness: denial, anger,
  bargaining, depression, and acceptance.*
Lo B, Jonsen AR: Ethical decisions in the care of a patient terminally ill
  with metastatic cancer. Ann Intern Med 92:107–111, 1980.
  *A case study analyzing ethical and legal considerations of patient refusal of
  therapy, euthanasia, and the side-effects of treatment. A good reference list is
  provided.*
Meyerowitz BE, Sparks FC, Spears IK: Adjuvant chemotherapy for breast
  carcinoma: Psychosocial implications. Cancer 43:1613–1618, 1979.
  *A prospective study of 50 patients receiving adjuvant chemotherapy. Interviews
  revealed that almost all experienced some emotional distress and behavioral
  disruption but 74% would still recommend adjuvant treatment to others.*
Morris T, Greer HS, White P: Psychological and social adjustment to mastec-
  tomy: A two-year follow-up study. Cancer 40:2381–2387, 1977.
  This is a prospective study of 160 patients adjusting to mastectomy.
Vanderpool HY: The ethics of terminal care. JAMA 239:850–852, 1978.
  This essay proposes ethical guidelines.
Yalom ID, Greaves C: Group therapy with the terminally ill. Am J Psychi-
  atry 134:396–400, 1977.
  Describes the experience of psychotherapy with cancer patients.
McKegney FP, Visco G, Yates J, Hughes J: An exploration of cancer staff
  attitudes and values. Med Pediatr Oncol 6:325–337, 1979.
  *This article provides a profile of a multidisciplinary team caring for cancer
  patients.*

105. PAIN

Pain, a symptom that usually occurs late in the course of malignant diseases, is
dreaded by all cancer patients. Pain in a patient with cancer may be due to
benign, unrelated causes, may be referred, and may be very difficult to control.

There are multiple components in the perception of pain, beginning with the
original stimulus. Initially a skin receptor is stimulated and pain sensations
are transmitted through smaller (A, delta, and c) fibers to the dorsal root
ganglion, where they traverse the spinal cord and ascend in the lateral
spinothalamic tract (which transmits pain and temperature sensations) to pain
centers in the thalamus. The pain sensation is finally perceived at the cortical
level. Visceral pain perception is always referred pain since sympathetic nerves
enter the spinal cord at many levels. Two types of pain exist; the first sensation
is sharp and localized, while a more diffuse, poorly localized pain perception
also occurs, probably transmitted over such alternative pathways as the dorsal
columns. The pain sensation may be modified by both the intensity of the initial
stimulus and by central processing, including sensory feedback. Pain tolerance
is also modified by cultural variables.

Pain caused by a malignant disease may be due to infection or inflammation,
to tissue or organ destruction by the cancer, to pressure on or invasion of
adjacent organs or tissues, or to dilatation of viscera and organs.

In some instances, pain may be produced by benign causes that obscure the
detection of an underlying malignancy. To use head and neck sites as an
example, pain referred to the ear may be produced by primary malignancies of
the oral cavity (trigeminal nerve), oropharynx (glossopharyngeal nerve), or
hypopharynx (vagus nerve). The lack of pain at the primary site may delay the

diagnosis of head and neck cancers. Painful associated infections may respond dramatically to antibiotics. However, a continual sore throat in patients with advanced larynx or hypopharyngeal cancers often signifies deep invasion by the tumor. In the thorax, superior or medially located lung cancers may cause pain by invasion of the chest wall, brachial plexus, or esophagus. Infection and pneumonia distal to obstructed bronchi may also produce chest pain or discomfort. Pain of cardiac origin is usually referred to the T_{1-4} dermatomes. In the abdomen, such benign processes in cancer patients as retroperitoneal, splenic, or hepatic hemorrhage in those with thrombocytopenia or other bleeding disorders; appendicitis; diverticulitis; benign bowel obstructions; renal and biliary colic; gastroduodenal ulcers; and pancreatitis may all produce chronic or colicky abdominal pain. In general, gastric pain is referred to T_{5-7}, biliary to T_{6-8}, small bowel to T_{8-10}, kidney to $T_{10}-L_1$, and bladder and rectal pain to S_{2-4} dermatomes.

In the treatment of chronic pain due to cancer, many individuals, including oncologists, family physicians, neurologists, neurosurgeons, psychiatrists, social workers, and the patient's family, may be involved. The patient must cope with the fear, anxiety, and depression of chronic pain; the patient must also deal with the loss of independence, the possible need for long-term medications, and the eventuality of terminal hospitalization with painful carcinomatosis.

Obtaining pain relief includes local therapy, the use of analgesic drugs, and interruption of pain pathways. Symptomatic, localized tumor masses may be treated by radiotherapy, surgery, and/or chemotherapy for local control and pain relief. Co-existing infections, which often occur in patients with head and neck carcinomas, should also be treated to reduce pain, but the underlying malignancy usually must be controlled to eradicate infections completely. The colicky pain from gastrointestinal obstruction due to malignancies may require tube decompression, parenteral nutrition, or surgical correction. Painful osseous lesions may require splinting, immobilization, or fixation to achieve comfort and optimum palliation.

Analgesic drugs are a mainstay in the control of pain caused by malignancies, but if nerve blocks or mechanical interruption of pain pathways are required, these manipulations should be performed prior to narcotic addiction. Effective, nonaddictive drugs for mild to moderate pain are aspirin and acetaminophen (Tylenol). The potential gastric irritative or anticoagulative effects of aspirin should be considered, however. More potent analgesics for greater degrees of pain are codeine (which may produce constipation) and pentazocine (Talwin), which may result in an altered sensorium. More potent, addictive narcotics such as morphine sulfate and meperidine (Demerol) may be required. Oral Dilaudid or methadone with its prolonged effects may also be used. Drugs such as aspirin and Compazine (a tranquilizer and antiemetic) may be combined with narcotics to produce more profound, long-lasting relief. Brompton's mixture, consisting of gin, morphine, cocaine, and chloroform water, is an excellent analgesic, antitussive, and mood-elevating regimen for patients with advanced, symptomatic cancers.

Pain control may also be attempted through the interruption of pain pathways. These may be blocked anywhere along the chain of transmission from the skin receptors to the central nervous system. In general the simplest procedure is performed first, followed by more difficult, potentially morbid methods, if the initial treatment fails to provide pain relief. Nerve blocks are performed (usually in specialized anesthesia pain clinics) only after full evaluation by cancer specialists, often including neurologists, neurosurgeons, and psychiatrists. Local anesthetic toxicity is prevented by avoiding either intravenous injections or an overdose of the anesthetic and by preventing rapid absorption of the drug. Incisional pain, if other causes such as herpes zoster, intrathoracic or intraabdominal diseases, and peripheral nerve tumors have been ruled out, may be controlled by injecting a trigger point with lidocaine and following it by phenol or alcohol blocks if the local anesthetic effectively produces pain relief. *Chest or abdominal wall pain* in a dermatomal distribution may also be relieved initially by procaine or lidocaine intercostal blocks and permanently by injections of such neurolytic agents as 100% alcohol or 10% phenol and water. Cutaneous blocks for postherpetic neuralgia are usually ineffective, since anesthesia of the skin may be produced without affecting the painful neuralgia. *Retroperitoneal or abdominal pain* from gastric, pancreatic, liver, and biliary malignancies may be diminished or completely abolished by percutaneous bilateral celiac ganglion blocks. Usually a lidocaine test dose is given, and if temporary pain relief is obtained, permanent celiac ganglion blocks with alcohol or phenol blocks are performed. Thoracic barbotage, in which spinal fluid is aspirated and reinjected at the thoracic level 10 or 20 times, has often given satisfactory pain relief and may be repeated as often as needed.

Special surgical techniques are used for various cancers. Multiple head and neck sites are innervated by either the trigeminal, glossopharyngeal, or vagus nerves. Head and neck pain may be due to dural, bone, or soft tissue invasion by recurrent or primary carcinomas, by nerve irritation, or by associated infections. Postirradiation osseous or soft tissue necroses should be ruled out before pain is attributed to recurrent carcinoma. Following radical neck dissections, neuromas may occasionally occur; excision or local anesthetic injections may be required to produce pain relief. Stellate ganglion blocks may diminish cervical pain from recurrent or persistent carcinomas in this region. Craniotomy, with rhizotomy of the fifth, ninth, and tenth cranial nerves and the upper posterior cervical nerves, has been performed in selected patients with severe pain who were expected to live more than 3 months and were able to tolerate the surgery. For this radical pain procedure, the best results were obtained when the most tracts were sectioned. Other, more morbid and less commonly used procedures are medullary tractotomy and frontal lobotomy. Other head and neck pains that may be confused with those due to recurrent neoplasms result from primary brain tumors, tic douloureux, subarachnoid hemorrhage, and cluster headaches.

When lower extremity and back pain occurs, herniated intervertebral discs or other benign causes of back pain such as lumbosacral strain, degenerative arthritis, or chronic adhesive arachnoiditis must be differentiated from primary spinal cord tumors or metastases. The presence of a primary tumor may indicate metastases as the cause of back pain. Spinal cord tumors produce focal, increasingly severe, and persistent radicular back pain. Pain in patients with spinal cord neoplasms is usually not relieved by rest; patients with disc disease, however, usually improve after a period of bed rest. Intradural, intramedullary spinal cord tumors often produce an early neurologic defect, followed by pain, whereas intradural, extramedullary neoplasms result in more severe pain and milder deficits. Extradural, extramedullary tumors (metastases) rapidly cause severe pain. Patients with intrinsic spinal cord or metastatic neoplasms usually note severe pain with hip flexion and internal or external rotation, whereas patients with a herniated disc develop severe pain with straight leg raising (which stretches the sciatic nerve). These patients also experience paravertebral muscle spasms and commonly have associated neurologic deficits. Spinal cord compression by malignancies may be treated by radiotherapy or surgery as indicated (see Part I, Chapter 5). Chronic pain in this region, if unresponsive to radiotherapy, surgical, or chemotherapeutic manipulations, may often be controlled by local nerve blocks or spinal fluid barbotage. More invasive procedures include rhizotomy, open cordotomy, and, recently, percutaneous cordotomy. Fifty percent of patients treated by cordotomy lose their pain relief in approximately 12 months. Experiments with operative placement of posterior column nerve stimulators have also been carried out; a drawback to this procedure is that laminectomy is needed to implant the stimulating device, which appears to be less effective in controlling pain due to metastatic neoplasms. Central procedures independent of those developed for head and neck cancers have also been used for the treatment of chronic pain. Transsphenoidal hypophysectomy is an accepted, effective form of hormonal manipulation in patients with metastatic breast and prostate carcinomas. Patients with advanced malignancies and a short life expectancy may benefit transiently from frontal lobotomy, while other procedures such as stereotactic cingulectomy are also under investigation.

D.G.

Bunney WE, Pert CB, Klee W, Costa E, Pert A, Davis GC: Basic and clinical studies of endorphins. Ann Intern Med 91:239–250, 1979.
This article discusses the role of endorphins in pain modulation.

Janetta P, Selker R, Albin M, Tenicela R, et al: The neurosurgical approach to the relief from pain. Curr Probl Surg 1973:1–72, 1973.
This 72-page issue covers the surgical aspects of pain relief.

Keats A, Lane M: The symptomatic therapy of pain. DM 1–40, June, 1963.
Review article.

Lewis BJ: The use of opiate analgesics in cancer patients. Cancer Treat Rep 63:341–342, 1979.
This is an editorial with a table of useful pharmacokinetic data.

Marks MD, Sachar EJ: Undertreatment of medical in-patients with narcotic analgesics. Ann Intern Med 78:173–181, 1973.
73% of patients studied received inadequate pain relief.

Olson K: Pain. *In* JF Holland and E Frei (Eds), Cancer Medicine. Philadelphia, Lea & Febiger, 1974. Pp. 1022–1035.
This chapter gives a brief description of pain neurophysiology.

Oster MW, Vizel M, Turgeon LR: Pain in terminal cancer patients. Arch Intern Med 138:1801–1802, 1978.
A study of pain patterns prior to death in 90 patients with and without cancer is made in this article.

Shimm DS, Logue GL, Maltbie AA, Dugan S: Medical management of chronic cancer pain. JAMA 241:2408–2412, 1979.
A good review of analgesics and psychoactive drugs which are useful in the medical management of chronic pain.

106. ANOREXIA AND ALIMENTATION

Malnourishment is defined as a 10% loss of weight associated with a serum albumin of less than 3.4 gm/100 ml. Such weight losses are commonly noted in cancer patients, in whom a negative nitrogen balance results in decreased wound healing, further reduction in caloric intake, and protein starvation. The goal of hyperalimentation in cancer patients is to maintain and restore nitrogen balance and anabolism, thus improving tolerance for surgery, radiotherapy, and/or chemotherapy. Proper alimentation is especially important in patients with gastrointestinal fistulae, bowel obstructions, and primary carcinomas of the bowel, and in those receiving abdominal irradiation. The acute side-effects from gastrointestinal radiation (nausea, vomiting, diarrhea, and crampy abdominal pain) may be decreased in severe cases by hyperalimentation; the overall tolerance to radiation and/or chemotherapy may also be improved by maintaining optimal nutrition.

Organ and muscle atrophy, poor wound healing, increased risk of developing severe infections, malabsorption, increased surgical risk, and poor tolerance for radiotherapy or chemotherapy all occur in anorectic, starved patients. Some form of maintenance alimentation may even be needed by healthy patients when surgery, chemotherapy, or radiotherapy is planned. Patients expected to be NPO for more than 7 to 14 days will probably need more calories than can be provided by routine peripheral intravenous maintenance. Preoperative patients; those with prolonged unconsciousness; those whose bowel must be put at rest because of fistulae, pancreatitis, or inflammatory bowel diseases; and those requiring nutritional support following burns, severe trauma, or cancer chemotherapy may need hyperalimentation for optimal therapeutic results.

To maintain proper weight, approximately 30 cal/kg/day are required, but 45 to 90 cal/kg may be necessary when there are fistulae or severe burns. 1 to 1.5 cc of fluid per calorie, plus replacement of abnormal fluid losses, is also necessary. These fluid requirements must be reduced in patients with renal disease or congestive heart failure. Twenty-eight essential nutrients, including essential amino and fatty acids, carbohydrates, vitamins, and trace elements, are also required. Patients ingesting fewer than 1000 cal/day and fewer than 30 gm of protein experience rapid malnutrition. To adequately replace the total caloric requirement *parenterally* in these patients, central venous alimentation must be used, since the hyperosmotic solutions that are needed are poorly tolerated by small peripheral veins.

The diagnosis of malnutrition is obvious when a weight loss of more than 10% has occurred in a patient with an underlying malignancy. If surgery, chemotherapy, or radiotherapy is planned, and if a gastrointestinal problem such as obstruction, fistula, or inflammatory bowel process is diagnosed, alimentation may be necessary. Physical examination of a malnourished patient reveals muscle wasting, milk edema with or without ascites, liver enlargement, cutaneous pallor, and a dry, scaly dermatitis, with decreased arm circumference and triceps fold measurements (normal are 25.3 and 23.2, 12.5 mm and 16.5 mm, respectively, for males and females). The most important laboratory test for diagnosing malnutrition is the creatinine-height index; normal values (mg/cm) are 10.2 for males and 5.8 for females. Decreased albumin, folate, vitamins A and C, calcium, magnesium, phosphorus, potassium, and lymphocyte counts may all be noted. Cell-mediated immunity may also be diminished.

When the decision has been made to begin maintenance feedings or hyperalimentation, an appropriate route for increasing caloric intake must be decided upon. Sufficient calories for hyperalimentation cannot be infused through peripheral veins, since the required hyperosmolar solutions produce intense phlebitis. Large lumen nasogastric tubes can be used for enteral supplementation but often result in such complications as pharyngorhinitis, parotitis, otitis media, aspiration and atelectasis, esophageal reflex and stricture, and decreased cough reflex. More recently, techniques of enteral alimentation, with or without peripheral supplements or central venous hyperalimentation (total parenteral nutrition, TPN) have all been used. Approximately two-thirds of malnourished cancer patients may need enteral alimentation alone or enteral alimentation with peripheral supplements, while one-third require TPN.

Enteral Alimentation

Feedings through a small diameter nasogastric tube can provide successful enteral hyperalimentation. The tube can be used for 6 weeks or more. If a longer period of alimentation is required, esophagostomy, gastrostomy, or jejunostomy may be necessary. This form of alimentation is contraindicated in the presence of bowel obstruction, acute gastrointestinal bleeding, or intractable vomiting. Small tube alimentation or hyperalimentation is simple, physiologic, well-tolerated, relatively inexpensive, and safer and less cumbersome than TPN, since no sterile fluid preparation or special alimentation teams are required. It also preserves the integrity and function of the gastrointestinal tract by providing nutrients intraluminally. Enteral alimentation may be used either as maintenance or for hyperalimentation.

Three types of diets may be used with enteral feedings. These for the most part are bulk-free, require minimal digestion, and do not need total pancreatic, gastric, or biliary secretions for absorption. They also have minimal fat content, are readily absorbed in the jejunum, and do not increase gastrointestinal motility.

Polymeric diets such as Vivonex, Ensure, Flexical, and Precision use high molecular weight carbohydrates, protein, and fat, provide 1 calorie/ml, are inexpensive, but require absorptive enzymes. They do not contain lactose. *Monomeric* diets such as Hycal and Contralyte contain amino acids and mono- or oligosaccharides but not starch or triglycerides. They also contain 1 calorie/ml but require little proteolytic or lipolytic activity and may be used in chronic diarrheal states when a low residue diet is desired. They are also useful when little fat or protein digestion can be expected, as in conditions such as fistulae and inflammatory bowel diseases. *High density* diets can provide high calories (2/ml) in limited volumes for patients with heart or renal disease who require fluid restrictions.

These diets should be administered continuously either by gravity flow or with small pumps. Bolus infusions increase the risk of developing crampy abdominal pain, nausea, or diarrhea. The gastrointestinal symptoms of nausea and vomiting, diarrhea, and cramps may be minimized by either decreasing the concentration of infusate, decreasing the volume, or using intravenous supplementation. The small tubes cause fewer complications than the large-bore nasogastric tubes that were used formerly, but tube obstruction, posterior pharyngeal irritation, and aspiration may occasionally occur. Hyperosmolar coma may develop if insufficient water is provided with the infusate. Patients with heart or renal disease may require volume restriction and high density diets. Patients should also be monitored so that weight gain is less than 1 pound a day. Greater daily weight gains represent edema rather than increased muscle mass. Weekly creatinine-height ratios, arm and triceps measurements, albumin, electrolytes, BUN, and serum glucose determinations should be obtained. The urine glucose should be measured twice daily. Peripheral alimentation may be used as a supplement to enteral alimentation for either hyperalimentation or maintenance feedings.

Total Parenteral Nutrition

If either or both enteral or peripheral infusions are inadequate to provide hyperalimentation, or if the gastrointestinal status of the patient precludes enteral feedings, central hyperalimentation (TPN) is then required. At the M.D. Anderson Hospital, over 400 patients received TPN for an average of 23.9 days, with a range of 10 to 147 days. Forty-three percent of these patients received TPN while undergoing chemotherapy, 24% were general surgical patients, 10% had head and neck surgery, 10% were undergoing radiotherapy, 6% were being treated for fistulae, and 7% were receiving general supportive care. With a TPN line in the superior vena cava, 25% hyperosmolar dextrose solutions, providing 4 calories/gm and 1 calorie/cc may be used. TPN has been successfully carried out through subclavian vein infusions, through arterial-venous fistulae and in the SVC with surgically inserted Silastic indwelling catheters.

The best TPN results have been obtained with aseptic catheter insertions, including careful skin preparation and the use of antibacterial ointment at the catheter site. A chest radiograph is obtained after insertion to document catheter tip position in the superior vena cava. To decrease the risks of fibrin deposition, infection, or cardiac trauma, the catheter should neither enter the heart nor cross the tricuspid valve. No blood products are infused and no blood is drawn through the catheter; the 45 μ filter and intravenous tubing are changed daily. The dressings covering the catheter entrance site in the skin are changed at least 3 times a week, using glove and mask technique, and additional antiseptic is applied at the catheter entrance site.

Solutions are prepared daily with the use of a laminar flow hood. Amino acid substrates and 50% glucose solutions are used to produce a 1000 cc solution containing 1000 calories and 5 or 6 gm of nitrogen, with a concentration of 1800 to 2400 milliosmoles/liter. Electrolytes, fat- or water-soluble vitamins, and trace elements are also added to the mixture. Serum albumin concentrations lower than 3.5 gm/ml are corrected by daily albumin infusions until effective liver production resumes, usually in 10 to 14 days. TPN is usually begun at a rate of 1000 ml daily by continuous infusion and increased 2000 to 3000 ml (and calories) per day. Cachectic cancer patients should receive a total of 2000 calories per day until positive nitrogen balance is restored, when the daily caloric intake may be increased. Insulin may be necessary to ensure proper glucose use, while glucosuria may result from fluctuating rates of fluid administration.

Septic complications develop in approximately 7% of patients receiving TPN, but only in 3% of cases in which strict aseptic technique is used. Blood cultures should be performed and the catheter removed if unexplained fevers occur. Such catheter changes are needed in approximately 9% of patients. Other complications, such as thrombosis of the superior vena cava, pneumothorax or hemothorax or mediastinum, air embolism, thoracic duct trauma, cardiac tamponade, arrythmias, or perforation all can occur.

Patients should be weighed daily. The weight gain after an initial rapid 3- to 4-pound increment should be ½ to 1 pound per day. The TPN infusion rate should be decreased if a more rapid weight gain ensues (due to edema). Fluid retention may be managed either by diuretics or by decreasing the infusion rate. Electrolytes and BUN are determined three times weekly, while urine glucose determinations are made several times daily. Liver function studies, serum albumin, phosphorus, calcium, magnesium, and creatinine determinations are made weekly. A specific TPN team manages these patients.

Alimentation may improve tolerance to both chemotherapy and radiotherapy. Surgical complications may be decreased if these techniques are used preoperatively and postoperatively rather than after severe complications have occurred. Hyperalimentation may also improve a patient's chances to undergo cancer surgery successfully.

D.G.

Copeland E, Dudrick S: Nutritional aspects of cancer. Curr Prob Cancer 1:1–51, 1976.
This complete review includes a technique of SVC catheterization.
Copeland E, MacFadyen B Jr, MacComb W, et al: Intravenous hyperalimentation in patients with head and neck cancer. Cancer 35:606–611, 1975.
Of 23 patients who underwent hyperalimentation 20 gained weight and recovered from their malnutrition; complications (sepsis or subclavian vein

thrombosis) occurred in 3 patients. An average of 17 days of hyperalimentation was needed to convert patients to surgical candidates.

Copeland E, Souchon E, MacFadyen B Jr, et al: Intravenous hyperalimentation as an adjunct to radiation therapy. Cancer 39:609–616, 1977.
Article gives results of TPN (total parenteral nutrition) in 39 irradiated patients.

Costa G, Donaldson SS: Current concepts in cancer: Effects of cancer and cancer treatment on the nutrition of the host. N Engl J Med 300:1471–1474, 1979.
A brief discussion of the nutritional effects of cancer and cancer treatment as well as management of the malnourished patient.

Dietel M, Vasic V, Alexander M: Specialized nutritional support in the cancer patient: Is it worthwhile? Cancer 41:2359–2363, 1978.
In this prospective study of TPN given preoperatively and postoperatively there were no deaths or significant complications. When TPN was started after complications occurred a 17% mortality was noted.

Dudrick S, Wilmore D: Long term total parenteral nutrition with growth, development and positive nitrogen balance. Surgery 64:134–142, 1967.
In this classic article hypertonic glucose was used primarily.

Heatley RV, Williams RHP, Lewis MH: Preoperative intravenous feeding—a controlled trial. Postgrad Med J 55:541–545, 1979.
74 patients with gastric or esophageal cancers randomly received either oral supplementation or oral feeding plus 7 to 10 days of IV alimentation preoperatively. Fewer wound infections were noted in the latter group.

Heymsfield S, Bethel R, Ansley J, et al: Enteral hyperalimentation: An alternative to central venous hyperalimentation. Ann Intern Med 90:63–71, 1979.
An excellent review. Recommends use of small bore, flexible nasoenteral tube and constant flow delivery of nutrient solution.

Jiejeebhoy K, Langer B, Tsallas G, Chu R, et al: Total parenteral nutrition at home: Studies in patients surviving 4 months to 5 years. Gastroenterology 71:943–953, 1976.
In 12 patients total parenteral nutrition was given at home through a Silastic, surgically placed SVC catheter.

Law D: Current concepts in nutrition: Total parenteral nutrition. N Engl J Med 297:1104–1107, 1977.
A brief but clearly written review article.

Ryan J Jr, Abel R, Abbott W, et al: Catheter complications in total parenteral nutrition. N Engl J Med 290:757–761, 1974.
Article reports on aseptic catheter management; there was a 3% sepsis rate, with a 29% rate if breaks in strict aseptic protocol occurred. Superior vena caval thrombosis was also noted.

Soeters PB, Ebeid AM, Fischer JE: Review of 404 patients with gastrointestinal fistulas. Impact of parenteral nutrition. Ann Surg 190:189–202, 1979.
In this retrospective review parenteral nutrition possibly improved spontaneous closure of fistulas.

107. HEMOPTYSIS

Hemoptysis commonly represents hemorrhage from the bronchial arteries, which arise from the systemic, rather than the pulmonary, circulation. The most common causes of hemoptysis are lung neoplasms, bronchiectasis, tuberculosis, and necrotizing pneumonia. Hemoptysis may occur with (1) infections: In tuberculosis there is usually cough productive of occasionally blood-streaked mucoid sputum; massive hemoptysis is rare. Other infectious causes of hemoptysis are fungal infections, pneumonia (with cough and bloody sputum), lung abscesses, and acute or chronic bronchitis and bronchiectasis (blood-streaked sputum or massive intermittent hemoptysis). It may also arise with (2) neoplasms such as bronchogenic carcinomas, bronchial adenomas, and, less commonly, pulmonary metastases. It may develop with (3) vascular abnormalities, such as pulmonary infarcts (hemoptysis occurs in 11%); mitral stenosis— hemorrhage occurs after the rupture of collateral vessels connecting engorged bronchial and pulmonary veins; pulmonary hemosiderosis, hypertension, and pulmonary arterial-venous malformations; and (4) with such *miscellaneous* disorders as hemorrhagic diatheses, pulmonary foreign bodies, trauma, and Goodpasture's syndrome; hemoptysis has also been noted 7 to 10 days after the pulmonary embolization of Ethiodol, which occurs routinely during lymphangiography.

When hemoptysis is not readily attributable to infection, recurs, or is persistent, the underlying cause should be determined. In the evaluation of a patient with minimal hemoptysis, a careful history describing the amount and frequency of bleeding; other pulmonary symptoms such as cough, fever, and productive sputum; and complaints suggesting hemorrhage from other head and neck sites should be elicited. Physical examination should include pulmonary and cardiac auscultation, examination of regional lymph nodes for evidence of metastatic neoplasm, estimation of vocal cord mobility, and a careful head and neck examination to rule out nasal, nasopharyngeal, or other upper airway sites of bleeding. A chest radiograph is mandatory; tomograms, bronchograms, or fluoroscopy may provide additional information. Multiple sputum samples should be obtained for cytologic evaluation, acid-fast stain and culture, and bacterial and fungal smears and cultures. An assessment for possible bleeding diatheses should also be made. Fiberoptic bronchoscopy and systematic segmental bronchial lavage during the bleeding episode may establish the site of bleeding in at least two-thirds of patients. A selective bronchial arteriogram may also allow a bleeding point to be localized. Ventilation function may often be determined at the bedside by performing a single breath forced vital capacity maneuver. If massive hemoptysis occurs (>600 cc of blood in 24 to 48 hours), vital signs should be closely monitored, a careful rapid physical examination performed, a chest radiograph obtained, and multiple units of blood typed and cross-matched. A tracheostomy may also be necessary. The bleeding site may be identified endoscopically and selective bronchial intubation carried out preoperatively.

Mild hemoptysis may be treated by bed rest and sedation, with the affected side dependent to minimize aspiration of blood, along with cough suppression and blood transfusions, if necessary. With massive hemoptysis, the rate of bleeding is the most important factor. The prognosis is grave if more than 600 ml of blood are produced in 16 hours. In one series, the mortality rate in operable patients who underwent emergency pulmonary surgery was 23% but increased to over 70% if operable patients did not receive surgery and in those who were inoperable. With massive hemoptysis, a bleeding point is identified by fiberoptic bronchoscopy if possible, the bleeding bronchus is intubated, and pulmonary resection is carried out. A Carlen double lumen tube may be necessary during surgery (to occlude the bleeding bronchus). Relative contraindications to surgery are advanced bilateral pulmonary disease, a poorly localized bleeding site, unresectable metastatic bronchogenic carcinomas, vital capacity less than 40% of normal, massive invasion of the mediastinum or great vessels, and recurrent hemoptysis after massive pulmonary resections.

If a patient is a poor surgical candidate or if surgery is not contemplated, the bleeding orifice may be identified by endoscopy and a balloon catheter inserted into the bleeding bronchus, either through the bronchoscope or percutaneously through the cricothyroid membrane, to prevent aspiration or asphyxiation. An emergency bronchial arteriogram is then performed. If a bleeding point is identified, it may be controlled by embolizing clots or other absorbable material. Care must be taken to avoid embolizing the distal aorta.

The best results after embolization therapy of hemoptysis were obtained with tuberculosis, bronchiectasis, and the pneumonoconioses. In one series 35 of 49 patients (76%) had no further hemoptysis for periods of 2–30 months after treatment by embolization during the acute bleeding episode. Embolic therapy of hemoptysis is palliative. Since the underlying cause is not treated, revascularization and recanalization of occluded vascular channels occurs, and the embolized material is eventually reabsorbed. Retrosternal pain occurs in 10% of embolized patients, while segmental small bowel necrosis requiring laparotomy has also been reported. Embolization should not be performed if the anterior spinal artery has an anomalous origin, since transverse myelitis may result from insertion of clots into such a vessel. Radiation doses of 3000 rads in 2 weeks or more produce excellent palliation of hemoptysis in 75% to 80% of patients. Radiation therapy is indicated for inoperable patients or for those with malignant pulmonary neoplasms for whom surgery is contraindicated. The radiation volume depends on the size, anatomic location, and extent of the neoplasm and the presence or absence of regional lymph node involvement.

D.G.

Crocco J, Rooney J, Fankushen D, et al: Massive hemoptysis. Arch Intern Med 121:495–498, 1968.
In this analysis of 67 patients with massive hemoptysis (600 ml in 48 hours) the bleeding site was localized in 65 of the 67. The prognosis was grave for patients who bled more than 600 ml in 16 hours.

Farina A, Alderman S, Carella R: Radiotherapy for bronchogenic carcinoma. Postgrad Med 63(2):117–123, 1978.
Reviews the role of radiation therapy in management of lung cancer; hemoptysis improved in 80% with 3000 rads in 2 weeks.

Gourin A, Garzon A: Control of hemorrhage in emergency pulmonary resection for massive hemoptysis. Chest 68:120–121, 1975.
Alternatives to the Carlen double lumen tube are described.

Remy J, Arnaud A, Fardou H, Giraud R, Voisin C: Treatment of hemoptysis by embolization of bronchial arteries. Radiology 122:33–37, 1976.
Forty-one of 49 patients treated during hemoptysis had immediate cessation of bleeding; 6 rebled; permanent control was therefore obtained in 35 of 49 (76%) for 2 to 30 months.

Wagner R, Baeza O, Stewart J: Active pulmonary hemorrhage localized by selective pulmonary angiography. Chest 67:121–123, 1975.
This article consists of a case report and a good discussion of pulmonary hemorrhage.

Wholey M, Chamorro H, Rao G, Ford W, Miller W: Bronchial artery embolization for massive hemoptysis. JAMA 236:2501–2504, 1976.
Article consists of case reports and a review of management of massive hemoptysis.

Pleural fluid may affect pulmonary function by restricting lung expansion and altering the parameters of ventilation and perfusion. These effects depend not only on the size of the effusion, but on whether it is unilateral or bilateral, as well as on the functional status of both lungs. Because symptoms of respiratory compromise may result from the presence of pleural fluid, and because of potential complications of atelectasis and/or pulmonary infection, proper management of the effusion and prevention of its recurrence are important. Not only can removal of the fluid promptly relieve symptoms, but prevention of its recurrence may sustain good quality of life and perhaps prolong survival.

As discussed in Part II, chapter 20, numerous benign conditions result in the formation of pleural fluid. When caused by malignancy, the effusion is usually secondary to metastatic carcinomas of the lung or breast or to lymphoma or leukemia. An initial thoracentesis is performed to establish the fluid's etiology, ascertain the palliative benefits of fluid removal (since some patients, for example, with extensive parenchymal lung disease may have little respiratory improvement), and document the recurrent nature of the effusion. Since the average time interval for malignant fluid reaccumulation is only 4 days, definitive therapy is usually necessary. Factors that should be considered in determining the nature of such therapy include the patient's general medical condition, the degree of respiratory disability and the underlying pulmonary status, the extent and location of malignant disease and its histology, the etiology of pleural fluid formation, prior or concurrent tumor therapy, and the patient's life expectancy.

Successful local treatment of a recurrent malignant pleural effusion depends upon full expansion of the lung and production of mesothelial fibrosis to obliterate the pleural space. Repeated thoracenteses may palliate symptoms temporarily but do not prevent fluid reaccumulation and may result in fluid loculation and lung entrapment. Closed tube thoracostomy is a more effective means of removing fluid, but it may not oppose the pleural surfaces sufficiently to produce obliteration of the pleural space. A variety of agents may be instilled into the pleural space to produce mesothelial fibrosis and obliteration of small pleural blood vessels. The effectiveness of these agents does not rely on their antineoplastic activity but on their ability to obliterate the pleural space. Nitrogen mustard, Thiotepa and 5-FU may all be systemically absorbed, resulting in varying degrees of myelosuppression. Bleomycin, quinacrine, and tetracycline are not myelosuppressive; but like the myelosuppressive agents, they may cause pleural pain and fever. In addition, quinacrine requires multiple instillations. Radioactive isotopes (^{198}Au, ^{32}P) have also been used, as has external hemithoracic irradiation. Instillation therapy requires complete pleural fluid evacuation and homogeneous distribution of the sclerosing agent in order to be effective. Consequently, percutaneous thoracentesis and drug instillation is inadequate. The most successful method is to drain the pleural space dry, using a closed tube thoracostomy, and then to instill a sclerosing agent, which is distributed over the pleural surface by changing the patient's position. The chest tube is removed only when no further fluid collection is documented. When this procedure is used, at least 50% of patients will be successfully treated. The sclerosing agent of choice appears to be tetracycline (which yielded an 80% response rate in one study), since it is nonmyelosuppressive and has the least morbidity.

Parietal pleurectomy is a definitive procedure that should be reserved for patients in good physical condition with good life expectancy. Indications include failure of thoracostomy tube drainage plus drug instillation, trapped luug, and diffuse mesothelioma. Although fluid control is virtually 100%, substantial morbidity and mortality (10% in one study) are associated with the procedure.

In patients with responsive tumors it may be appropriate to consider systemic chemotherapy or hormonal therapy of the pleural effusion prior to local pleural treatment. And in those patients with mediastinal lymphoma and negative pleural cytologic findings, mediastinal irradiation alone may relieve the pleural effusion.

C.P.

Bayly TC, Kisner DL, Sybert A, et al: Tetracycline and quinacrine in the control of malignant pleural effusions: A randomized trial. Cancer 41:1188–1192, 1978.
  Complete control was obtained in more than 80% of instillations with either drug; tetracycline produced significantly less pain and fever.
Friedman MA, Slater E: Malignant pleural effusions. Cancer Treat Rev 5:49–66, 1978.
  Article is a summary of pathophysiological concepts, diagnostic procedures, and therapeutic approaches.
Greenwald DW, Phillips C, Bennett JM: Management of malignant pleural effusion. J Surg Oncol 10:361–368, 1978.
  Describes a modified technique of thoracostomy and sclerosis.
Izbicki R, Weyhing BT III, Baker L, et al: Pleural effusion in cancer patients: A prospective randomized study of pleural drainage with the addition of radioactive phosphorus to the pleural space vs. pleural drainage alone. Cancer 36:1511–1518, 1975.
  Both methods controlled approximately 50% of the effusions in women with breast cancer.
Leff A, Hopewell PC, Costello J: Pleural effusion from malignancy. Ann Intern Med 88:532–537, 1978.
  A complete clinical discussion of diagnosis and therapy is provided.
Legha SS, Muggia FM: Pleural mesothelioma: Clinical features and therapeutic implications. Ann Intern Med 87:613–621, 1977.
  An excellent and comprehensive review.
Martini N, Bains MS, Beattie EJ Jr: Indications for pleurectomy in malignant effusion. Cancer 35:734–738, 1975.
  Article provides a retrospective analysis of 106 patients with malignant effusion.

109. PERICARDIAL EFFUSION

Approximately 10% to 20% of patients with malignant disease develop neoplastic involvement of the pericardium and/or heart, yet few (10% to 25% of such patients) have clinically apparent cardiac disease prior to death. The most common problem encountered in those patients who do become symptomatic is the development of cardiac tamponade secondary to pericardial effusion and/or constriction. When tumor is documented in the pericardium, it rarely represents primary disease (such as mesothelioma); rather, it is almost always secondary to metastatic spread via local extension, lymphatic invasion, or hematogenous dissemination. Those malignancies most frequently associated with pericardial disease include lung cancer, breast cancer, lymphoma, and leukemia. There is also a high incidence of cardiac disease in patients with metastatic melanoma, in which tumor often involves the visceral pericardium and myocardium. A cytologically benign pericardial effusion may result from mediastinal lymphatic obstruction, as often seen in patients with lymphoma. Some other causes of pericardial disease include infectious diseases (viral, bacterial, tuberculous, fungal), connective tissue disorders (systemic lupus erythematosus, rheumatoid disease, scleroderma), myxedema, radiation injury, drugs (procainamide, hydralazine, anthracyclines), Dressler's syndrome, trauma, and uremia.

Making the clinical diagnosis of malignant pericardial disease is often difficult. Although the symptoms and signs of pericardial involvement are similar to those for other etiologies, the cancer patient usually has other intrathoracic disease and systemic illness, which complicates the presenting manifestations. The typical features of cardiac tamponade include complaints of dyspnea, orthopnea, cough, chest pain; physical findings of tachycardia, increased venous pressure with pleural effusions and hepatic engorgement, decreased systemic blood pressure with narrow pulse pressure and pulsus paradoxus, and normal or distant heart sounds; and laboratory studies that demonstrate a normal or enlarged cardiac silhouette and an electrocardiogram revealing elevated ST segments or nonspecific T-wave changes, decreased voltage, and, occasionally, electrical alternans. The size of the pericardial effusion and its hemodynamic significance depend on such factors as the rate of fluid accumulation and the elastic properties of the pericardium (as modified by the presence of tumor or prior radiation injury, for example). Clinically apparent malignant effusions tend to be large and easily quantified by echocardiography.

Pericardiocentesis is used to relieve cardiac tamponade secondary to effusion and to establish the etiology of pericardial fluid formation. Although the hemodynamic compromise may be dramatically improved with removal of less than 50 ml of fluid, it is important to remove as much of the effusion as possible (for diagnostic studies and to assess fluid reaccumulation). Malignant pericardial fluid is typically a serosanguineous exudate. In addition to the usual fluid studies of specific gravity, protein, cell count, stains, and cultures, there must be cytologic analysis to document the neoplastic etiology of the fluid. With metastatic carcinoma, the pericardial fluid cytologic analysis is more than 80% accurate with virtually no false-positive results. The yield with lymphoma or mesothelioma is considerably less. A positive cytology establishes the presence of malignant pericardial disease and may define the tumor's histopathology but does not always identify the primary.

Occasionally the elevated venous pressure attributed to pericardial effusion with tamponade will not be relieved by pericardiocentesis alone. This may be the case with superior vena cava syndrome, congestive heart failure, and subacute effusive-constrictive pericardial disease. The latter condition is most often found months to years following radiation therapy to the mediastinum, including the heart (at least 4000 rads), or may be caused by tuberculosis or extensive neoplastic disease. Its diagnosis may be made by simultaneous pressure measurements in the right atrium and pericardial sac.

The treatment of neoplastic pericardial disease depends upon its etiology, its hemodynamic significance, the patient's general medical condition, and the extent and histologic characteristics of the metastatic malignancy. Pericardiocentesis usually relieves the signs and symptoms of cardiac tamponade; however, the fluid may reaccumulate in 24 to 48 hours. Multiple taps or indwelling catheter placement has been reported to be effective in controlling fluid formation. It is frequently necessary to combine this procedure with other local or systemic measures, however. In responsive tumors (such as lymphomas or breast cancer) systemic chemotherapy may be initiated. When local therapy is needed, various agents (5-FU, thiotepa, nitrogen mustard, quinacrine, ^{198}Au, ^{32}P, tetracycline) may be instilled into the pericardial sac, or external radiation therapy may be delivered (at least 3000–4000 rads for solid tumors). The response rate with these local modalities is at least 50%, with remission durations of more than 4 to 6 months.

Surgical procedures that may be considered include pericardial window (partial pericardiectomy) and pericardiectomy. Pericardial window is usually reserved for those patients with rapid fluid reaccumulation or failure of other local measures, and may be highly effective. Visceral pericardiectomy is the treatment of choice for patients with subacute effusive-constrictive pericardial disease secondary to radiation therapy. It is usually not advisable for those patients with extensive metastatic disease but is indicated for those with pericardial mesothelioma.

The prognosis for patients with neoplastic pericardial disease depends upon its etiology, its hemodynamic significance, the effectiveness of therapy, the patient's general medical condition, and the extent and histologic character of the metastatic malignancy. Average survivals have been reported to be as long as 12 to 16 months in responsive patients.

C.P.

Cham WC, Freiman AH, Carstens PHB, et al: Radiation therapy of cardiac and pericardial metastases. Radiology 114:701–704, 1975.
In 38 patients radiation therapy resulted in 60% showing clinical improvement.
Cohen JL: Neoplastic pericarditis. Cardiovasc Clin 7:257–269, 1976.
Article reviews incidence, clinical manifestations, and therapy of neoplastic pericarditis.
Flannery EP, Gregoratos G, Corder MP: Pericardial effusions in patients with malignant diseases. Arch Intern Med 135:976–977, 1975.
Short-term indwelling catheter drainage in 6 patients is described.
Fowler NO: Diseases of the pericardium. Curr Probl Cardiol 2:1–38, 1978.
This is an excellent presentation of pathophysiology, clinical features, and diagnostic considerations.
Hill GJ II, Cohen BI: Pleural pericardial window for palliation of cardiac tamponade due to cancer. Cancer 26:81–93, 1970.
A report is made of 4 patients in whom a pleural pericardial window was made.
Krikorian JG, Hancock EW: Pericardiocentesis. Am J Med 65:808–814, 1978.
This is a retrospective review of 123 patients undergoing pericardiocentesis.
Mann T, Brodie BR, Grossman W, McLaurin L: Effusive-constrictive hemodynamic pattern due to neoplastic involvement of the pericardium. Am J Cardiol 41:781–786, 1978.
Findings in 8 patients with this pattern are discussed.
Martini N, Freiman AH, Watson RC, Hilaris BS: Intrapericardial instillation of radioactive chromic phosphate in malignant pericardial effusion. Am J Roentgenol 128:639–641, 1977.
Article reports on therapy in 28 patients with malignant pericardial effusion.
Theologides A: Neoplastic cardiac tamponade. Semin Oncol 5:181–192, 1978.
A comprehensive literature review.
Zipf RE Jr, Johnston WW: The role of cytology in the evaluation of pericardial effusions. Chest 62:593–596, 1972.
Of 15 patients with later documented pericardial tumor, 12 had positive pericardial fluid cytology.

Liver metastases are often a major source of morbidity and mortality for patients with cancer. Symptoms may include right upper quadrant pain, which is made worse by breathing, coughing, or changes in position, and diffuse or focal tenderness to palpation. Hepatomegaly is present in the majority of patients and may be associated with jaundice, ascites, palpable abdominal masses, friction rubs, and/or bruits. The diagnosis is usually made without difficulty, as described in Part II, Chapter 23.

Local strategies that have been used singly or in combination to palliate hepatic metastases include intra-arterial chemotherapy, hepatic artery ligation, and external hepatic irradiation. Although all may be transiently effective in relieving symptoms or producing tumor regressions, none has been shown to be clearly superior to systemic chemotherapy. In addition there is little evidence that survival is prolonged by these approaches. The rationale for intra-arterial chemotherapy is that the liver may be the only clinically apparent site of metastatic disease, that progression of disease in the liver leads to early death, that higher local drug concentrations can be obtained, and that systemic chemotherapy toxicity may be avoided if drugs are used that are metabolized by the liver. Intra-arterial (IA) 5-fluorouracil has been used most often in patients with metastatic colon carcinoma. Generally patients have previously received 5-FU systemically prior to initiation of IA therapy. In spite of this prior chemotherapy exposure, the objective response rate is approximately 50%, albeit transient. The median survival of responders is 7 months compared to 2 months for patients who do not respond. The toxic side-effects (leukopenia) of 5-FU are usually minimal in most patients; however, the morbidities of intra-arterial therapy remain, including inhospital infusion, percutaneous or surgical catheter placement, potential infection and/or hemorrhage, possible thrombus formation in the infused vessels (up to 28% in one series) with subsequent vessel occlusion and downstream embolization, and displacement of the intra-arterial catheter.

Hepatic artery ligation has been combined with IA infusion therapy without obvious improvement in results. Although ligation should theoretically lead to selective tumor anoxia, responses are brief and probably due to the rapid development of extensive collateralization. External hepatic irradiation has also been used to palliate hepatic metastases. In one series objective responses were seen in 44% of patients, with symptomatic improvement in an additional 40%. The median survival of responders was 9 months. The treatment was well tolerated, and radiation hepatitis was not seen with 2400 rads in 300 rad fractions. Recent data suggest that combined chemotherapy and irradiation approaches may improve the palliative benefits of either modality alone.

Surgical resection of hepatic metastases has also been used in selected patients. With solitary metastases the operative mortality is low, and the 5-year survival was as high as 30% in one series. On the other hand, with multiple metastases, the operative mortality may be as high as 15% to 20%, and the 5-year survival only 13% in one series.

C.P.

Ansfield FJ, Ramirez G, Davis HL Jr, et al: Further clinical studies with intrahepatic arterial infusion with 5-fluorouracil. Cancer 36:2413–2417, 1975.
Of 293 patients who could be evaluated, 55% showed objective improvement with a median survival of 7 months.

Foster JH: Survival after liver resection for secondary tumors. Am J Surg 135:389–394, 1978.
A literature review.

Friedman M, Cassidy M, Levine M, Phillips T, Spivack S, Resser KJ: Combined modality therapy of hepatic metastasis. Cancer 44:906–913, 1979.
Intra-arterial chemotherapy plus irradiation resulted in objective regressions in 10 of 21 patients who could be evaluated.

Garnick MB, Ensminger WD, Israel M: A clinical-pharmacological evaluation of hepatic arterial infusion of adriamycin. Cancer Res 39:4105–4110, 1979.
A study of 5 patients who showed higher hepatic venous vs. peripheral venous drug levels is reported.

Goldman ML, Bilbao MK, Rosch J, Dotter CT: Complications of indwelling chemotherapy catheters. Cancer 36:1983–1990, 1975.
Article provides evaluation of intra-arterial infusion in 39 patients.

Grage TB, Vassilopoulos PP, Shingleton WW, et al: Results of a prospective randomized study of hepatic artery infusion with 5-fluorouracil versus intravenous 5-fluorouracil in patients with hepatic metastases from colorectal cancer: A Central Oncology Group study. Surgery 86:550–555, 1979.
The response rate (23% vs. 34%), median time to progression (23 vs. 26 weeks), and median survival (13 vs. 10 weeks) were comparable in both groups (a total of 61 patients were studied).

McDermott WV Jr, Paris AL, Clouse ME, Meissner WA: Dearterialization of the liver for metastatic cancer: Clinical, angiographic and pathologic observations. Ann Surg 187:38–46, 1978.
In this description of 5 cases palliation of symptoms was obtained in 3 patients.

Meyer JE, Messer RJ, and Patel VC: Diagnosis and treatment of obstructive jaundice secondary to liver metastases. Cancer 41:773–775, 1978.
This report of 3 cases illustrates the utility of local field irradiation for extrahepatic biliary obstruction.

Patt YZ, Mavligit GM, Chuang VP, et al: Percutaneous hepatic arterial infusion (HAI) of mitomycin C and floxuridine (FUDR): An effective treatment for metastatic colorectal carcinoma of the liver. Cancer 46:261–265, 1980.
Objective responses were documented in 10 of 12 patients with a median remission duration of 6 months.

Ramming KP, Sparks FC, Eilber FR, Morton DL: Management of hepatic metastases. Semin Oncol 4:71–80, 1977.
A review of the literature and experience at the University of California at Los Angeles is provided in this article.

Sherman DM, Weichselbaum R, Order SE, et al: Palliation of hepatic metastasis. Cancer 41:2013–2017, 1978.
Hepatic irradiation in 55 patients is analyzed in this article.

111. BOWEL OBSTRUCTION

Bowel obstruction is one of the most common gastrointestinal surgical problems, resulting in at least 9000 deaths in the United States yearly. The mortality from bowel obstruction decreased from 60% in the 1900s, to 20% by the 1930s, and to 10% from the 1950s to the present. Two-thirds of bowel obstructions involve the small bowel, one-third the colorectum.

Approximately one-third of small bowel obstructions are caused by adhesions. Other frequent causes of bowel obstructions are hernias, either external or internal (herniation into the epiploic foramen, around ostomies, or through areas of adhesions), and intra-abdominal malignancies. Less frequently, inflammatory bowel diseases, postirradiation strictures, impaction, volvulus, intussusception and diverticulitis may also produce bowel obstructions.

Abdominal pain, emesis, obstipation, and abdominal distention are all present in varying degrees in patients with bowel obstruction. In complete obstruction of the proximal bowel, vomiting is the most important symptom. Abdominal pain also occurs but is poorly localized and noncolicky. Because of the massive emesis, hydrogen ion and potassium are lost, resulting in metabolic alkalosis. In distal, complete bowel obstruction, colicky pain, vomiting, distention, constipation, and ultimately obstipation all occur. When the large bowel is obstructed, obstipation and distention are commonly noted. Pain and vomiting occur late in the course. Ileus, characterized by ineffective bowel propulsion, may also occur because of smooth muscle fatigue during prolonged mechanical obstruction. Ileus may also be noted in the postoperative period, after trauma, or with abdominal inflammatory processes, intestinal ischemia, or ureteral colic.

The history in patients with bowel obstructions may reveal the above symptoms, the presence of an intra-abdominal neoplasm, prior abdominal surgery, a hernia, or prior abdominal irradiation. The physical examination may reveal hyperperistalsis in early complete obstruction of the distal small bowel; but late in the course, as fatigue of the gut smooth muscle occurs, the bowel sounds may be decreased or absent. Abdominal distention, tenderness, rigidity, or rebound tenderness should be noted. The presence of a mass, enlarged lymph nodes, or hernias should also be elicited. A rectal examination is mandatory. The vital signs are usually normal in early bowel obstruction, but if infarction or perforation have occurred, fever, shock, and dehydration may all be noted. Laboratory studies should include a complete blood and platelet count; BUN; urinalysis with specific gravity, amylase, and electrolyte determinations; and coagulation parameters. A chest radiograph and four-way abdominal x-rays should also be performed. Dilated bowel loops with air-fluid levels are commonly noted in acute obstruction. However, air-fluid levels may be decreased in early proximal, or closed loop bowel obstruction, or with diminished gas volume in the loops. Barium or gastrografin gastrointestinal studies, either through a tube or peroral (or a barium enema), may be necessary when the diagnosis of intestinal obstruction is in doubt. Intravenous urograms may also be indicated when retroperitoneal abnormalities are suspected. Occasionally such special procedures as cystograms and fistula tract injections are also indicated. An abdominal paracentesis should be considered but is contraindicated in patients with massive abdominal distention. In bowel infarction the aspirated fluid is usually foul-smelling and reddish brown, contains increased amylase concentrations, and is often infected with coliform bacteria. In pancreatitis, however, the amylase is also elevated, but *E. coli* is not cultured from the fluid, which is neither foul nor reddish brown in color.

Strangulation obstruction may be confused with hemorrhagic pancreatitis or mesenteric vascular occlusion. In this severe disorder, abdominal tenderness is the most common complaint, followed by tachycardia, leukocytosis, severe abdominal pain, fever, muscle guarding, a palpable abdominal mass, shock, hypothermia, and bloody diarrhea. Late in the course the hematocrit and urine specific gravity are elevated, hypokalemia and decreased chloride both occur, and the serum amylase may be elevated.

With ileus, diffuse, constant pain is usually noted, there are few or no bowel sounds, and radiographs reveal uniform gas distribution. A gastrointestinal series may be necessary to confirm the diagnosis. Acute ileus may also result from acute appendicitis, gastroenteritis, and pancreatitis.

In radiation small bowel injury, a small bowel series may be abnormal, demonstrating atrophic ulcerated mucosa in areas of rigid, narrow bowel. Adhesions, bowel wall thickening, nondistensibility, mucosal effacement, and bowel dilatation and ulceration may also be prominent x-ray findings.

The initial therapy of bowel obstruction includes the administration of intravenous fluids and electrolytes. Antibiotics and hyperalimentation may also be necessary. Nasogastric tube decompression should be performed to decrease emesis, distention, and the possibility of aspiration. In most cases the central venous pressure should be monitored, and if moderate or severe bowel obstruction has occurred, bladder catheterization and monitoring of urine output should be initiated. Immediate surgery is required for strangulation obstruction. In patients with complete obstruction, the preoperative preparation should not be unduly delayed, since strangulation may occur. Exceptions to immediate operation occur in patients with postoperative obstruction, those with prior operations for obstruction in whom strangulation is not suspected, when abdominal carcinomatosis is present, or early in the course of radiation enteritis and obstruction. With postirradiation bowel obstruction, such medical therapy as dietary manipulation, parenteral steroids, and tube decompression may lead to resolution of the problem, but if surgery is necessary, it should be performed electively, if possible, rather than on an emergency basis late in the course of complete obstruction. If, however, obstruction due to radiation enteritis progresses after intensive medical management or if gastrointestinal bleeding or fistulization occurs, surgical exploration and resection or bypass of the diseased bowel should be performed. Surgical procedures for relief of bowel obstructions include lysis of adhesions; resection of obstructing neoplasms; resection or bypass of affected bowel and creation of anastomoses to uninvolved intestinal segments; consideration of proximal diversion with massive obstruction or in the presence of perforation or strangulation; resection of foreign bodies; and exteriorization of anastomoses when the remaining bowel is marginally viable. When multiple adhesions or areas of radiation injury are present, the entire bowel should be examined to rule out potential sites of distal obstruction. When bowel obstruction is due to such radiosensitive neoplasms as lymphomas, abdominal irradiation may be considered. With complete obstruction, however, resection or bypass of the affected area may still be necessary if conservative treatment and radiotherapy fail to resolve the problem.

The average hospital stay for patients with mechanical small bowel obstruction is 17 to 21 days, with a 6% to 25% risk of developing a postoperative infection. The operative mortality alone approximates 10%, with an overall mortality of 10% to 20%. Patients with intra-abdominal neoplasms and bowel obstruction, however, have an operative mortality of 50% to 60%. When bowel infarction occurs, an overall mortality of 35% may be expected. If both a temperature greater than 39°C and shock are present, however, an 85% mortality rate has been noted. The causes of death in mechanical small bowel obstruction are irreversible shock, 45%; cardiovascular causes, 40% (myocardial infarction, cerebrovascular accidents, congestive heart failure or cardiac arrest); pneumonia, 9%; and emboli, 6%.

D.G.

Fielding LP, Stewart-Brown S, Blesvosky L: Large-bowel obstruction caused by cancer: A prospective study. Br Med J 2:515–517, 1979.
  Hospitalizations were shorter for patients who had primary, rather than staged, resections.
Guiffre J: Intestinal obstruction: Ten year experience. Dis Colon Rectum 15:426–430, 1972.
  Article provides a review of causes and treatment of small bowel obstruction.

Mason R: Small bowel obstruction. *In* Rhodes Textbook of Surgery. Philadelphia, J.B. Lippincott, 1977. Pp. 1115–1121.
   *A short review of pathophysiology, causes, and treatment of small bowel
   obstruction is found in this chapter.*

Mason R, Guernsey J, Hanks G, Nelsen T: Surgical therapy for radiation
enteritis. Oncology 22:241–257, 1968.
   *In 35 irradiated patients most who needed resection required it within 12
   months of XRT. There was a 20% operative mortality.*

Nadrowski L: Pathophysiology and current treatment of intestinal obstruction. Rev Surg 31:381–407, 1974.
   A comprehensive review.

Sufran S, Matsumoto T: Intestinal obstruction. Am J Surg 130:9–14, 1975.
   *In 171 patients who had intestinal obstructions the most common causes were
   adhesions, hernias, and neoplasms.*

112. RENAL FAILURE

Renal failure may develop in cancer patients as a consequence of the disease
and/or its treatment. Rarely, there may be direct tumor infiltration of the
kidneys; more commonly, there is postrenal ureteral or bladder outlet obstruction. Bilateral renal infiltration is most often reported in acute lymphoblastic
leukemia and diffuse lymphoma, in which it causes bilaterally enlarged kidneys with elongated calyces. Unlike postrenal causes, it has no associated hydronephrosis. Bilateral ureteral obstruction may be due to extrinsic compression
of the ureters by a large mass; or to multiple retroperitoneal lymph nodes,
intrinsic ureteral metastases, or obstruction at the ureteral orifices by bladder
tumor masses.

Ultrasound studies may document hydronephrosis, while it may be necessary
to use infusion or retrograde pyelography to demonstrate the level of ureteral
obstruction. Bladder outlet obstruction is most commonly encountered in carcinoma of the prostate but may also be due to urethral metastases from other
malignancies. It is most readily documented through cystoscopy. Lymphomatous or leukemic involvement of the kidneys and ureters may be treated with
radiation and/or chemotherapy. On the other hand, solid tumor ureteral
obstruction may require surgical urinary diversion followed by high-dose irradiation. In such instances the aggressiveness of therapy should be balanced
by extent of disease, potential for palliative benefit, and overall prognosis.

Another tumor-related cause of renal failure is the presence of myeloma
paraproteins. There is both associated glomerular and tubular damage, with
the tubular precipitation of proteinaceous material. Such patients may have
poorly reversible acute renal failure with dehydration and hypotension (as for
intravenous pyelography or venography).

Acute uric acid nephropathy results from massive tumor cell lysis, the release of intracellular nucleoproteins, and the subsequent excess production of
uric acid. It occurs most often in newly treated patients with lymphoma or
leukemia. There is rapid development of hyperuricemia and uricosuria with
precipitation of uric acid crystals within the renal collecting tubules and collecting ducts, leading to an intrarenal obstructive nephropathy. Oliguria and renal
shutdown may ensue because of the mechanical obstruction of uric acid
sludge. Once this has occurred, it may be necessary to initiate hemodialysis in
order to reduce the excretory load of plasma urate.

Fortunately, uric acid nephropathy can usually be avoided by anticipating its development in patients with leukemia, lymphoma, or bulky responsive solid tumors. Allopurinol, given prophylactically prior to the initiation of antitumor therapy (at least 12 hours), can reduce endogenous production of uric acid by inhibiting the conversion of xanthine to uric acid. Alkalinization to pH > 7.4 ensures that more than 95% of the uric acid filtered is in a soluble ionized form; and, with concurrent hydration, minimizes the risk of intrarenal uric acid precipitation.

Rarely, xanthine production itself may be so excessive that a similar obstructive nephropathy develops due to xanthine intratubular precipitation. Like uric acid, methotrexate can cause intrarenal obstruction due to precipitation of the drug within the renal tubules and collecting ducts. An amorphous yellow tubular precipitate may be identified on renal biopsy and elevated methotrexate drug levels found in the renal parenchyma. Like uric acid, methotrexate is more soluble at alkaline pH, so that alkalinization and vigorous hydration aid in reducing this complication. Hemodialysis is an effective means of clearing methotrexate if there is complete renal shutdown.

Other antitumor drugs that have associated nephrotoxicity are *cis*-diamminedichloroplatinum (Part VI, Chapter 99) and streptozotocin (Part VI, Chapter 98). Antimicrobial agents may also lead or contribute to acute renal failure. Other causes of renal failure in cancer patients include hypercalcemia (Part I, Chapter 10), disseminated intravascular coagulation (Part I, Chapter 8), radiation nephritis (Part I, Chapter 2), and pyelonephritis.

C.P.

Ahmad S, Shen F, Bleyer WA: Methotrexate-induced renal failure and ineffectiveness of peritoneal dialysis. Arch Intern Med 138:1146–1147, 1978.
This case report describes the inability to effectively remove methotrexate by peritoneal dialysis in acute renal failure.

Appel GB, Neu HC: The nephrotoxicity of antimicrobial agents. N Engl J Med 296:663–670; 722–728; 784–787, 1977.
Article provides a comprehensive summary of the nephrotoxicity of antimicrobial agents.

Djerassi I, Ciesielka W, Kim JS: Removal of methotrexate by filtration-absorption using charcoal filters or by hemodialysis. Cancer Treat Rep 61:751–752, 1977.
A brief report is given of effective hemodialysis in 6 patients.

Garnick MB, Mayer RJ: Acute renal failure associated with neoplastic disease and its treatment. Semin Oncol 5:155–165, 1978.
An excellent summary.

Kanfer A, Vandewalle A, Morel-Maroger L, Feintuch M-J, Sraer JD, Roland J: Acute renal insufficiency due to lymphomatous infiltration of the kidneys: Report of six cases. Cancer 38:2588–2592, 1976.
Bilaterally enlarged kidneys and mild proteinuria suggest the diagnosis of lymphomatous infiltration.

Kelton J, Kelley WN, Holmes EW: A rapid method for the diagnosis of acute uric acid nephropathy. Arch Intern Med 138:612–615, 1978.
A urinary uric acid to creatinine concentration ratio of greater than 1.0 appeared to distinguish acute uric acid nephropathy in 5 patients from other causes of acute renal failure.

Lundberg WB, Cadman ED, Finch SC, Capizzi RL: Renal failure secondary to leukemic infiltration of the kidneys. Am J Med 62:636–642, 1977.
Article includes a case report and literature review.

Madias NE, Harrington JT: Platinum nephrotoxicity. Am J Med 65:307–314, 1978.
A literature review.
Robinson RR, Yarger WE: Acute uric acid nephropathy. Arch Intern Med 137:839–840, 1977.
This editorial discusses the etiology of this syndrome.

113. BONE METASTASES

Neoplasms most likely to produce bone metastases are carcinoma of the lung, breast, kidney, thyroid, and prostate. Bone lesions also occur with multiple myeloma, melanomas, other genitourinary cancers, gastrointestinal neoplasms, and lymphomas. The bone lesions of Hodgkin's disease and the non-Hodgkin's lymphomas are usually blastic.

The most common symptom of bone metastases is pain. Pain can result from expansile osseous lesions, from pathologic fractures, or from spinal cord or nerve root compression following epidural extension of neoplasm from an involved bone.

A careful history and physical examination should be performed, including a neurologic examination to rule out spinal cord compression. Appropriate radiographs of painful areas should be obtained to demonstrate the lesions. Since bone metastases are rarely solitary, a Tc 99m bone scan may be useful in showing other sites of osseous involvement. However, with lytic bone disease caused by myeloma, the bone scan is rarely positive, whereas a bone survey may reveal widespread bony destruction. A serum calcium determination should also be obtained to rule out hypercalcemia in a patient with multiple osseous metastases.

The diagnosis of bone metastases is not difficult when a primary carcinoma has been diagnosed. In the rare instance of an isolated osseous lesion without a known source of origin, however, a tissue diagnosis should be obtained if possible, either through a fluoroscopically guided cutting needle biopsy or by an open procedure, if the site is inaccessible percutaneously. The important differentiation between postirradiation osteitis secondary to prior irradiation and bone metastases must also be made when a patient has received prior high-dose irradiation to the area of involvement. A history of prior radiotherapy to the area and the presence of irregular, lytic lesions confined to the irradiated volume should allow the correct diagnosis to be established. Metastases usually give rise to localized lytic, blastic, or mixed lesions in an otherwise normal-appearing bone, whereas in postirradiation osteitis diffuse, mixed lesions closely conform to the prior radiation treatment volume.

If a pathologic fracture has occurred in a long bone, fixation and stabilization should be performed prior to irradiation of the lesion. When there is more than 25% involvement of the cortex of a weight-bearing long bone, fixation should be considered the initial treatment of choice. Fixation may diminish the pain experienced with weight-bearing, may avoid a pathologic fracture, and allows the patient to be mobilized earlier so that treatment may be given without producing a pathologic fracture.

For patients with either painful localized bone lesions or with lytic long bone or vertebral metastases, radiotherapy is the treatment of choice. The irradiation should produce control of pain without causing such sequelae as severe skin reactions, radiation pneumonitis, carditis or myelitis, and injury to the gastrointestinal tract. The radiotherapy course should not be unduly prolonged;

however, patients with bone metastases have a mean survival of at least 14 months, so late injury to normal tissues (especially the spinal cord) is possible. Radiation therapy doses ranging from 1000 rads in two 500-rad fractions to 5000 rads in 5 weeks to the site of bone involvement should produce permanent relief of pain in approximately 85% of patients. There appears to be no difference in the frequency of palliation for the most common neoplasms, which metastasize to bone-prostate, breast and lung cancers, myeloma, and lymphoma. Pain relief can be expected to occur as early as 2 weeks after the radiotherapy is initiated and should be obtained in most patients by 1 to 3 months. The addition of systemic chemotherapy may be indicated for patients with myeloma, testicular or small cell lung cancers, or the lymphomas. Patients with breast carcinomas, depending on menopausal status and the extent of prior treatment, may be managed subsequently by chemotherapy, ablative procedures, or hormonal manipulation. Endocrine ablation or hormonal therapy may also produce long remissions in patients with prostatic carcinomas.

D.G.

Allen K, Johnson T, Hibbs G: Effect of bone palliation as related to various treatment regimens. Cancer 37:984–987, 1976.
A high percentage of permanent pain relief (85%) was gained both in patients with breast cancer and those with other malignancies with radiation doses ranging from 1000 rads in 2 days to 4000 rads in 3 weeks. There were no differences in results between dose regimens, retrospectively analyzed.

Boland J, Glicksman A, Vargha A: Single dose radiation therapy in the palliation of metastatic disease. Radiology 93:1181–1184, 1969.
Single doses, 500 rads to 1200 rads, provided good to excellent pain relief in 90% of patients, with high percentage responses in both those with breast and with prostate cancers.

Fiddler M: Prophylactic internal fixation of secondary neoplastic deposits in long bones. Br Med J 1:341–343, 1973.
There were no pathological fractures with less than 25% cortical involvement. The article lists the advantages of prophylactic internal fixation; 19 patients with pathological fractures were studied.

Gilbert H, Kagan A, Nussbaum H, et al: Evaluation of radiation therapy for bone metastases: Pain relief and quality of life. Am J Roentgenol 129:1095–1096, 1977.
In 158 patients the median survival from first symptoms of bone metastases was 14 months. In 73% of sites treated patients obtained pain relief in 3 months, and approximately 60% sustained relief up to 1 year or death.

Hendrickson F, Shehata W, Kirchner A: Radiation therapy for osseous metastases. Int J Radiat Oncol Biol Phys 1:275–278, 1976.
In this article short course radiotherapy, prospective study, ranged from a single dose of 900 rads to 300 rads times 10. There were no observed differences in this dose range; 85% of patients improved with decreased pain. It is notable that prostate cancer responded more slowly than other metastases.

Howland W, Loeffler R, Starchman D, Johnson R: Post-irradiation atrophic changes of bone and related complications. Radiology 117:677–685, 1975.
This is a good review of postirradiation bone changes and differential diagnosis of these lesions.

Schutte HE: The influence of bone pain on the results of bone scans. Cancer 44:2039–2043, 1979.
When bone pain was present in patients with primary cancer, 82 of 130 had positive scans. Without bone pain, only 13 of 97 patients had positive studies and 10 of the 13 had osteoblastic lesions.

Viral infections that may be serious in the compromised cancer patient are herpes varicella-zoster, herpes simplex, cytomegalovirus, vaccinia, and rubeola. Other viral infections appear to have the same frequency and clinical course in the cancer patient as in the normal population.

The primary infection of herpes varicella (chickenpox) in adults is probably more severe in those with malignancies. The typical maculopapular eruption on the trunk spreads centrifugally to involve the entire skin. The papules become vesicles, then crust, scab, and heal. Superimposed bacterial infections (*Staphylococcus aureus, Streptococcus pyogenes, Escherichia coli,* and *Pseudomonas aeruginosa*) of the lesions occur in almost 10% of patients. However, fatalities are usually attributable to the development of viral pneumonitis or meningoencephalitis, whereas visceral involvement of the liver or pancreas is not fatal. The diagnosis of varicella-zoster may be established by immunofluorescence study of scraped lesions and serial serologies. Treatment of herpes varicella is limited to supportive care, discontinuance of immunosuppressive drugs, and protective isolation. No effective means of active immunization is available. Passive immunization with zoster immune globulin or plasma may modify or prevent infection if given within 72 hours of exposure, whereas pooled gamma globulin is ineffective. Antiviral therapies (adenine arabinoside, interferon) remain investigational.

Herpes zoster presents with skin lesions like those of varicella, but the distribution is usually dermatomal and only later generalized. It is seen only in patients who have previously acquired varicella and is due to the reactivation of latent virus residing in the sensory ganglia. In the normal population its incidence is only 1% to 5%, increasing with age. On the other hand it may be seen in up to 25% of patients with Hodgkin's disease. Predisposing factors include recent radiation and/or chemotherapy, advanced or recurrent disease, and probably splenectomy. Skin dissemination occurs 6 to 10 days after the primary dermatomal infection, and, although morbid, it is not life-threatening. In the normal population skin dissemination is seen in fewer than 2%, while it may occur in up to 25% of affected patients with Hodgkin's disease. Visceral dissemination (involving the gastrointestinal tract, myocardium, lungs, and nervous system) is unusual, even in the compromised host. Antiviral therapies that appear to be effective in diminishing primary dermatomal infection and the incidence of skin dissemination are interferon and adenine arabinoside. Both agents must be administered early in the course of the disease and are ineffective once the disease is established. Other measures include supportive care, protective isolation, pain relief for neuralgia, and discontinuance of immunosuppressive therapy.

Clinically significant cytomegalovirus (CMV) infections are rarely seen in the normal host. In cancer patients the disease is probably due to the reactivation of latent virus rather than exogenous exposure. CMV can be transmitted by blood transfusion, and the risk of acquiring the virus by this route is proportional to the amount of blood transfused. Clinical manifestations of the disease include a heterophil-negative mononucleosis-like syndrome, fever with morbilliform rash, overt or subclinical hepatitis, hemolytic anemia, diffuse or focal pneumonitis, gastroenteritis, and azotemia. The diagnosis is best established by identifying the typical intranuclear inclusions of infected cells on biopsy material. The presence of these cells in urine does not necessarily have a correlation with symptomatic infection, however. Serial serologies and viral cultures may also be helpful. There is no established antiviral therapy. Treatment is symptomatic.

Smallpox vaccinations may be hazardous in the immunosuppressed patient. There may be a severe local reaction ("vaccinia necrosum") or, occasionally, development of generalized vaccinia. Vaccinia immune globulin and marboran (1-methylisatin 3-thiosemicarbazone) may be helpful in selected patients.

C.P.

Dolin R, Reichman RC, Mazur MH, Whitley RJ: Herpes zoster-varicella infections in immunosuppressed patients. Ann Intern Med 89:375–388, 1978.
Article discusses clinical manifestations, neurological complications, immunodiagnosis, and therapy with adenine arabinoside.
Feldman S, Cox F: Viral infections and haematological malignancies. Clin Haematol 5:311–328, 1976.
Article outlines clinical presentations and diagnostic considerations.
Hirsch MS, Swartz MN: Drug therapy: Antiviral agents. N Engl J Med 302:903–907 and 949–953, 1980.
An excellent review of antiviral agents.
Ho M: Cytomegalovirus infections and diseases. DM 24:1–61, 1978.
An excellent summary of all aspects of these infections and diseases.
Merigan TC, Rand KH, Pollard RB, et al: Human leukocyte interferon for the treatment of herpes zoster in patients with cancer. N Engl J Med 298:981–987, 1978.
High-dosage interferon significantly reduced the frequency of cutaneous dissemination and progression within the primary dermatome when compared to placebo.
Pazin GJ, Armstrong JA, Lam MT, et al: Prevention of reactivated herpes simplex infection by human leukocyte interferon after operation on the trigeminal root. N Engl J Med 301:225–230, 1979.
This prospective double-blind study demonstrates the significant benefit of interferon when compared to a placebo.
Rosen PP: Cytomegalovirus infection in cancer patients. Pathol Annu 13:175–208, 1978.
This article provides a complete pathological description of cytomegalovirus infection.
Ruckdeschel JC, Schimpff SC, Smyth AC, Mardiney MR Jr: Herpes zoster and impaired cell-associated immunity to the varicella-zoster virus in patients with Hodgkin's disease. Am J Med 62:77–85, 1977.
In vitro lymphocyte responsiveness was measured in 32 patients and compared to 12 normal donors.
Whitley RJ, Ch'ien LT, Dolan R, et al: Adenine arabinoside therapy of herpes zoster in the immunosuppressed: NIAID collaborative antiviral study. N Engl J Med 294:1193–1199, 1976.
This prospective randomized study in 87 patients demonstrates the significant efficacy of Ara-A in early infection.
Whitley RJ, Soong S-J, Dolin R, et al: Adenine arabinoside therapy of biopsy-proved herpes simplex encephalitis. N Engl J Med 297:289–294, 1977.
Ara-A significantly reduced mortality when compared to a placebo (28% vs. 70%); the drug must be administered early, however.

115. FUNGAL AND PROTOZOAL INFECTIONS

Opportunistic infections with fungi or protozoa are increasingly common in patients with malignant disease. As many as 30% of cancer patients may have documented *Candida* infection at autopsy, and in certain leukemic populations the incidence of *Pneumocystis carinii* may be as high as 25%. These diseases rarely occur in the normal host and are associated with immunosuppressive states (leukemias, lymphomas, corticosteroid and antitumor therapy, neutropenia and antibacterial therapy). An aggressive diagnostic approach is warranted, since these may be rapidly fatal diseases that require early institution of specific antimicrobial therapy. In general the diagnosis of invasive fungal or protozoal infection requires demonstration of organisms in biopsy specimens of viable tissue. Fungal serologies may be suggestive, but negative titers do not exclude infection; and a positive *Pneumocystis* titer may be found in the normal host. Isolation of fungus from sputum, blood, or urine does not necessarily indicate invasive infection, whereas positive cultures of cerebrospinal, intraocular, or pleural fluid do.

The most common invasive fungal infection in cancer patients is *Candida albicans,* accounting for almost three-quarters of all infections. Other fungi encountered are aspergillus, mucormycosis, cryptococcosis, histoplasmosis, and coccidioidomycosis. Because the symptoms and signs of disseminated candidiasis may be nonspecific, fewer than 10% of infections are identified before death. Consequently the diagnosis should be considered in any case of a high-risk febrile patient who does not respond to adequate antibacterial therapy for an unidentified infection. The portals of entry are usually the mouth, oropharynx, and gastrointestinal tract, although surgical wounds or indwelling catheters may also provide a source. Invasive lesions may be identified in virtually any organ but are most often found in the esophagus, intestine, lung, and kidney. Microscopy reveals both pseudohyphae and yeast forms. Amphotericin B is the standard therapy; resistance to 5-fluorocytosine may develop early; and experience with miconazole is limited.

Aspergillus accounts for 5% to 30% of invasive fungal infections, and its incidence appears to be increasing. In cancer patients the disease is characterized by a necrotizing pneumonia with associated pulmonary infarction. The patient may have hemoptysis and a pleural friction rub, and the chest x-ray reveals a diffuse patchy infiltrate. It is uncommon to see a localized segmental or lobar infiltrate or a cavitary lesion. Sputum cultures are usually negative for fungi, as are serologies, and the diagnosis rests on finding characteristic hyphae of invasive aspergillus. Although usually limited to the lungs, the disease may disseminate to involve the brain and gastrointestinal tract. Amphotericin B, 5-fluorocytosine, and aerosolized nystatin have all been used in treatment.

Pneumocystis carinii is an acute, rapidly progressive, diffuse pulmonary infection that is usually fatal without prompt, specific antimicrobial therapy. The disease probably results from reactivation of latent organisms rather than from exogenous exposure, since high antibody titers are present in the majority of normal people. Typically patients present with the abrupt onset of fever to 38° to 40°, a dry nonproductive cough, and tachypnea to more than 40 respirations per minute. There may also be cyanosis, nasal flaring, and intercostal retraction. Upon physical examination the lungs may be clear or may reveal scattered dry rales. The chest x-ray demonstrates diffuse bilateral alveolar infiltrates; however, occasional patients may have solitary lesions, lobar infiltrates, or unilateral disease processes. Arterial blood gases reveal hypoxemia and respiratory alkalosis. The diagnosis can rarely be established by demonstrating organisms on sputum or transtracheal aspiration. Usually invasive procedures, such as percutaneous lung aspiration, bronchial brush biopsy, and open lung biopsy, are required to obtain adequate tissue. The organism in tissue or on imprints may be stained with Gomori's methenamine silver nitrate or toluidine blue O. These techniques identify organisms in approximately 60% of patients with the typical clinical presentation of *Pneumocystis.* Pentamidine

Isethionate is an effective treatment for the disease, reducing mortality to less than 25%; however, it is highly toxic, with a multitude of side-effects. An equally effective regimen with minimal toxicity is trimethoprim (TMP, 20 mg/kg)-sulfamethoxazole (SMZ, 100 mg/kg), administered daily by mouth in four divided doses for 14 days. Serum levels should be obtained to guide drug dosage. In addition to antimicrobial therapy, patients require close monitoring of hypoxemia, oxygen therapy, and often assisted or controlled ventilation. Because TMP-SMZ is so effective for active infection it has also been studied for prophylaxis of *Pneumocystis* in high-risk patients. Administered during the period of susceptibility, it has been shown to be highly effective in preventing active infection as compared to a placebo (TMP, 5 mg/kg, and SMZ, 20 mg/kg, daily in two divided doses).

C.P.

Hoeprich PD: Chemotherapy of systemic fungal diseases. Annu Rev Pharmacol Toxicol 18:205–231, 1978.
  Amphotericin B, 5-fluorocytosine, and miconazole are discussed in depth.
Hughes WT: *Pneumocystis carinii* pneumonia. N Engl J Med 297:1381–1383, 1977.
  Article summarizes data on biology, clinical manifestations, therapy, and prophylaxis.
Hughes WT: Protozoan infections in haematological diseases. Clin Haematol 5:329–345, 1976.
  Report reviews clinical features and therapy of Pneumocystis carinii *and* Toxoplasmosis gondii.
Hughes WT, Kuhn S, Chaudhary S, et al: Successful chemoprophylaxis for *Pneumocystis carinii* pneumonitis. N Engl J Med 297:1419–1426, 1977.
  In this randomized, double-blind study 17 of 80 patients receiving a placebo acquired Pneumocystis carinii *pneumonia, whereas none of 80 receiving trimethoprim-sulfamethoxazole prophylaxis did (p < 0.01).*
Krick JA, Remington JS: Opportunistic invasive fungal infections in patients with leukaemia and lymphoma. Clin Haematol 5:249–310, 1976.
  Article is an excellent comprehensive clinical review of fungal infections in patients with leukemia and lymphoma.
Rosen PP: Opportunistic fungal infections in patients with neoplastic diseases. Pathol Annu 11:255–315, 1976.
  A comprehensive review of the pathology involved in opportunistic fungal infections.
Stevens DA: Miconazole in the treatment of systemic fungal infections. Am Rev Resp Dis 116:801–806, 1977.
  Article provides a review of the treatment experience in coccidioidomycosis.
Winston DJ, Lau WK, Gale RP, Young LS: Trimethoprimsulfamethoxazole for the treatment of *Pneumocystis carinii* pneumonia. Ann Intern Med 92:762–769, 1980.
  Reviews experience with intravenous administration in 11 patients and presents guidelines for treatment of Pneumocystis *pneumonia.*

PART VIII. STAGING

Currently used staging classifications for common tumor sites are presented here. Alternative classifications in common use are also listed (e.g., bladder and colorectum). *The Manual for Staging of Cancer 1978,* available from the American Joint Committee (AJC), 55 E. Erie St., Chicago, Illinois 60611, is an excellent source for the TNM (T = primary tumor; N = regional lymph nodes; M = distant metastatic sites) staging system.

D.G.

116. HEAD AND NECK CANCER (AJC, 1977)

Cervical Lymph Nodes
(applicable to all head and neck sites)
N_0: Nodes clinically uninvolved.
N_1: Single clinically positive homolateral node, tumor <3 cm.
N_{2a}: Single clinically positive homolateral node 3–6 cm.
N_{2b}: Multiple clinically positive homolateral nodes, all <6 cm.
N_{3a}: Clinically positive homolateral node(s), at least one >6 cm.
N_{3b}: Bilateral clinically positive nodes.
N_{3c}: Contralateral clinically positive nodes only.

Oral Cavity
T Categories
T_{1s}: Carcinoma in situ.
T_1: Tumor 2 cm or less.
T_2: Tumor 2–4 cm.
T_3: Tumor >4 cm.
T_4: Massive tumor >4 cm with deep invasion of antrum, pterygoid muscles, root of tongue, or skin of neck.

Stage Groupings
Stage   I: $T_1N_0M_0$
Stage II: $T_2N_0M_0$
Stage III: $T_3N_0M_0$
$\quad\quad\quad\quad$ $T_{1,2,or3}$ N_1M_0
Stage IV: $T_4N_0M_0$
$\quad\quad\quad\quad$ Any T, N_2M_0
$\quad\quad\quad\quad$ Any T, any N, M_1

Supraglottis
T_{1s}: Carcinoma in situ.
T_1: Tumor confined to site of origin with normal mobility.
T_2: Tumor extension to adjacent supraglottic sites or glottis without fixation.
T_3: Tumor limited to larynx with fixation and/or extension to postcricoid area, medial wall of pyriform sinus, or preepiglottic space.
T_4: Massive tumor extending beyond larynx to involve oropharynx, soft tissues of neck, or destruction of thyroid cartilage.

Glottis
T_{1s}: Carcinoma in situ.
T_1: Tumor confined to vocal cords with normal mobility.

T_2: Supraglottic and/or subglottic tumor extension with normal or impaired vocal cord mobility.

T_3: Tumor confined to larynx with vocal cord fixation.

T_4: Massive tumor with thyroid cartilage destruction and/or extension beyond confines of larynx.

Subglottis

T_{1s}: Carcinoma in situ.

T_1: Tumor confined to subglottic region.

T_2: Tumor extension to vocal cords with normal or impaired vocal cord mobility.

T_3: Tumor confined to larynx with vocal cord fixation.

T_4: Massive tumor with cartilage destruction and/or extension beyond larynx.

Stage Groupings

Stage   I: $T_1N_0M_0$

Stage II: $T_2N_0M_0$

Stage III: $T_3N_0M_0$

$T_{1,2,or3} N_1M_0$

Stage IV: $T_4N_0M_0$

Any T, N_2M_0

Any T, any N, M_1

Paranasal Sinuses

T Classification

T_0: No evidence of primary tumor.

T_1: Tumor confined to antral mucosa of infrastructure without bone erosion or destruction.

T_2: Tumor confined to suprastructure mucosa without bone destruction, or to infrastructure with destruction of medial or inferior bony walls only.

T_3: Extensive tumor invading skin or cheek, orbit, anterior ethmoid sinuses, or pterygoid muscle.

T_4: Massive tumor with invasion of pterygoid plate, posterior ethmoids, nasopharynx, pterygoid plates, or base of skull.

Stage Groupings

Stage   I: $T_1N_0M_0$

Stage II: $T_2N_0M_0$

Stage III: $T_3N_0M_0$

$T_{1,2,or3} N_1M_0$

Stage IV: $T_4N_{0,1}M_0$

Any T, $N_{2,3} M_0$

Any T, any N, M_1

Pharynx

Nasopharynx

T_{1s}: Carcinoma in situ.

T_1: Tumor confined to one nasopharyngeal site or no tumor visible (biopsy positive).

T_2: Tumor involving two nasopharyngeal sites.

T_3: Tumor extension into nasal cavity or oropharynx.

T_4: Skull invasion, cranial nerve involvement, or both.

Oropharynx

T_{1s}: Carcinoma in situ.

T_1: Tumor 2 cm or less.

T_2: Tumor 2-4 cm.
T_3: Tumor >4 cm.
T_4: Massive tumor >4 cm with invasion of bone, soft tissues of neck, or root of tongue.

Hypopharynx
T_{1s}: Carcinoma in situ.
T_1: Tumor confined to site of origin.
T_2: Tumor extension to adjacent site or region without fixation of hemilarynx.
T_3: Tumor extension to adjacent site or region with fixation of hemilarynx.
T_4: Massive tumor with invasion of bone or soft tissues of neck.

Stage Groupings
Stage   I: $T_1N_0M_0$
Stage II: $T_2N_0M_0$
Stage III: $T_3N_0M_0$
            $T_{1,2,or3} \, N_1M_0$
Stage IV: $T_4N_0M_0$
            Any T, N_3M_0
            Any T, any N, M_1

117. BREAST CANCER (UICC, 1974)

TNM Classification
T—Primary Tumor
TIS—carcinoma in situ
(*Note:* Paget's disease with a demonstrable tumor is classified according to the size of the tumor.)
T_0: No demonstrable tumor.
T_1: Tumor 2 cm or less in greatest dimension.
T_{1a}: No fixation to underlying fascia and/or muscle.
T_{1b}: Fixation to underlying fascia and/or muscle.
T_2: Tumor 2-5 cm in greatest dimension.
T_{2a}: No fixation to underlying fascia and/or muscle.
T_{2b}: Fixation to underlying fascia and/or muscle.
T_3: Tumor >5 cm in greatest dimension.
T_{3a}: No fixation to underlying fascia and/or muscle.
T_{3b}: Fixation to underlying fascia and/or muscle.
T_4: Tumor of any size with direct extension to chest wall or skin.
T_{4a}: Chest wall fixation.
T_{4b}: Edema, infiltration, or ulceration of skin of breast (including peau d'orange), or satellite skin nodules confined to the same breast.
T_{4c}: Both of the above.
T_{4d}: Inflammatory carcinoma (AJC Committee, 1977).

N—Regional Lymph Nodes
N_0: No palpable homolateral axillary nodes.
N_1: Movable homolateral axillary nodes.
N_{1a}: Nodes not considered to contain growth.
N_{1b}: Nodes considered to contain growth.
N_2: Homolateral axillary nodes fixed to one another or to other structures.
N_3: Homolateral supraclavicular or infraclavicular nodes or edema of the arm.

M—Distant Metastases
M_0: No evidence of distant metastases.
M_1: Distant metastases present.

Stage Groupings
Stage   I: $T_{1a} N_0$ or $N_{1a} M_0$
$T_{1b} N_0$ or N_{1a}
Stage II: $T_0 N_{1b} M_0$
$T_{1a} N_{1b} M_0$
$T_{1b} N_{1b} M_0$
$T_{2a} N_0$ or N_{1a} or $N_{1b} M_0$
$T_{2b} N_0$ or N_{1a} or $N_{1b} M_0$
Stage III: Any T_3 with any N M_0
Any T_4 with any N M_0
Any T with $N_2 M_0$
Any T with $N_3 M_0$
Stage IV: Any T, any N with M_1

118. LUNG CANCER (AJC, 1977)

T Classification
T_X: Positive cytology only or tumor that cannot be assessed.
T_0: No evidence of primary tumor.
T_{1s}: Carcinoma in situ.
T_1: Tumor <3.0 cm, surrounded by lung or visceral pleura; without invasion proximal to a lobar bronchus at bronchoscopy.
T_2: Tumor >3.0 cm or a tumor of any size that either invades visceral pleura or has associated atelectasis or obstructive pneumonitis extending to hila. Proximal extent of tumor must be in a lobar bronchus or 2.0 cm distal to the carina. No pleural effusion. Atelectasis or obstructive pneumonitis must involve an entire lung.
T_3: Direct extension into an adjacent structure; or tumor involving a main bronchus <2.0 cm from carina; or any tumor with atelectasis or obstructive pneumonitis involving an entire lung or a pleural effusion.

Nodal Involvement
N_0: No demonstrable nodal metastases.
N_1: Peribronchial and/or ipsilateral hilar nodal metastases, including direct extension.
N_2: Mediastinal lymph node metastases.

Distant Metastases
M_X: Not assessed.
M_0: No known distant metastases.
M_1: Distant metastases present.

Stage Groupings
Stage   I: $T_{1s} N_0 M_0$
$T_1 N_0 M_0$
$T_1 N_1 M_0$
$T_2 N_0 M_0$
Stage II: $T_2 N_1 M_0$

Stage III: T_3, and N, any M
N_2 with any T or M
M_1 with any T or N

119. COLORECTAL CANCER (AJC, 1977)

T Classification

T_X: Depth of penetration not specified.
T_0: No demonstrable tumor.
T_{1S}: Carcinoma in situ.
T_1: Clinically benign lesion, or lesion confined to mucosa or submucosa.
T_2: Involvement of muscular wall or serosa.
T_3: Involvement of all layers of colon or rectum with extension to adjacent structures and/or organs. No fistula present.
T_4: Fistula present with any of above.
T_5: Direct extension beyond immediately adjacent organs or tissues.

Nodal Involvement

N_X: Nodes not assessed.
N_0: Nodes not involved.
N_1: Regional nodes involved (distal to inferior mesenteric artery).

Metastases

M_X: Not assessed.
M_0: No known distant metastases.
M_1: Distant metastases present.

Stage Groupings

Stage 0: $T_{1S}N_0M_0$
Stage I: $T_0N_0M_0$
I_A: $T_{0,1}N_0M_0$
$T_{0,1}N_XM_0$
I_B: $T_2N_0M_0$
Stage II: $T_{3-5}N_0M_0$
$T_{3-5}N_XM_0$
Stage III: Any T, N_1M_0
Stage IV: Any T, and N, M_1

Duke's (Astler-Collier)

A: Lymph nodes negative. Limited to mucosa.
B_1: Extension through mucosa but still within bowel wall; nodes negative.
B_2: Extension through entire bowel wall; nodes negative.
C_1: Lesion limited to bowel wall; nodes positive.
C_2: Extension through entire bowel wall; nodes positive.

120. RENAL CARCINOMA (AJC, 1977)

T Classification

T_X: Minimum requirements cannot be met.
T_0: No evidence of primary tumor.

T_1:   Small tumor, minimal renal and calyceal distortion or deformity. Circumscribed neovasculature surrounded by normal parenchyma.
T_2:   Large tumor with deformity and/or enlargement of kidney and/or collecting system.
T_3:   Tumor may extend into perinephric tissues, renal vein and/or vena cava.
T_{3a}: Tumor involving perinephric tissues.
T_{3b}: Tumor involving renal vein.
T_{3c}: Tumor involving renal vein and infradiaphragmatic vena cava.
T_4:   Tumor involving neighboring structures or supradiaphragmatic vena cava.
T_{4a}: Tumor invasion of neighboring structures (muscle, bowel).
T_{4b}: Tumor involving supradiaphragmatic vena cava.

Lymph Nodes
N_X: Minimum requirements cannot be met.
N_0: No evidence of involvement of regional nodes.
N_1: Single, homolateral regional nodal involvement.
N_2: Involvement of multiple regional, contralateral, or bilateral nodes.
N_3: Fixed regional nodes (assessable only at surgical exploration).
N_4: Involvement of juxtaregional nodes.

If lymphography is used, add "1" between N and the above number; if there is surgical confirmation add $(+)$ positive and $(-)$ negative histopathology. For example, N_{11+} means positive lymphogram with surgical confirmation.

Metastases
M_X: Not assessed.
M_0: No known distant metastases.
M_1: Distant metastases present.

No stage grouping recommended.

121. BLADDER CANCER (AJC, 1977)

T Classification   **Jewett-Marshall Classification**

T_X: Minimal requirements cannot be met.
T_a: Papillary noninvasive carcinoma.
T_{1s}: Carcinoma in situ (sessile).
T_0:   No evidence of primary tumor.   0
T_1:   Microscopic invasion beyond muscularis mucosa.   A
T_2:   Superficial muscle invasion. B_1
T_{3a}: Deep muscle invasion. B_2
T_{3b}: Invasion through full thickness of bladder wall.   C
T_{4a}: Tumor invading prostate, uterus or vagina.   D
T_{4b}: Tumor fixed to pelvic wall and/or invading the abdominal wall. D_1: pelvic lymph node metastases.

D_2: para-aortic lymph node metastases.

Lymph Nodes
N_X: Minimum requirements cannot be met.
N_0: No involvement of regional lymph nodes.
N_1: Involvement of a single homolateral regional lymph node.
N_2: Involvement of contralateral, bilateral, or multiple regional lymph nodes.
N_3: Fixed pelvic wall mass with a free space between mass and bladder tumor.
N_4: Involvement of juxtaregional lymph nodes.

Metastases
M_X: Not assessed.
M_0: No known distant metastases.
M_1: Distant metastases present.

No stage grouping recommended.

122. PROSTATE CANCER

T Classification (AJC 1977)   Urologic Staging
T_X: Minimum requirements cannot be met.
T_0: No tumor palpable.
T_1: Tumor intracapsular, surrounded by normal gland.   } A
T_2: Tumor confined to gland, deforming contour and invading capsule, but lateral sulci and seminal vesicles not involved.   } B
T_3: Tumor extends beyond capsule with or without involvement of lateral sulci and/or seminal vesicles.
T_4: Tumor fixed or involving neighboring structures.   } C

Nodal Involvement
N_X: Minimum requirements cannot be met.
N_0: No involvement of regional lymph nodes.
N_1: Involvement of a single regional lymph node.
N_2: Involvement of multiple regional lymph nodes.
N_3: Free space between tumor and fixed pelvic sidewall mass.
N_4: Involvement of juxtraregional nodes.

Distant Metastases
M_X: Not assessed.
M_0: No known distant metastases.   } D
M_2: Distant metastases present.

No stage grouping recommended.

T Classification (AJC 1977)
T_X: Minimum requirements cannot be met.
T_0: No evidence of primary tumor.
T_1: Limited to body of testis.
T_2: Extension beyond the tunica albuginea.
T_3: Involvement of the rete testis or epididymis.
T_{4a}: Invasion of spermatic cord.
T_{4b}: Invasion of scrotal wall.

N Classification
N_X: Minimum requirements cannot be met.
N_0: No evidence of involvement of regional lymph nodes.
N_1: Involvement of a single homolateral regional lymph node, which, if inguinal, is mobile.
N_2: Involvement of contralateral, bilateral, or multiple regional lymph nodes, which, if inguinal, are mobile.
N_3: Palpable abdominal mass present or fixed inguinal lymph nodes.
N_4: Involvement of juxtaregional nodes.

Distant Metastases
M_X: Not assessed.
M_0: No known distant metastases.
M_1: Distant metastases present.

No stage grouping recommended.

Walter Reed Staging (Maier, *J. Urol.* 101:356–359, 1969)
I_A: Tumor confined to one testis. No evidence for spread beyond testis.
I_B: Positive iliac or para-aortic nodes at lymphadenectomy.
II: Clinical or radiographic evidence of metastases to inguinal, iliac, or para-aortic lymph nodes. No demonstrable visceral or supradiaphragmatic metastases.
III: Supradiaphragmatic or distant metastases.

124. OVARIAN CANCER (AJC, 1977—FIGO)

T Classification

Stage I: Growth limited to ovaries.		T_1
I_A: Limited to one ovary; no ascites.		T_{1a}
I_{Ai}: Capsule intact.		
I_{Aii}: Capsule ruptured and/or tumor on external surface.		
I_B: Growth limited to both ovaries; no ascites.		T_{1b}
I_{Bi}: Capsule intact.		
I_{Bii}: Capsule ruptured and/or tumor on external surface.		
I_C: Either I_A or I_B with ascites, or peritoneal washings.		T_{1c}
Stage II: Growth involving one or both ovaries with pelvic extension.		T_2
II_A: Extension to uterus and/or tubes.		T_{2a}
II_B: Extension to other pelvic tissues.		T_{2b}
II_C: Either II_A or II_B with ascites or + peritoneal washings.		T_{2c}

Stage III: Extrapelvic intraperitoneal metastases and/or positive retroperitoneal nodes. Tumor limited to pelvis with biopsy-proved small bowel or omental extension. T_3

Stage IV: Distant metastases, liver metastases, or cytologically positive pleural fluid. T_4

Lymph Nodes
N_X: Not assessed.
N_0: Not involved.
N_1: Regional nodes involved.

Metastases
M_X: Not assessed.
M_0: No known distant metastases.
M_1: Distant metastases present.

Stage Groupings
Stage I_{Ai}: $T_{1ai}N_0M_0$
$\quad I_{Aii}$: $T_{1aii}N_0M_0$
$\quad I_{Bi}$: $T_{1bi}N_0M_0$
$\quad I_{Bii}$: $T_{1bii}N_0M_0$
$\quad I_C$: $T_{1c}N_0M_0$
Stage II_A: $T_{2a}N_0M_0$
$\quad II_B$: $T_{2b}N_0M_0$
$\quad II_C$: $T_{2c}N_0M_0$
Stage III: $T_3N_{0-1}M_0$
$\quad\quad\quad T_{1,2}N_1M_0$
$\quad\quad\quad T_4N_{0-1}M_0$
Stage IV: Any M_1

125. CERVICAL CANCER (AJC, 1977; incorporates FIGO)

T Classification
Stage 0: Carcinoma in situ, intraepithelial carcinoma. T_{1s}
Stage I: Carcinoma strictly confined to cervix.
$\quad I_A$: Microinvasive carcinoma (early stromal invasion). T_{1a}
$\quad I_B$: All other cases of stage I. T_{1b}
Stage II: Extension beyond cervix, but not to pelvic sidewall. Vaginal involvement, but not to distal third.
$\quad II_A$: No obvious parametrial involvement. T_{2a}
$\quad II_B$: Obvious parametrial involvement. T_{2b}
Stage III: Extension to pelvic sidewall and/or to lower third of vagina. All cases with hydronephrosis or a nonfunctioning kidney are included, unless they are known to be due to another cause.
$\quad III_A$: No extension to pelvic sidewall. T_{3a}
$\quad III_B$: Extension to pelvic sidewall and/or hydronephrosis. T_{3b}
Stage IV: Extension beyond true pelvis or clinical involvement of bladder or rectal mucosa.
$\quad IV_A$: Extension to adjacent organs. T_{4a}
$\quad IV_B$: Extension to distant organs. T_{4b}

Nodal Involvement

N_X: Not possible to assess nodes.
N_0: No nodal involvement.
N_1: Evidence of regional node involvement.
N_2: Pelvic sidewall mass not in continuity with parametrial mass.
N_3: Fixed or ulcerated regional nodes.
N_4: Juxtaregional lymph node involvement.

Distant Metastases

M_X: Not assessed.
M_0: No known distant metastases.
M_1: Distant metastases present.

Stage Groupings

Stage   0: T_{1s}
Stage I_A: $T_{1a}N_XM_0$
         I_B: $T_{1b}N_XM_0$
Stage II_A: $T_{2a}N_XM_0$
        II_B: $T_{2b}N_XM_0$
Stage III_A: $T_{3a}N_XM_0$
       III_B: $T_{3b}N_XM_0$
Stage IV_A: $T_{4a}N_XM_0$
        IV_B: $T_{4a}N_XM_0$
               Any M_1

126. ENDOMETRIAL CANCER (AJC, 1977 and FIGO)

T Classification

Stage 0: Carcinoma in situ.	T_{1s}
Stage I: Confined to uterus.	T_1
I_A: Uterine length 8 cm or less.	T_{1a}
I_B: Uterine length 8 cm.	T_{1b}

Recommended: Subgrouping stage I cases by histologic grade.
    G_1: Highly differentiated adenocarcinoma.
    G_2: Moderately differentiated adenocarcinoma.
    G_3: Predominantly solid or undifferentiated carcinoma.

Stage II: Extension to cervix.	T_2
Stage III: Extrauterine extension but not outside the true pelvis.	T_3
Stage IV: Extrapelvic extension or involvement of bladder or rectal mucosa.	T_4

Lymph Nodes

N_X: Not assessed.
N_0: No regional lymph node involvement.
N_1: Regional lymph nodes involved.

Distant Metastases

M_X: Not assessed.
M_0: No distant metastases.
M_1: Distant metastases present.

Stage Groupings
Stage   0: T_{1s}
Stage I_A: $T_{1a}N_XM_0$
          I_B: $T_{1b}N_XM_0$
Stage   II: $T_2N_XM_0$
Stage   III: $T_3N_XM_0$
          $T_{1-3}N_1M_0$
Stage IV_A: $T_{4a}N_{X-1}M_0$
        IV_B: $T_{4b}N_{X-1}M_0$
        Any M_1

---

127. SOFT TISSUE SARCOMAS (AJC, 1977)

Primary Tumor
T_X: Minimum requirements cannot be met.
T_0: No demonstrable tumor.
T_1: Tumor <5 cm.
T_2: Tumor >5 cm.
T_3: Bone, major vessel, or nerve invasion.

Tumor Grade
G_1: Well differentiated.
G_2: Moderately well differentiated.
G_{3-4}: Poorly to very poorly differentiated.

Nodal Involvement
N_X: Minimum requirements cannot be met.
N_0: No histologically verified lymph node metastases.
N_1: Histologically verified regional lymph node metastases.

Distant Metastases
M_X: Not assessed.
M_0: No known distant metastases.
M_1: Distant metastases present.

Stage Groupings
Stage I_A: $G_1T_1N_0M_0$
          I_B: $G_1T_2N_0M_0$
Stage II_A: $G_2T_1N_0M_0$
         II_B: $G_2T_2N_0M_0$
Stage III_A: $G_3T_1N_0M_0$
        III_B: $G_3T_2N_0M_0$
        III_C: Any G, $T_{1,2}N_1M_0$
Stage IV_A: Any G, T_3 any N, M_0
        IV_B: Any G, any T, any N, M_1

---

128. LYMPHOMAS

Clinical Staging (CS)
(Determined by history, physical examination, radiologic studies, isotopic scans, urine and blood tests, and the initial biopsy)

Stage   I: Involvement of a single lymph node region (I) or of a single ex-
            tralymphatic organ or site (I_E).
Stage II: Involvement of two or more lymph node regions on the same side of
            the diaphragm (II) or localized involvement of an extralymphatic
            organ or site and of one or more lymph node regions on the same side
            of the diaphragm (II_E).
Stage III: Involvement of lymph node regions on both sides of the diaphragm
            (III), which may also be accompanied by localized involvement of
            extralymphatic organ or site (III_E) or by involvement of the spleen
            (II_S) or both (III_{S-E}).
Stage IV: Diffuse or disseminated involvement of one or more extralymphatic
            organs or tissues with or without associated lymph node enlarge-
            ment. The reason for classifying the patient stage IV is identified by
            symbols:

N—Lymph nodes	S—Spleen
H—Liver	L—Lung
M—Marrow	O—Bone
P—Pleura	D—Skin

Systemic Symptoms

A: None present
B: Any or all of these three:
    1. Unexplained weight loss >10% of body weight in 6 months prior to
       admission.
    2. Unexplained fever with temperatures >38°C.
    3. Night sweats.

Pathologic Staging (PS)

Involvement found at laparotomy or by any further removal of tissue for histologic examination other than that taken for the original diagnosis.

N+ or −	other lymph node biopsies
H+ or −	liver biopsy
S+ or −	splenectomy
L+ or −	lung biopsy
M+ or −	marrow biopsy
P+ or −	pleura or pleural fluid cytology
O+ or −	bone biopsy
D+ or −	skin biopsy

BIBLIOGRAPHY

American Joint Committee for Cancer Staging and End Results Reporting [AJCCS]: Manual for Staging of Cancer, 1978. AJCCS, Chicago, 1977.

Astler V, Colles F: The prognostic significance of direct extension of carcinoma of the colon and rectum. Ann Surg 139:846–852, 1954.

Gabriel W, Dukes C, Bussey H: Lymphatic spread in cancer of the rectum. Br J Surg 23:395–413, 1935.

Suit H, Russell W, Martin R: Sarcoma of soft tissue: Clinical and histopathologic parameters and response to treatment. Cancer 35:1478–1483, 1975.

UICC: TNM Classification of Malignant Tumors. UICC, Geneva, 1973.

INDEX

Lymphoma(s)—*Continued*
  T-cell, mycosis fungoides and, 78–81
  treatment
    aggressive tumors, 204–205
    delay and mode choice, 203
    indolent tumors, 202
    kidney, 280
    relapse-related tumors, 202, 204, 205

Malignant melanoma. *See* Melanoma
Malnutrition, 265, 266. *See also* Alimentation
Mammography in breast cancer, 51, 97
Mandibular osteoradionecrosis, 231
Mastectomy in breast cancer, 97–98
Mediastinal masses, 4, 55
Mediastinoscopy
  esophageal cancer, 105
  superior vena cava syndrome, 5
Medullary tractotomy for pain, 264
Medulloblastomas, brain, 85, 87
Melanoma, 82–84
  amelanotic, 83
  classification and prognosis, 82–83, 148
  diagnosis and clinical signs, 83
  metastatic, 148–149, 274
  regional relapse, 148
  treatment and follow-up, 83–84, 148–149
Meninges
  leukemia, 13, 14, 207
    chemotherapy plus radiation and, 256
    prophylaxis, 13
  tumor infiltration, 13–15
    diagnosis and symptoms, 14
    incidence and types, 13–14
    treatment, 14–15
Meningiomas, brain, 85
Metastases. *See also* Metastatic malignancy
  bladder cancer, 120, 177
  bone tumors, 138
  brain tumors, 150
  breast cancer
    palliation, 158, 159
    sites and incidence, 157, 282, 283
    treatment, 98, 158–159
  cervical carcinoma, 131–133
  colorectal cancer, 108, 109, 169
  endometrial carcinoma, 134, 135, 187
  esophageal cancer, 105, 106
  gastric cancer, 59, 107, 166
  head and neck cancer, 153
  liver cancer, 37, 52, 54–55, 166, 169, 173, 276. *See also* Liver cancer, metastatic
  lung cancer, 101, 102
    non-small cell, 163–164
    small cell, 100, 160, 161–162
    treatment, 103
  melanoma, 148, 149, 274
  ovarian cancer, 130, 183–184

pancreatic cancer, 112, 113, 171–172
prostatic cancer, 122, 123, 124, 283
renal cancer, 118, 174, 175
soft tissue sarcomas, 140, 191–192, 301
spinal tumors, 264
testicular cancer, 126, 127
thyroid cancer, 95, 155, 156
uterine sarcomas, 135
Metastatic malignancy
  adrenals, 27
  bladder, 177, 297
  bone
    bladder cancer and, 120
    breast cancer and, 282, 283
    diagnosis, 282
    incidence, 137
    prostatic cancer and, 122, 178, 179, 283
    treatment, 282–283
  brain, 9, 85, 149, 161
  breast, 24, 293
    staging, 294
  carcinoid, 115, 116
    diagnosis and symptoms, 172–173
    treatment, 173–174
  cardiopathy and, 274
  cervix
    diagnosis, 185
    staging, 300
    treatment, 185–186
  chemotherapy, from unknown site, 147
  colorectal, 168, 169, 295
  combination therapy, 145
  diabetes insipidus and, 27, 28
  endometrium, 300
  esophagus, 165
  general management principles, 145–146
  head and neck, 152, 153
  liver
    carcinoid syndrome and, 173
    gastric cancer and, 166
  lung, 138
    staging, 294
    treatment, 47–48
  lymph node
    breast cancer and, 293
    cervical cancer and, 132
    colorectal cancer and, 169
    endometrial cancer and, 135
    esophageal cancer and, 105, 106
    ovarian cancer and, 183
    prognosis and, 77
    prostatic cancer and, 122, 123, 124
    renal cancer and, 296
    squamous cell carcinoma and, 146
    staging cervical, 291
    testicular cancer and, 126–127
    thyroid cancer and, 95
    unknown primary sites, 146
  lymph node aspiration cytology in, 39
  melanoma, 148–149

meninges, 13–15
osteogenic sarcoma, 189–190
ovary, 299
pancreas, 171
pericardial effusion and, 273–274
pituitary, 27, 28
pleural effusion and, 49, 272, 273
prostate
    diagnosis, 178
    hormone manipulation in, 265
    staging, 297
pulmonary nodule as, 47
renal, 296
risk, postoperative radiation therapy
    and, 251
skin, 41, 42, 149
soft tissue sarcoma, 191–192
    staging, 301
spinal cord compression and, 11
staging, 145. *See also under specific
    condition*
stomach, 166
testis, 125
thyroid, 154–155
unknown primary sites, 146–147
ureteral obstruction and, 177
Methotrexate, 239–240
high-dose, 239–240
intrathecal, 15, 240
intraventricular via Ommaya reservoir,
    15
in meningeal disease, 14
in recurrent head and neck cancer, 153
toxicities, 15, 153, 240
    kidney, 281
    radiation plus, 256
Methyl-CCNU, 247
Mohs chemosurgery in skin cancer, 80
MOPP, 200
Mouth cancer
incidence and prognosis, 90
staging, 291–292
symptoms and treatment, 91–92
Multiple myeloma, 22, 215–216
Mumps orchitis, 68
Myasthenia gravis, 73
Myasthenic (Eaton-Lambert) syndrome, 73
Mycosis fungoides, 42, 78, 81
Myelitis, postirradiation, 232
Myelogenous leukemia
acute, 200, 216
chronic, 212–214
Myelography, 12, 86
Myeloma(s)
bone, 137
multiple, 22, 215–216
paraproteins, renal failure and, 280
Myelosuppression
anthracycline antibiotics, 242–243
cyclophosphamide, 237
cytosine arabinoside, 241
vinblastine, 246

Narcotics for pain, 263
Nasogastric tube
decompression in bowel obstruction, 279
in enteral alimentation, 266–267
Nasopharyngeal cancer, 90, 92, 292
Neck cancer. *See* Head and neck cancer
Needle biopsy, 5
Nephrectomy in renal cancer, 118, 175
Nephropathy
radiation nephritis, 256
uric acid and xanthine, 280–281
Nephrotoxicity
cis-diamminedichloroplatinum, 248, 281
methotrexate, 240, 281
streptozotocin, 248, 281
Nephro-ureterectomy in renal cancer,
    118
Nerve blocks for pain, 263–264
Neurofibrosarcomas, soft tissue, 140
Neuromas, postoperative, 264
Neuromuscular disorders, associated
    malignancies, 72–73
Neurotoxicity of chemotherapeutic agents,
    238, 246
Neutropenia
antibiotic prophylaxis in adrenal in-
    sufficiency with, 27
diagnosis and management of, 17–18
Nevi, melanoma and, 82
Nitrogen mustard and radiation in
    superior vena cava syndrome, 5
Nitrosoureas, 236, 247–248
in melanoma, 83
nephrotoxicity, 281
Nodular goiter, 43–44
Non-Hodgkin's lymphomas. *See* Lym-
    phoma(s)
Nonlymphocytic leukemia, 210–211

Oligodendrogliomas, brain, 85, 87
Oliguria, postoperative, 221–222, 224
Oophorectomy in breast cancer, 158
Opportunistic infections
fungal or protozoan, 285–287
in leukemia, 286
Orchiectomy
prostatic cancer, 123, 179
testicular cancer, 69, 125
Orchitis, 68
Oropharyngeal cancer, 292–293
Osteogenic sarcoma, relapsing or meta-
    static, 189–190
Osteopathy
hypertrophic pulmonary osteoar-
    thropathy (HPO), 72
malignancy associated with, 72
postirradiation mandibular os-
    teoradionecrosis, 231
Osteosarcomas
bone, 137–139
combination therapy, 138
soft tissue, 140